EXPERT GUIDE TO
RHEUMATOLOGY

OTHER TITLES IN THE ACP EXPERT GUIDES SERIES

ALLERGY AND IMMUNOLOGY
Edited by Raymond G. Slavin and Robert E. Reisman

INFECTIOUS DISEASES
Edited by James S. Tan

ONCOLOGY
Edited by Jacob D. Bitran

OTOLARYNGOLOGY
Edited by Karen H. Calhoun
Associate Editors: David E. Eibling and Mark K. Wax

For a catalogue of publications available from ACP, contact:

Customer Service Center
American College of Physicians
190 N. Independence Mall West
Philadelphia, PA 19106-1572
215-351-2600
800-523-1546, ext. 2600

Visit our Web site at www.acponline.org

Expert Guide to

RHEUMATOLOGY

Arthur M.F. Yee, MD, PhD

Weill Medical College of Cornell University
Hospital for Special Surgery and
New York–Presbyterian Hospital

Stephen A. Paget, MD, FACP, FACR

Weill Medical College of Cornell University
Hospital for Special Surgery and
New York–Presbyterian Hospital

AMERICAN COLLEGE OF PHYSICIANS
PHILADELPHIA

Clinical Consultant: David R. Goldmann, MD, FACP
Manager, Book Publishing: Diane McCabe
Developmental Editor: Victoria Hoenigke
Production Supervisor: Allan S. Kleinberg
Senior Production Editor: Karen C. Nolan
Interior Design: Kate Nichols
Cover Design: Elizabeth Swartz
Index: Nelle Garrecht

Manufactured in the United States of America
Printed by Versa Press
Composition by UB Communications

Library of Congress Cataloging-in-Publication Data

Rheumatology / [edited by] Arthur M.F. Yee, Stephen A. Paget.
    p. cm.—(ACP key diseases series)
    Includes bibliographical references and index.
    ISBN 1-930513-55-0
    1. Rheumatology. 2. Rheumatism. 3. Arthritis. 4. Connective tissues—Diseases. I. Yee,
Arthur M.F. II. Paget, Stephen A. III. Series.

RC927.R4822 2004
616.7'23—dc22

2004057476

The authors and publisher have exerted every effort to ensure that drug selection and
dosage set forth in this book are in accordance with current recommendations and practice at the time of publication. In view of ongoing research, occasional changes in govern-
ment regulations, and the constant flow of information relating to drug therapy and drug
reactions, the reader is urged to check the package insert for each drug for any change in
indications and dosage and for added warnings and precautions. This care is particularly
important when the recommended agent is a new or infrequently used drug.

05 06 07 08 09 / 9 8 7 6 5 4 3 2 1

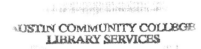

Acknowledgments

The invaluable contributions of many individuals have brought this project to completion. Deepest appreciation is sincerely given to Dr. Flavia Golden for her unwavering support, to Ms. Margaret Quan for her able assistance in research and production, and to Ms. Lisa Yee for her illustrations. We also thank Ms. Vicki Hoenigke, Ms. Karen Nolan, and the entire production team at the American College of Physicians for their tireless and efficient efforts.

Contributors

Helen E. Bateman, MD, FACR, FACAAI
Clinical Assistant Professor of Medicine, Division of Rheumatology
University of Medicine and Dentistry of New Jersey-Robert Wood Johnson Medical School
Overlook Hospital
Westfield, New Jersey

Kristina B. Belostocki, MD
Instructor of Medicine, Division of Rheumatology
Weill Medical College of Cornell University
Hospital for Special Surgery and New York-Presbyterian Hospital
New York, New York

Jessica R. Berman, MD
Instructor of Medicine, Division of Rheumatology
Weill Medical College of Cornell University
Hospital for Special Surgery and New York-Presbyterian Hospital
New York, New York

Mathias P.G. Bostrom, MD
Associate Professor, Department of Orthopedic Surgery
Weill Medical College of Cornell University
Hospital for Special Surgery
New York, New York

Barry D. Brause, MD, FACP
Clinical Professor of Medicine, Division of International Medicine and Infectious Diseases
Weill Medical College of Cornell University
Hospital for Special Surgery and New York-Presbyterian Hospital
New York, New York

David J. Chang, MD
Adjunct Assistant Professor of Medicine, Division of Rheumatology
University of Pennsylvania School of Medicine
Hospital of the University of Pennsylvania
Philadelphia, Pennsylvania

Scott M. Cook, MD
Fellow, Department of Orthopaedic Surgery
Weill Medical College of Cornell University
Hospital for Special Surgery
New York, New York

Stephen J. DiMartino, MD, PhD
Fellow, Department of Medicine, Division of Rheumatology
Weill Medical College of Cornell University
Hospital for Special Surgery and New York-Presbyterian Hospital
New York, New York

Petros Efthimiou, MD
Fellow, Department of Medicine, Division of Rheumatology
Weill Medical College of Cornell University
Hospital for Special Surgery and New York-Presbyterian Hospital
New York, New York

Doruk Erkan, MD
Instructor of Medicine, Division of Rheumatology
Weill Medical College of Cornell University
Hospital for Special Surgery and New York-Presbyterian Hospital
New York, New York

Theodore R. Fields, MD, FACP, FACR
Associate Professor of Clinical Medicine, Division of Rheumatology
Weill Medical College of Cornell University
Hospital for Special Surgery and New York-Presbyterian Hospital
New York, New York

Allan Gibofsky, MD, JD, FACP, FACR, FCLM
Professor of Medicine and Public Health, Division of Rheumatology
Weill Medical College of Cornell University
Hospital for Special Surgery and New York-Presbyterian Hospital
New York, New York

Susan Goodman, MD
Assistant Professor of Clinical Medicine, Division of Rheumatology
Weill Medical College of Cornell University
Hospital for Special Surgery and New York-Presbyterian Hospital
New York, New York

Melanie J. Harrison, MD, MS
Assistant Professor of Medicine, Division of Rheumatology
Weill Medical College of Cornell University
Hospital for Special Surgery and New York-Presbyterian Hospital
New York, New York

Lionel Ivashkiv, MD
Associate Professor of Medicine and Immunology, Division of Rheumatology
Weill Medical College of Cornell University
Hospital for Special Surgery and New York-Presbyterian Hospital
New York, New York

Lawrence J. Kagen, MD
Professor of Medicine, Division of Rheumatology
Weill Medical College of Cornell University
Hospital for Special Surgery and New York-Presbyterian Hospital
New York, New York

Stuart S. Kassan, MD, FACP
Clinical Professor of Medicine
University of Colorado Health Sciences Center
Denver, Colorado

Leah Lande, MD
Fellow, Department of Medicine, Division of Pulmonary and Critical Care Medicine
Weill Medical College of Cornell University
New York-Presbyterian Hospital
New York, New York

Michael D. Lockshin, MD, FACP
Professor of Medicine and Obstetrics-Gynecology, Division of Rheumatology
Weill Medical College of Cornell University
Hospital for Special Surgery and New York-Presbyterian Hospital
New York, New York

Steven K. Magid, MD, FACP, FACR
Associate Professor of Clinical Medicine, Division of Rheumatology
Weill Medical College of Cornell University
Hospital for Special Surgery and New York-Presbyterian Hospital
New York, New York

Joseph A. Markenson, MD, FACP, FACR
Professor of Clinical Medicine, Division of Rheumatology
Weill Medical College of Cornell University
Hospital for Special Surgery and New York-Presbyterian Hospital
New York, New York

Charis F. Meng, MD, LAc
Instructor of Medicine, Division of Rheumatology
Weill Medical College of Cornell University
Hospital for Special Surgery and New York-Presbyterian Hospital
New York, New York

Haralampos M. Moutsopoulos, MD, FACP, FACR
Professor and Director, Department of Pathophysiology
University of Athens School of Medicine
Athens, Greece

Stephen A. Paget, MD, FACP, FACR
Professor of Medicine, Chief of the Division of Rheumatology
Physician-in-Chief, Hospital for Special Surgery
Weill Medical College of Cornell University
Hospital for Special Surgery and New York-Presbyterian Hospital
New York, New York

Daniel F. Rosberger, MD, PhD
Clinical Assistant Professor of Ophthalmology
Weill Medical College of Cornell University
New York-Presbyterian Hospital
New York, New York

Linda A. Russell, MD
Assistant Professor of Clinical Medicine, Division of Rheumatology
Weill Medical College of Cornell University
Hospital for Special Surgery and New York-Presbyterian Hospital
New York, New York

Lisa R. Sammaritano, MD, FACP, FACR
Associate Professor of Clinical Medicine, Division of Rheumatology
Weill Medical College of Cornell University
Hospital for Special Surgery and New York-Presbyterian Hospital
New York, New York

Sergio Schwartzman, MD
Associate Professor of Medicine, Division of Rheumatology
Weill Medical College of Cornell University
Hospital for Special Surgery and New York-Presbyterian Hospital
New York, New York

Robert F. Spiera, MD, FACP, FACR
Assistant Professor of Medicine, Division of Rheumatology
Albert Einstein College of Medicine
Beth Israel Medical Center
New York, New York

Ioannis Tassiulas, MD
Instructor of Medicine, Division of Rheumatology
Weill Medical College of Cornell University
Hospital for Special Surgery and New York-Presbyterian Hospital
New York, New York

Athanasios G. Tzioufas, MD
Assistant Professor, Department of
  Pathophysiology
University of Athens School of
  Medicine
Athens, Greece

Eduardo Wainstein, MD
Assistant Professor of Medicine
University of Chile School of Medicine
Hospital Salvador
Santiago, Chile

Seth A. Waldman, MD
Clinical Assistant Professor,
  Department of Anesthesiology
Weill Medical College of Cornell
  University
Hospital for Special Surgery
New York, New York

Yusuf Yazici, MD
Clinical Assistant Professor of
  Medicine, Division of
  Rheumatology
State University of New York Health
  Science Center at Brooklyn
Long Island College Hospital
Brooklyn, New York

Arthur M.F. Yee, MD, PhD
Assistant Professor of Medicine,
  Division of Rheumatology
Weill Medical College of Cornell
  University
Hospital for Special Surgery and New
  York-Presbyterian Hospital
New York, New York

Introduction

Rheumatology is a rapidly evolving field. During the past several years, many exciting discoveries and insights into the etiology and pathogenesis of rheumatic disorders have been made. This has led to the development of innovative therapies and novel approaches to the management of these conditions that are at once safer and more effective.

This book was written to provide an accessible reference to the state-of-the-art practice of rheumatology. The intended audience is practicing internists and medical subspecialists, but individuals at all levels of medical training will find this text useful. Although the clinical aspects of rheumatology are highlighted, special emphasis is also given to those current concepts of etiology and pathogenesis that are pertinent to the practical management of patients.

Arrangement of This Book

This volume is broadly divided into eight sections. Basic principles of rheumatology are outlined first, including the general clinical approach to rheumatic diseases, the immunology of rheumatological conditions, and the methodology behind evidence-based rheumatology. Individual diseases are addressed in the next five sections, which, although by no means exhaustive, include the major diseases and syndromes relevant to most internists. Several vignettes are then discussed as examples of problem-based approaches to the diagnosis and management of clinical problems in rheumatology. The final three chapters are devoted to describing the medicines used in the treatment of inflammatory rheumatic diseases.

The contributing authors were selected because of their specific interests and are all in some capacity directly involved with patient care, even those whose primary activities are in basic research. Many are regarded as international thought leaders in rheumatology. The contributors were charged with the task of providing the same information and guidance that they would give to physicians who refer patients to them. Simply stated, this expert guide hopes to offer the same advice and counsel as would a consulting rheumatologist.

Approaching Rheumatic Diseases

It is not an exaggeration to hold that a proficient rheumatologist needs first to be a proficient internist. The practice of modern rheumatology demands facility with all medical subspecialties. Although a patient may present with a seemingly localized or non-specific complaint, one of the first tasks facing a rheumatologist is to determine whether a problem is an isolated one or part of a broader systemic illness. Familiarity with the conditions described in this volume facilitates the gathering, filtering, and integrating of pertinent information.

Many rheumatic disorders are diagnosed clinically, and therefore a thorough history, a complete review of systems, and an observant physical examination are absolutely central in directing the clinician down the path towards arriving at the correct diagnosis. Laboratory and radiological findings can be helpful to support or to argue against possible diagnoses but are often inconclusive and should always be interpreted in the context of the entire clinical picture. Empiric treatment is commonly required even when laboratory or imaging studies are unrevealing, incomplete, or unavailable.

Pathological data can also sometimes be misleading. Unlike an infection or a malignancy that is treated based on the results of a microbial stain or culture or the histopathology of a biopsy specimen, rheumatic conditions frequently call upon the clinician to become comfortable with a substantial level of diagnostic uncertainty. This is especially true in circumstances where the illness is incompletely differentiated or not yet fully evolved and the patient cannot be easily "pigeon-holed" into a clear-cut diagnosis. Nevertheless, even in such cases, the clinician should always remember to treat the patient, *not* the diagnosis, and the patient should be managed according to what he or she brings to the bedside.

Also, rheumatological disorders are frequently chronic and unpredictable in course. Therefore, ongoing vigilance is necessary to ensure response to treatment, to prevent and monitor for toxicities due to therapy, and to promptly identify relapses or new disease manifestations.

The use of laboratory studies, especially immunological and serological testing, is of particular pertinence in the evaluation of rheumatological disorders. While extremely important, their usefulness is ultimately determined by the clinician's understanding of their individual properties and limitations. Moreover, immunological and serological tests are notorious for significant inter-laboratory variability. Some tests are extremely sensitive, such as antinuclear antibodies in systemic lupus erythematosus (SLE), and thus are useful for screening purposes; a negative result is reasonably strong evidence against the diagnosis of the disease. Other tests are helpful for their specificity, such as anti-proteinase 3 antibody in Wegener's granulomatosis, in which case a positive test is good evidence for the presence of the disease.

In all cases, however, the results of such tests must always be taken in the context of the entire clinical setting. Similarly, while changes in tests like the erythrocyte sedimentation rate or the C-reactive protein may correlate with disease activity in many instances, modifications in therapeutic management should at all times address the clinical picture and not be directed merely towards the laboratory findings. Care must be taken to avoid being led astray by laboratory testing and to always treat the patient and not the test results.

Future Prospects

The last decade of the twentieth century marked the advent of groundbreaking achievements in rheumatology. The recognition of the central role of specific cytokines such as tumor necrosis factor-α and interleukin-1 in a variety of inflammatory rheumatic diseases led to the development of effective therapeutic agents that specifically target these proteins. Specific inhibitors of cyclooxygenase-2 are now widely available as the direct result of the discovery of this isozyme as an inducible producer of pro-inflammatory prostaglandins. Elucidation of pathophysiological processes in osteoporosis and Paget's disease resulted in the use of bisphosphonates to inhibit the bone-resorption activities of osteoclasts in these and other conditions. These are but a few examples of bench science translated to clinical application.

The new century brings even greater promises. With logarithmic progress in immunology, molecular biology, genetics, genomics, and biotechnology, further seminal advances into the pathogenesis of rheumatic diseases are inevitable and will foster innovative approaches to treatment. An even more exciting and challenging prospect will be the discovery of early prognostic indicators that will enable the clinician to more finely tailor therapeutic plans for individual patients. Finally, as is increasingly being recognized, many rheumatological conditions are characterized by fundamental pathophysiological pathways that also occur in non-rheumatological disorders. New therapeutic approaches may progressively cross disciplinary boundaries and lead to even greater understanding of basic pathogenic processes.

Arthur M.F. Yee, MD, PhD
Stephen A. Paget, MD

Contents

SECTION VI: DEGENERATIVE DISEASES AND REGIONAL PAIN SYNDROMES

SECTION VII: COMMON SYMPTOMS AND COMORBIDITIES

SECTION I

GENERAL ISSUES

1

■ ■ ■

Clinical Implications and Applications of Immunity and Inflammation

Stephen J. DiMartino, MD, PhD

Lionel Ivashkiv, MD

Patients often ask questions such as "Why did I get rheumatoid arthritis?" or "What exactly is this drug doing for my lupus?" Unfortunately, typical responses are often complex, vague, and imprecise because despite the hundreds of articles that are published monthly advancing understanding of immune and inflammatory processes, fundamental questions regarding the etiology of many rheumatic diseases remain unanswered. Moreover, the exact therapeutic mechanisms of action of most anti-rheumatic medications are unknown, even in the face of proven efficacy.

During the past few years, however, an increasing number of seminal scientific discoveries have revolutionized the clinical practice of rheumatology. Specific components of both the cellular and the molecular arms of the immune system have been deliberately and effectively targeted for the treatment of systemic autoimmune and inflammatory diseases. While not intended to be a comprehensively detailed discussion of immunology, this chapter gives a brief overview of normal immune processes and of how derangements in these processes might lead to autoimmunity and inappropriate inflammation. In addition, examples will be given of how new insights into the pathogenesis of rheumatic diseases are being exploited for therapeutic purposes.

Overview of the Immune Response and Autoimmunity

The immune system is a complex network of cells (lymphocytes, macrophages/monocytes, neutrophils, and dendritic cells) and soluble factors (antibodies, complement, and cytokines) that can identify and eliminate invading microorganisms and cancerous cells. Deficiencies of the immune system can make a host susceptible to infection, and inappropriate activity or over-activity can result in systemic autoimmune and inflammatory diseases.

The immune system can be conceptually divided into two arms: 1) innate immunity and 2) acquired or adaptive immunity. However, this division is largely academic because both arms usually work simultaneously and cooperatively to prevent disease.

Innate Immunity

Innate immunity provides constitutive protection and immediate response against invading microorganisms that are not dependent on previous exposure to a particular pathogen. It refers to the part of the immune system intrinsic to a given species and, in humans, includes the following components: 1) physical barriers such as skin and mucosa as first-line defense against penetration by microorganisms; 2) physiological barriers such as temperature (e.g., development of fever) and pH (e.g., gastric acid) that can inhibit the growth of invading pathogens; 3) soluble factors found in serum and extracellular fluid (e.g., complement and lysozyme) that are toxic to microorganisms; and 4) phagocytic cells such as macrophages and neutrophils that possess evolutionarily determined pattern-recognition receptors (receptors specific for common components of bacteria [e.g. endotoxin], viruses, and fungi) which, when activated, enable these cells to engulf and destroy microorganisms.

Adaptive Immunity

Adaptive or acquired immunity refers to the immune response that can specifically recognize, neutralize, and eradicate foreign pathogens. Upon first encounter with any microorganism or vaccine, the components of the adaptive immune response involved in initial recognition become amplified and then fine-tuned for enhanced specificity. Afterwards, the adaptive immune response establishes long-lived memory for the specific microorganism. Later, subsequent re-exposure to the same microorganism results in an even quicker and more effective immune response.

The immune system is able to develop an adaptive specific response against antigens to which it has had no prior exposure through random and unique genetic rearrangements that occur within the DNA of each lymphocyte. These rearrangements enable individual lymphocytes to express cell surface receptors (i.e., the B cell receptor in B lymphocytes and the T cell receptor in T lymphocytes) that recognize specific antigens. Because billions of lymphocytes are circulating at any given moment, billions of potential targets can be recognized. When a microorganism invades, lymphocytes recognizing different antigens of the microorganism become activated, multiply, and differentiate into long-lived memory cells.

Major components of the adaptive immune response include B lymphocytes, helper T lymphocytes, cytotoxic T lymphocytes, antigen-presenting cells (APCs), cytokines, and antibodies. Helper T lymphocytes play the central role in regulating the activation state of all lymphocytes and macrophages. B lymphocytes express membrane-bound antibodies (i.e., the B cell receptors) on their cell surfaces and when activated can differentiate into plasma cells that produce large quantities of soluble antibodies bearing unique specificity. Cytotoxic T lymphocytes can seek out and specifically destroy virally infected and cancerous cells.

APCs include macrophages, dendritic cells, and B cells, and they engulf, degrade, and process foreign material for presentation to lymphocytes. This mechanism is an important regulatory step for the selection of antigens to which the immune system will respond.

Cytokines and antibodies are soluble factors integral to immune responses. Cytokines are a highly diverse group of small proteins (typically smaller than 30 kDa) secreted by leukocytes and other cell types that regulate the immune system by either stimulating or inhibiting the development and activation of immune cells. Antibodies are large proteins produced by plasma cells that ostensibly recognize one specific target. Binding of antibody to its target can initiate various inflammatory processes, including activation of the complement cascade, induction of phagocytosis, and stimulation of toxic metabolite production by phagocytic cells.

Although many events occur simultaneously when a foreign microbe and its human host interact, the following scenario is a brief example of a generic adaptive immune response: Microbe X gains access and entry into host tissue via a breach in the skin or mucosa. Ensuing tissue damage and components of the organism itself activate the complement cascade, which results in increased local blood flow and vascular permeability and causes tissue infiltration by circulating neutrophils and monocytes/macrophages from peripheral blood. Cytokines produced by these inflammatory cells stimulate local APCs (e.g., tissue macrophages and resident dendritic cells) to engulf whole or partially destroyed Microbe X and to process microbial components into peptide fragments that are loaded into the cell surface major histocompatability complex (MHC) molecules. The APCs then migrate to a nearby lymph node where the peptide-MHC complex is presented to helper T cells.

For an individual helper T cell to become activated, two events must take place (Figure 1-1). First, foreign material in the form of oligopeptides or other small molecules is presented by APCs to lymphocytes packaged within the specialized cell surface receptors called MHC molecules. The helper T cell, through its T cell receptor, must strongly recognize the peptide-MHC complex presented by the APC. Second, the helper T cell must receive the appropriate co-stimulatory signals from the APC that interact

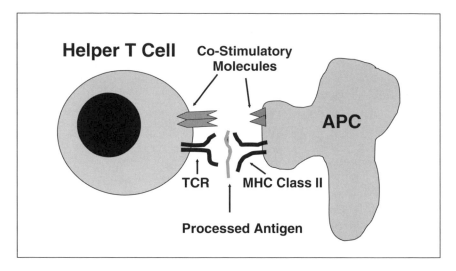

Figure 1-1   Activation of a helper T lymphocyte. An antigen-presenting cell (APC) packages processed antigens within major histocompatibility complex (MHC) class II molecules and presents them to the helper T cell, which specifically recognizes the MHC-antigen complex through its unique T cell receptor (TCR). At the same time, cognate co-stimulatory molecules on the two cells interact, resulting in activation of the T cell. If no interaction between co-stimulatory molecules occurs, the immune response may become aborted. (Courtesy of Dr. Mary K. Crow.)

with corresponding molecules on the lymphocyte; otherwise, the immune response may be aborted. Once activated, however, the helper T cell proliferates, generates long-lived memory cells, and produces cytokines that can stimulate B cells, which are themselves specific for the presented peptide. Activated B cells will multiply, generate memory cells, and differentiate into plasma cells producing large quantities of antibodies, thereby conferring humoral immunity specific for Microbe X.

Autoimmunity

The immune system evolved to defend against foreign microorganisms. Dysregulation of the immune system can lead to an inappropriate immune response against components of the self, a phenomenon generically termed *autoimmunity*. Many autoimmune disorders are characterized by the presence of highly specific antibodies that react to host components, implicating an aberration in immune response that results in the flawed recognition of self-antigens as being foreign. This interaction typically results in tissue damage or altered function. Autoimmune disorders can be organ-specific or systemic (Table 1-1). However, many other systemic inflammatory diseases (e.g., sarcoidosis) are not associated with autoantibodies, suggesting aberrations in non-humoral arms of the immune system in these disorders.

Table 1-1   Selected Autoimmune Diseases and Associated Autoantibodies

Disease	Target of Autoantibody
Organ-specific diseases	
Graves' disease	Thyroid-stimulating hormone receptor
Myasthenia gravis	Acetylcholine receptor
Goodpasture's syndrome	Basement membrane of kidney and lung
Autoimmune hemolytic anemia	Erythrocyte membrane constituents
Pernicious anemia	Intrinsic factor
Idiopathic thrombocytopenia purpura	Platelet membrane constituents
Systemic diseases	
Rheumatoid arthritis	Immunoglobulin G
Systemic lupus erythematosus	dsDNA and other nuclear constituents
Wegener's granulomatosis	Neutrophil proteolytic enzymes
Diffuse scleroderma	Topoisomerase I
Limited scleroderma (CREST syndrome)	Centromere
Poly/Dermatomyositis	tRNA synthetases

How the immune system is perturbed to lead to autoimmunity and inflammation remains under investigation, but data point to the contribution of both environmental and genetic factors. Infectious triggers are clearly implicated for some rheumatological disorders (e.g., viral polyarthritis after parvovirus B19 infection, group A beta-hemolytic streptococci in acute rheumatic fever, reactive arthritis after enteric or genitourinary infections, or *Borrelia burgdorferi* in Lyme disease), but for most systemic autoimmune diseases, definitive infectious etiologies have yet to be identified. On the other hand, it is evident that genetic factors play a crucial role in the development of inflammatory rheumatic diseases. The HLA-B27 haplotype has long been strongly linked to ankylosing spondylitis and the other spondylo-arthropathies, even though only a minority of individuals with HLA-B27 will develop disease. Other HLA markers are associated with predisposition to, or the expression of, other illnesses such as rheumatoid arthritis (RA), Lyme disease, and acute rheumatic fever. In systemic lupus erythematosus (SLE), studies have shown a 25% concordance rate in identical twins compared with a 10% concordance rate in fraternal twins. Clearly, then, environmental and heritable influences are both important determinants in the clinical manifestations of inflammatory rheumatic diseases.

Targeting the Immune System in the Treatment of Autoimmune and Inflammatory Diseases

Because of the premise that systemic rheumatological disorders are immunologically mediated diseases, it should not be surprising that many of the medications historically used for the treatment of these diseases are immunosuppressive drugs "borrowed" from oncology and transplant medicine. Methotrexate, azathioprine, mycophenylate, and cyclophosphamide are among the numerous drugs commonly used for rheumatic illnesses that globally suppress the activation, differentiation, and proliferation of different immune cell types. However, although clinically useful, the precise beneficial mechanisms of action of these agents on the molecular and cellular levels are usually not clear. Moreover, because of their potent and pleiotropic properties, they are also associated with many adverse effects, and the therapeutic window of these drugs in the treatment of rheumatic disease can be quite narrow. Thus, dosages tend to be much lower than those used by the oncologist, with the aim of always trying to strike an acceptable balance between the control of the disease and the risk of unwanted side effects.

Among the goals in refining therapeutic approaches is developing more precisely targeted therapies through an increased understanding of the immunology of rheumatic diseases. It is hoped that more focused therapy will simultaneously increase efficacy while reducing toxicities. Some examples of how specific components of the immune system are targeted by current and investigational therapies are given below (Table 1-2).

Cytokines

Cytokines are a large and diverse group of proteins produced predominantly (although not exclusively) by leukocytes that play critical roles in regulating the activation, proliferation, and differentiation of immune cells. Many cytokines such as tumor necrosis factor (TNF)-α, interleukin (IL)-1, IL-6 and interferon-γ, are considered pro-inflammatory, while others such as IL-4, IL-10 and transforming growth factor-β are thought to be predominantly anti-inflammatory. A current paradigm in rheumatology holds that an imbalance between the relative activities of "pro-inflammatory" and

Table 1-2   Components of the Immune System and Selected Targeted Therapies

Cytokines	Etanercept, infliximab, adalimumab, anakinra
Autoantibodies	Intravenous immunoglobulin, plasmapheresis, protein A immunoadsorption
T cells	Cyclosporin A
B cells	Rituximab, LJP-394
Neutrophils	Colchicine
Complement system	Eculizumab
Co-stimulatory molecules	CTLA-4-Ig

"anti-inflammatory" cytokines weighted towards the former can result in the development of inflammatory and autoimmune diseases. Although a useful construct, this paradigm is nonetheless an oversimplification, as it is clear that whether a particular cytokine is pro- or anti-inflammatory depends greatly upon the timing and context of its appearance during the immune response.

TNF-α Inhibitors

An excellent example of how scientific discovery can directly lead to advances in patient care is the development of TNF-α antagonists (1). Three agents produced by recombinant DNA technology are available: etanercept, infliximab, and adalimumab. It is known that macrophages and T cells from RA patients overexpress TNF-α and that blockade of TNF-α not only markedly improves clinical status and retards tissue destruction but significantly reduces production of other pro-inflammatory cytokines. These observations place TNF-α at a critical regulatory point at the top of the pro-inflammatory cytokine "pyramid." Currently, although TNF-α inhibitors are formally approved for only a handful of conditions (i.e., RA, juvenile RA, Crohn's disease, psoriatic arthritis), rheumatologists have found promise for their use in other inflammatory conditions such as sarcoidosis, vasculitis, and spondyloarthropathies.

Anakinra

IL-1β, another early-acting pro-inflammatory cytokine, can induce the production of a plethora of downstream inflammatory molecules and is implicated as an important factor in the destructive processes in the rheumatoid joint (2). IL-1 receptor antagonist (IL-1Ra) is a naturally occurring competitive inhibitor of IL-1β that binds to the IL-1 receptor, thereby blocking the activity of IL-1β. Anakinra, a recombinant form of human IL-1Ra, has been shown to prevent or retard the progression of joint erosions in RA and is approved for the treatment of this disease.

Autoantibodies

Many autoantibodies have been implicated in contributing to inflammation and organ damage in autoimmune diseases. In SLE, immune complexes containing antibodies to dsDNA deposit in glomeruli, leading to glomerulonephritis. In the antiphospholipid antibody syndrome, antibodies to a phospholipid-binding protein called β_2-glycoprotein-1 may activate endothelial cells and trigger inappropriate thrombosis in both arteries and veins. In Wegener's granulomatosis, anti-neutrophil cytoplasmic antibodies bind to cell surface enzymes on neutrophils and may cause dysregulated activation of these cells as they circulate. In autoimmune hemolytic anemia and immune thrombocytopenia purpura, antibodies bind to cell surface proteins on erythrocytes and platelets, respectively, resulting in their destruction and/or clearance by the immune system. Intravenous immunoglobulin, plasmapheresis, and protein A immunoadsorption (Prosorba Column) have been used to reduce the titers or effects of autoantibodies.

Intravenous Immunoglobulin

Intravenous immunoglobulin is obtained from pooled human plasma from thousands of donors and consists of whole IgG molecules. Clinical benefit has been shown in dermatomyositis, anti-phospholipid antibody syndrome, certain manifestations of SLE, immune thrombocytopenia pupura, Guillain-Barré syndrome, and Kawasaki's disease (3). The mechanism of action is probably multifaceted and is thought to include 1) blockade of Fc receptors, 2) binding to and inhibition of complement components, 3) direct neutralization of the autoantibodies themselves, and 4) shortening the half-lives of autoantibodies by saturation of the IgG salvage receptor known as FcRn.

Plasmapheresis

In plasmapheresis, plasma and its soluble constituents are removed from whole blood; the cellular components are left intact. Plasmapheresis is thought to remove pathogenic soluble factors such as autoantibodies and pro-inflammatory cytokines from circulation (4). However, it is not clear what effect plasmapheresis has on these molecules within tissues. Plasmapheresis is typically used in conjunction with pharmacological immunosuppressive therapies in situations such as severe manifestations of SLE (notably hemorrhagic alveolitis), catastrophic anti-phospholipid antibody syndrome, and severe vasculitis associated with hyperviscosity.

Protein A Immunoadsorption (Prosorba Column)

Staphylococcoccal protein A has high affinity for IgG and IgG-containing immune complexes. Using plasmapheresis technology, plasma can be filtered through a silica matrix containing protein A before being returned to the body, thereby removing putative pathogenic antibodies and immune complexes. Protein A immunoadsorption has shown some benefit in the treatment of various autoimmune diseases and is approved for the treatment of severe RA (5), but its use has been limited to a salvage role by the availability of generally more effective and less costly therapies.

T Lymphocytes

The central role that T cells play in the development of the acquired immune response together with the observation of T cells within the lesions of some inflammatory diseases have led to the therapeutic targeting of these cells.

Cyclosporin A

Cyclosporin A is a fungal metabolite that specifically inhibits T cell activation, proliferation, and cytokine production by suppressing the expression of early inflammatory genes at the transcriptional level (6). Its potent immunosuppressive properties have made it a first-line agent in the prevention of organ transplant rejection. Cyclosporin A has been shown to be beneficial in the treatment of RA and is approved for this indication, but predictable adverse effects have limited use. However, combination therapy with other immunosuppressive drugs may enable the use of lower dosages and thereby limit drug toxicities.

B Lymphocytes

B cells are the precursors of antibody-producing cells and can also function as APCs. Therefore they have become an attractive therapeutic target in autoantibody-mediated diseases.

Rituximab
CD20 is a cell surface molecule of unknown function that is specifically expressed on the surface of B cells. Rituximab is a chimeric monoclonal anti-CD20 antibody of human and mouse origin. In humans, the drug is well tolerated and has rapidly come to use as first-line therapy in the treatment of some B cell lymphomas. It effectively binds to, and causes the depletion of, B cells in peripheral blood and lymph nodes. The therapeutic benefit of rituximab in the treatment of autoimmune hemolytic anemia and immune thrombocytopenia purpura has led to its increased use in the management of other autoimmune diseases. Rituximab has shown benefit in RA and SLE in several encouraging investigations (7) and is being studied for use in many other conditions.

LJP-394
LJP-394 is currently in phase III trials for the treatment of SLE. This molecule specifically targets anti-dsDNA antibodies and the B cells that produce them. Structurally, LJP-394 is composed of four identical double-stranded 20-base DNA fragments, each attached to a central triethylene glycol core. This molecule is thought to bind to the B cell receptors on B cells that produce anti-dsDNA antibodies and in the absence of T cell "help" causes these B cells to become inactive. In addition, this drug may also directly bind to and neutralize soluble anti-dsDNA antibodies themselves. A recent study has shown LJP-394 therapy in SLE patients with circulating high-affinity antibodies for LJP-394 decreases the frequency of renal flares and lengthens disease-free intervals between flares (8).

Neutrophils

Neutrophils are the fastest moving and most abundant leukocytes and therefore are the first to appear during an acute inflammatory response. They are stockpiled with preformed degradative enzymes and proteinases.

Some of these enzymes are the actual target of autoantibodies known as anti-neutrophil cytoplasmic antibodies, which are seen in a variety of systemic inflammatory diseases.

When activated, neutrophils generate toxic oxygen radicals that destroy foreign pathogens and can also damage host tissue. Neutrophils are normally stimulated by pro-inflammatory cytokines, but as noted earlier, in certain inflammatory disorders such as Wegener's granulomatosis, there is evidence that circulating anti-neutrophil cytoplasmic antibodies can also activate neutrophils by binding to proteinases expressed on cell surfaces.

Colchicine

This ancient drug binds to the microtubules of neutrophils, inhibiting their migration into tissues and preventing the release of digestive enzymes from intracellular granules. Colchicine is now used predominantly in the treatment or prophylaxis of gout and pseudogout but also has been used for other inflammatory conditions including serositis in SLE, amyloidosis, familial Mediterranean fever, and Behçet's syndrome.

Complement System

The complement system is a cascade of plasma proteins that can be activated by immune complexes as well as bacterial cell surfaces and culminates in the generation of the membrane attack complex (a protein complex that literally pokes holes in cell membranes) and several anaphylatoxins (pro-inflammatory molecules that increase vascular permeability, attract leukocytes, and further stimulate the production of other pro-inflammatory molecules). The most potent anaphylatoxin, C5a, is formed during complement activation by cleavage of its parent molecule, C5. During SLE flares, there is evidence of extensive complement activation in the blood. In addition, complement activation products can be found in the synovial fluid in RA and in psoriatic skin lesions.

Eculizumab

This monoclonal murine antibody binds to and clears C5 and prevents the generation of both C5a and the membrane attack complex. Eculizumab has been shown to ameliorate disease in animal models of autoimmune disease (9). Currently, the drug is in clinical trials for RA and SLE.

Co-Stimulatory Molecules

Co-stimulatory molecules must be expressed on the surface of APCs during antigen presentation to the lymphocyte in order for activation of a lymphocyte to take place. If a lymphocyte strongly recognizes a peptide-MHC complex in the absence of co-stimulation, it will become inactive (i.e., anergic).

Conceptually then, blockade of the co-stimulatory signal should result in rendering the lymphocyte anergic to the presented antigen.

CTLA-4-Ig

B7-1 and B7-2 are co-stimulatory receptors expressed on APCs, which, upon interaction with cognate receptors on T cells, serve to activate the engaged T cells. CTLA-4-Ig is a genetically engineered fusion of the extracellular portion of cytotoxic T lymphocyte antigen-4 (CTLA-4) with the Fc portion of IgG designed to interfere with this interaction. In vitro and animal models have shown that the co-stimulatory signal is indeed blocked by CTLA-4-Ig, and in a recent placebo-controlled study CTLA-4-Ig has shown modest benefit in the treatment of RA (10).

REFERENCES

1. **Feldmann M, Maini RN.** Anti-TNF-alpha therapy of rheumatoid arthritis: what have we learned? Ann Rev Immunol. 2001;19:163-96.

2. **Dayer JM, Feige U, Edwards CK 3rd, Burger D.** Anti-interleukin-1 therapy in rheumatic diseases. Curr Opin Rheumatol. 2001;13:170-6.

3. **Kazatchkine MD, Kaveri SV.** Immunomodulation of autoimmune and inflammatory diseases with intravenous immune globulin. N Engl J Med. 2001;345:747-55.

4. **Madore F.** Plasmapheresis: technical aspects and indications. Crit Care Clin. 2002; 18:375-92.

5. **Matic G, Bosch T, Ramlow W.** Background and indications for protein A-based extracorporeal immunoadsorption. Ther Apher. 2001;5:394-403.

6. **Yocum DE.** T cells: pathogenic cells and therapeutic targets in rheumatoid arthritis. Semin Arthritis Rheum. 1999;29:27-35.

7. **Leandro MJ, Edwards JC, Cambridge G, et al.** An open study of B lymphocyte depletion in systemic lupus erythematosus. Arthritis Rheum. 2002; 46:2673-7.

8. **Alarcon-Segovia D, Tumlin JA, Furie RA, et al.** LJP-394 for the prevention of renal flare in patients with systemic lupus erythematosus: results from a randomized, double-blind, placebo-controlled study. Arthritis Rheum. 2003;48:442-54.

9. **Wang Y, Hu Q, Madri JA, et al.** Amelioration of lupus-like autoimmune disease in NZB/WF1 mice after treatment with a blocking monoclonal antibody specific for complement component C5. Proc Natl Acad Sci U S A. 1996;93:8563-8.

10. **Kremer JM, Westhovens R, Leon M, et al.** Treatment of rheumatoid arthritis by selective inhibition of T-cell activation with fusion protein CTLA-4-Ig. N Engl J Med. 2003;249:1907-15.

2

■ ■ ■

Outcomes Measures

Melanie J. Harrison, MD, MS

Rheumatology encompasses a large and broad spectrum of varied medical conditions, many of which share a significant overlap of clinical characteristics in terms of diagnosis, prognosis, and clinical course. Many conditions are systemic (not limited to involvement of the joints) and multi-systemic (affecting multiple organ systems). Such complexity makes meaningful and interpretable comparisons between individuals, groups of individuals, or even two points in time within the same individual difficult. The chronic, variable, fluctuating, and progressive nature of most of these conditions further compounds the difficulty that rheumatologists face in the evaluation of clinical outcomes, both at the level of an individual patient and for the purpose of assessing populations. For all these reasons, it has been imperative for the rheumatology community to define clinical diagnostic criteria and outcomes measures and establish their appropriate research use. Such clinical instruments reduce complex clinical problems to manageable proportions. However, although this simplification is necessary for purposes of generalization and measurement, caution should be taken to avoid oversimplification and consequent minimization of the details and nuances of a complicated condition.

Classification and Diagnosis

Unlike a malignancy that is diagnosed with a tissue biopsy or an infection that is identified through culture, rheumatic diseases frequently cover a spectrum of illness, are empirically recognized, and are rarely diagnosed by employing a single definitive test. In many ways, they may be considered syndromes or groups of signs and symptoms that collectively indicate a particular medical condition.

To assist in this categorization, classification criteria have been developed for many rheumatic diseases. These criteria were specifically designed for research purposes to establish standardization, thereby enabling different centers to investigate similar groups of patients and allowing comparisons between centers.

Classification criteria are empirically defined and usually established through consensus. They do not have 100% specificity or 100% sensitivity, but they have been developed to attain reasonable levels of each. It is important to emphasize that these classifications are biased toward accurate inclusion; their purpose is to guarantee that subjects selected for studies of a particular disease population truly have the condition. Moreover, the criteria are dynamic and may undergo periodic revisions as medical knowledge grows and understanding of the illnesses changes. For example, the well-established 1982 classification criteria for systemic lupus erythematosus (SLE) were recently re-evaluated and revised in 1997.

Because classification criteria include prominent and characteristic signs and symptoms by design, they are commonly used in the clinical setting as diagnostic guidelines. However, they were never meant for this purpose, and in clinical practice patients will often manifest some of the signs and symptoms suggestive of the illness even though they do not strictly fulfill classification criteria. For this reason, clinicians must take care not to allow diagnosis to be hindered or limited by these guidelines. Furthermore, because many rheumatic diseases are slow to evolve and do not appear in full form overnight, it is often only over time that individuals meet enough criteria to be classified into a specific disease category. Nevertheless, for the treating physician, this does not mean that the approach taken to manage a patient with an "incompletely evolved" illness should differ from that for a patient who exhibits the "full-blown" condition.

Choosing What to Measure: Disease Activity, Flare, Damage, and Remission

Once patients are diagnosed as having a particular rheumatic disease, monitoring and documenting of the clinical course and outcomes are needed. Disease "activity," "flare," "damage," and "remission" are expressions often used by practitioners to describe the state of the patient's illness. These terms carry clinical meanings that are generally understood but require further definition, clarification, and formalization for rheumatology research purposes.

In rheumatology, disease *activity* is the absolute value of the overall health status of a patient due to a specific condition at a particular point in time and has both qualitative and quantitative attributes. Qualitatively, disease activity can be described by which organs or systems are involved and in what ways. Quantitatively, activity refers to the degree to which this involvement is occurring. Over time, disease activity may increase, decrease, or stay the same. Disease activity reflects clinical manifestations attributable directly or indirectly to the pathogenesis of the disease and is a reversible phenomenon that can be corrected upon control or resolution of the underlying pathological process.

Disease *flare* differs from disease activity in that it is a perceived threshold above which disease activity becomes more clinically important. Metaphorically, it is the temperature at which we might consider a patient to have a fever. It is at this point that the level of concern, method of observation, therapeutic intervention, and perception of prognosis all change.

In contrast to disease activity, disease *damage* refers to irreversible injury to organs or tissue and does not need to be attributed solely to the disease itself. In SLE, for example, damage may include irreparable injuries caused by the disease, its treatment, or both. It is assumed that damage is more likely to be sustained with more severe, refractory, or prolonged illness, not only because of the disease per se but also because of increased exposure to the potential toxicities of treatments. The concept of damage thus incorporates the cumulative permanent effects of the disease and of attendant indirect costs.

Among practicing clinicians, *remission* often implies that disease activity is non-existent, with or without the need for ongoing treatment. However, for research purposes, the American College of Rheumatology (ACR) has defined remission (specifically for rheumatoid arthritis [RA]) as the absence of signs and symptoms of active disease without need for any treatment for the condition, an occurrence that is relatively rare for most common chronic rheumatic diseases (1). It should be noted, however, that this definition of remission is based on activity, not damage. Therefore, a patient may have suffered past disease damage (e.g., resulting in joint replacements) but have neither signs nor symptoms of active disease. While the surgical correction is evidence that the underlying condition had clear historical impact, the lack of need for ongoing immunosuppressive or anti-inflammatory therapy suggests that there are no active disease manifestations, and so this patient would be considered to be in disease remission.

Arthritis-Specific Measurement: Assessment of Function and Disability

A primary component of many rheumatic diseases is arthritis of one or more joints, and a significant consequence of arthritis is decreased or limited function, which can lead to permanent physical disability. Activities of daily living (ADL) are the basic behaviors representing "primary biological and psychosocial functions" and usually include fundamental functions such as dressing, feeding, and bathing oneself (2). More than 100 ADL scales have been developed, and they have been used in studies of various populations. Instrumental ADL (IADL) are more specific. They focus on the performance of specific activities that are required to execute ADL and to function within the community. Examples of IADL include shopping, cooking, and managing money. There are many IADL scales, some of which ask highly detailed information about performance ability. ADL and IADL scales are commonly used in clinical outcomes studies of arthritis because the potential for physical disability in these conditions is great.

The disability dimension of the Stanford Health Assessment Questionnaire (HAQ) is the most commonly used instrument within rheumatology for the evaluation of physical function and performance (3). Originally developed in 1980, the HAQ was designed for the clinical evaluation of adults with arthritis and has been translated into several languages, which allows for administration and comparison among different countries and cultures. It has also undergone multiple adaptations, revisions, and validation for use in varied settings and for different diseases, including spondylitis, acquired immunodeficiency syndrome, and pediatric rheumatic disease.

The disability dimension of the HAQ consists of 20 individual items describing activities commonly performed on a daily basis. The respondent is asked to grade his or her ability to perform each activity during the previous week. Scoring is based on a Likert scale ranging from zero ("without any difficulty") to four ("unable to do"). For example, requiring an assistive device such as a raised toilet seat, jar opener, or long-handled appliance for reach is scored two, "with much difficulty." The 20 items are then grouped into eight components: dressing and grooming, arising, eating, walking, maintaining hygiene, reaching, gripping, and performing outdoor activities. The average of the highest scores from each component area is the mean Functional Disability Index. Higher scores correspond to greater disability.

The HAQ has well-documented validity, reliability, and responsiveness (sensitivity to change). It has been shown to correlate with work disability, health services utilization, and mortality, especially in RA populations. The modified HAQ is a revised format of the original questionnaire that includes eight items from the functional disability scale in addition to items addressing patient satisfaction and self-perception of health and performance.

Other outcomes instruments of function and disability include the Arthritis Impact Measurement Scale (AIMS) and the revised and more frequently used form, AIMS2. These have a broader scope and examine physical, emotional, and social domains (4). Accordingly, questions included in these scales address not only physical function, activity, and well-being, but also issues of social support, psychological support, patient satisfaction, health perceptions, areas for improvement, and overall impact of disease.

Outcomes Assessment

Osteoarthritis: The WOMAC Index

Osteoarthritis (OA) is a localized degenerative arthritis. Its clinical manifestations vary depending on the joints that are involved. Because of patient-to-patient variability, generalized health status and functional ability instruments are often employed in order to evaluate global outcomes and compare them with various presentations of OA. Additional instruments, such as pain scales and measurements of radiographic progression, are also frequently used as independent outcomes measures or as an adjunct to these broader questionnaires.

The Western Ontario MacMaster Universities Osteoarthritis Index (WOMAC) was designed specifically to assess short-term outcomes in hip and knee OA and was developed to focus on the most common and problematic symptoms of OA that bring patients to seek medical attention (5). As such, the instrument has inherent clinical relevance. It consists of 24 items, is multi-dimensional and self-administered, and was derived from six previously developed and validated questionnaires, including the HAQ and the AIMS (Table 2-1). The WOMAC has three symptom domains or subscales (pain, stiffness, and physical function), each of which is potentially modifiable, giving the instrument significant sensitivity to change or responsiveness. Subscales can be evaluated as separate measures or summated to give a total score. Higher scores reflect more severe disease. The WOMAC has well-documented reliability, validity, and responsiveness, and has been used frequently in clinical trials assessing therapeutic modalities such as non-steroidal anti-inflammatory drugs, analgesics, physical therapy, educational interventions, and surgery.

At present, available therapy for OA offers only symptomatic relief, and current outcomes measures to evaluate therapeutic success concentrate on this clinical endpoint. However, as newer agents with the potential to alter the course and progression of OA (so-called disease-modifying drugs) are developed, novel outcomes instruments concentrating on the presence of disease modification will need to be developed.

Rheumatoid Arthritis: The ACR Response Criteria

Not long ago, clinical and research rheumatologists evaluated outcomes of RA predominantly by using anatomical and physiological measures, such as laboratory markers of inflammation (erythrocyte sedimentation rate [ESR] or C-reactive protein [CRP]) and radiographic changes (e.g., joint space narrowing or erosions). However, these measurements per se have limited relevance to patients and do not consistently correlate with self-reported well-being or functional status. It was apparent that the subjective evaluation of pain, stiffness, and related symptoms was obligatory not only for

---

Table 2-1   WOMAC Osteoarthritis Index, Version VA3.1

- All answers are given on a scale ranging from none to extreme.
- Patients are instructed to answer as per the condition of the study joint in the last 48 hours.

SECTION A - PAIN

How much pain have you had . . .

1. when walking on a flat surface?
2. when going up or down stairs?
3. at night while in bed?
4. while sitting or lying down?
5. while standing?

SECTION B - STIFFNESS

How severe has your stiffness been . . .

6. after you first woke up in the morning?
7. after sitting or lying down or while resting later in the day?

SECTION C - DIFFICULTY PERFORMING DAILY ACTIVITIES

How much difficulty have you had . . .

8. when going down the stairs?
9. when going up the stairs?
10. when getting up from a sitting position?
11. while standing?
12. when bending to the floor?
13. when walking on a flat surface?
14. getting in or out of a car, or getting on or off a bus?
15. while going shopping?
16. when putting on your socks or panty hose or stockings?
17. when getting out of bed?
18. when taking off your socks or panty hose or stockings?
19. while lying in bed?
20. when getting in or out of the bathtub?
21. while sitting?
22. when getting on or off the toilet?
23. while doing heavy household chores?
24. while doing light household chores?

From Bellamy N, Buchanan WW, Goldsmith CH, et al. Validation study of WOMAC: a health status instrument for measuring clinically important patient relevant outcomes to antirheumatic drug therapy in patients with osteoarthritis of the hip or knee. J Rheumatol. 1988;15:1833-40; with permission.

making individual treatment decisions but also for determining effectiveness of therapeutic regimens in clinical trials.

In practice, judgments about disease activity and subsequent clinical decision-making are based on a combination of bedside, laboratory, and radiographic findings, as well as the overall subjective presentation by the patient. No single sign or symptom alone dictates therapy for RA. Historically, endpoints commonly used in RA clinical trials were often poorly standardized, not comprehensive, insensitive to change, and overlapping in content. Furthermore, the use of different outcomes measures between trials prevented the comparison of therapeutic results against accepted standards.

In 1993, in order to resolve these issues, the ACR Response Criteria were developed to serve as a standardized composite index of outcomes measures that was comprehensive and specific and that captured the essence of overall positive change or improvement in the patient with active RA (6). Using this index, patients could be classified as improved or not improved after therapeutic intervention. The ACR recommendations include the following core measures for use in all clinical RA drug trials: tender joint count; swollen joint count; a measure of disability (usually the HAQ); patient and physician global assessments of disease activity; patient assessment of pain; and a physiological measure of inflammation such as the ESR or CRP (Table 2-2). Each individual component of this index is calculated as the degree of improvement in each component between two time points. A patient is said to be improved and reach an "ACR 20" if both the tender and swollen joint counts are at least 20% improved over the baseline assessment and if at least three of the five remaining component scores are also improved by at least 20%. "ACR 50" and "ACR 70" scores are similarly calculated, using 50% and 70% thresholds, respectively. Because these are response criteria, they require at least two assessments over time and can only be used in longitudinal studies.

This index has been validated and used extensively in most RA clinical trials to assess short-term outcome or improvement in disease activity. The individual components may also be viewed as separate outcomes measures to better understand the specific manifestations of RA. Furthermore, other outcomes measures such as fatigue and duration of morning stiffness are often added to the composite measure in order to assess other signs and

Table 2-2   Criteria and Calculation of ACR 20 (50, 70) Response

Tender joint count	MUST document an *improvement* in scores by
Swollen joint count	20% (50%, 70%) for BOTH of these measures;
Pain (visual analog scale)	**AND**
Patient's global assessment	
Physician's global assessment	MUST document a 20% (50%, 70%) *decline*
Assessment of function/disability (Health Assessment Questionnaire)	in ANY 3 of these 5 measures
Acute phase reactant (ESR or CRP)	

ESR = erythrocyte sedimentation rate; CRP = C-reactive protein.
From Felson DT, Anderson JJ, Boers M, et al. The American College of Rheumatology preliminary core set of disease activity measures for rheumatoid arthritis clinical trials. The Committee on Outcome Measures in Rheumatoid Arthritis Clinical Trials. Arthritis Rheum. 1993;36:729-40; with permission.

symptoms common to RA activity and to evaluate longer-term and key outcomes (e.g., radiographic damage).

Another composite set of outcome measurements called the Disease Activity Score is more frequently used in Europe than the ACR Response Criteria. This calculation requires the tender joint count, the swollen joint count, a patient global assessment of disease activity, and the ESR. Unlike the ACR Response Criteria, the Disease Activity Score reflects a single point in time, and scores taken at different times can be compared to quantify a clinical change. It has been validated, is sensitive to change, and has been found to correlate with functional disability and radiological progression.

Systemic Lupus Erythematosus: SLEDAI and SLICC/ACR

The between-patient and within-patient heterogeneity of SLE makes it extremely difficult to generalize about the disease for the purpose of evaluating and comparing outcomes. Several attempts to quantify different aspects of SLE, particularly disease activity, have resulted in the development and validation of numerous clinical instruments. Some of these instruments have been well accepted by clinical investigators and are frequently used to assess and document changes in the clinical status of lupus patients.

The Systemic Lupus Erythematosus Disease Activity Index (SLEDAI) was developed by a consensus committee and contains 24 items or "descriptors" (Table 2-3) (7). The descriptors include symptoms reported by the patient, signs found on physical examination, and laboratory test results that reflect disease activity in SLE. They fall into nine different organ systems and must be present during the 10 days before evaluation. Each descriptor

Table 2-3   Systemic Lupus Erythematosus Disease Activity Index (SLEDAI)

Weight	Descriptor	Weight	Descriptor
8	Seizure	4	Proteinuria
8	Psychosis	4	Pyuria
8	Organic brain syndrome	2	Rash
8	Visual disturbance	2	Alopecia
8	Cranial nerve disorder	2	Mucosal ulcers
8	Lupus headache	2	Pleurisy
8	Cerebrovascular accident	2	Pericarditis
8	Vasculitis	2	Low complement
4	Arthritis	2	Increased DNA binding
4	Myositis	1	Fever
4	Urinary casts	1	Thrombocytopenia
4	Hematuria	1	Leukopenia

Items are scored only if descriptor is present at the time of visit or in the preceding 10 days.
Modified from Bombardier C, Gladman DD, Urowitz MB, et al. Derivation of the SLEDAI: a disease activity index for lupus patients. The Committee on Prognosis Studies in SLE. Arthritis Rheum. 1992;35:630-40; with permission.

is weighted to reflect the clinical importance of the SLE-associated condition. For example, a seizure or vasculitis is assigned a value of 8, while pericarditis or alopecia is given a score of 2. SLEDAI scores are the sum of the weighted scores of all descriptors present. Therefore, a rise in total score presumably reflects an increase in activity, whereas a fall in total score suggests a decrease in activity. However, no absolute change has yet been validated as indicative of clinical improvement, flare, or remission.

Another disease activity instrument for SLE is the British Isles Lupus Activity Group, which, unlike the SLEDAI, was specifically developed for longitudinal use and is designed to evaluate clinically important changes in disease status over time (8). This system also accounts for the physician's intention to treat and includes not only measures of the severity of organ system involvement but also of the aggressiveness of therapy. For example, highest scores are given when disease-modifying therapy such as immunosuppressive agents or daily prednisone 20 mg (or equivalent) is required.

As survival in SLE has improved, morbidities secondary to recurrent exacerbations, ongoing disease activity, tissue damage, and treatment-related adverse events have become increasingly prevalent and salient features. In response, the Systemic Lupus International Collaborating Clinics/ACR (SLICC/ACR) Damage Index was developed to measure the cumulative long-term and irreversible effects of both ongoing disease and toxicities associated with treatment, especially corticosteroids (9). It is presumed that more severe or unremitting disease requires more intense or long-standing treatment. Accordingly, irreversible disease-related and iatrogenic injury are both regarded as important contributors to the overall health status of the patient. The SLICC/ACR Damage Index contains 39 different irreversible medical conditions caused by SLE, its treatment, or both (Table 2-4). Examples include cataracts, cerebrovascular accidents, shrinking lung syndrome, end-stage renal disease, avascular necrosis, premature gonadal failure, and malignancy. SLE-related organ damage has been shown to be associated with poor overall outcome.

Other Outcomes Measures and Comparisons Between Conditions

While the HAQ and AIMS are instruments specifically designed for use among arthritis patients and address common aspects of most chronic musculoskeletal conditions, more generic instruments such as the Medical Outcomes Survey-Short Form 36 (SF-36), the Sickness Impact Profile, and the Nottingham Health Profile are also often applied to rheumatic disease populations to evaluate overall health status.

The SF-36 is a generic instrument designed for use in the general population and contains 36 items that measure eight dimensions: physical functioning, role limitations caused by physical problems, role limitations caused by emotional problems, social functioning, mental health, vitality,

Table 2-4   Irreversible Conditions Included in the Systemic Lupus International Collaborating Clinics/American College of Rheumatology (SLICC/ACR) Damage Index

Ocular
Cataracts
Retinal changes or optic atrophy

Neuropsychiatric
Cognitive impairment or major
   psychosis
Chronic treatment for seizures
Cerebrovascular accident or
   resection (not for malignancy)
Cranial or peripheral neuropathy
Transverse myelitis

Renal
Chronic renal insufficiency
   (glomerular filtration rate <50%
   or proteinuria >3 g/d)
End-stage renal disease

Pulmonary
Pulmonary hypertension
Pulmonary fibrosis
Shrinking lung syndrome
Pleural fibrosis
Pulmonary infarction or resection
   (not for malignancy)

Cardiovascular
Angina or coronary artery bypass
   surgery
Myocardial infarction
Cardiomyopathy
Valvular disease
Chronic pericarditis or
   pericardiectomy

Peripheral vascular
Chronic claudication
Minor tissue loss (e.g., pulp space)
Significant tissue loss (e.g.,
   amputation)
Venous thrombosis, ulceration, or
   stasis

Gastrointestinal
Infarction or resection (not for
   malignancy) of bowel, spleen, liver,
   or gall bladder
Mesenteric insufficiency
Chronic peritonitis
Upper gastrointestinal tract stricture
   or surgery
Pancreatic insufficiency

Musculoskeletal
Atrophy or weakness
Deforming or erosive arthritis
Osteoporosis with fracture or
   vertebral collapse
Avascular necrosis
Osteomyelitis
Ruptured tendon

Skin
Alopecia
Extensive scarring or panniculum

Other
Premature gonadal failure
Diabetes
Malignancy

Modified from Gladman D, Ginzler E, Goldsmith C, et al. The development and initial validation of the Systemic Lupus International Collaborating Clinics/American College of Rheumatology damage index for systemic lupus erythematosus. Arthritis Rheum. 1996;39:363-9; with permission.

pain, and general health perceptions (10). It is often used in conjunction with more disease-specific outcome measures in rheumatic disease studies; many investigations have documented significant correlations between the SF-36 and arthritis-specific measures such as the HAQ patient and physician global assessments.

The Sickness Impact Profile and the Nottingham Health Profile examine patient perceptions of physical, social, and emotional aspects of health in order to evaluate overall status and limitations (11,12). The items are generically constructed, applicable to a diverse range of conditions, and practical for use in the study of patients with arthritis. Although these more generic instruments offer less sensitivity for detecting abnormalities specific for individual conditions, they do allow some comparison of outcomes of particular rheumatic diseases to other musculoskeletal and non-musculoskeletal conditions.

Use of Clinical Outcomes Instruments for Rheumatology in the Office Setting

The practice of rheumatology involves the management of many chronic, fluctuating, and progressive illnesses for which the use of appropriate clinical instruments is especially beneficial to both patient and practitioner. Small and gradual clinical changes, unnoticed in the short-term, may accumulate over time and become significant in the long-term. Longitudinal administration and review of outcomes instruments in clinical practice can help physicians accurately monitor change over the course of chronic illnesses. Clinical instruments or questionnaires can be utilized much like laboratory tests or radiographs with norms and expected variability over time because they are standardized and valid measures of otherwise subjective observations. Instruments used in the office setting should be easy to administer, understandable to respondents, and readily interpreted and applied to clinical decision-making.

Although many clinical instruments are designed for the evaluation of populations and not for the assessment of individuals, some may also be applicable to clinical practice, either in their original or in an adapted form. For example, simple visual analog scales (Fig. 2-1) measuring pain, fatigue, or global assessment of disease activity can be easily understood and completed by patients, rapidly quantified, and easily tracked for changes over time. These single-item evaluations are often used in research investigations. They are clinically relevant to patients and practitioners and have documented validity. Other more complex questionnaires can

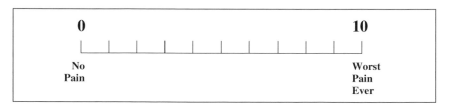

Figure 2-1 Visual Analog Scale. A simple line scale ranging from 0 (asymptomatic) to 10 (worst possible symptoms) can be used to serially follow a specific clinical feature such as pain, fatigue, or global assessment in individual patients.

also be quickly administered and interpreted for use in the clinical setting. These include the SF-36 to assess overall health and the HAQ to measure disability. A clinical HAQ has been developed for use specifically in clinical settings.

However, some clinical instruments, such as the ACR Response Criteria, are not appropriate for following individual patients. The ACR Response Criteria were developed to categorize active RA patients in clinical studies as responders or non-responders to particular treatment regimens but were not designed for use in individual RA patients, or to follow the course of disease. Only those individuals who attain the arbitrary threshold deemed 20% improvement are classified as responders. Thus, an individual who is only 19% improved, while still clinically better, would nonetheless not meet the ACR Response Criteria. Furthermore, at baseline assessment, individuals must be in a somewhat "poor" condition to allow for a significant percentage improvement. Patients with only mild signs and symptoms of disease have minimal room for improvement, and it is therefore difficult for them to meet ACR Response Criteria at any level.

Summary

Rheumatology comprises a vastly heterogeneous group of medical conditions, many of which are systemic or multisystemic, difficult to diagnose, and challenging to evaluate with respect to clinical outcomes. Rheumatological diseases are also frequently chronic and unpredictable in course. Developing diagnostic criteria and outcomes measurements for clinical use is therefore necessary to help identify and monitor complex clinical problems. However, because of the complexities in disease course, some imprecision in measurements should be expected. As with laboratory test results, outcomes measurements in patients with rheumatic disease must be considered in the context of the individual patient's overall clinical picture.

Outcomes instruments have been developed to assess disease activity, disease flare, disease damage, and remission. Several such instruments are designed to measure outcomes for specific disorders, including arthritis-specific measurements, which primarily assess function and disability. Generic instruments that are applicable to most chronic musculoskeletal conditions may also be used, although these are less sensitive for detecting condition-specific abnormalities. Most of these instruments were originally instituted to facilitate comparisons between study populations. For diseases such as systemic lupus erythematosus, where the between-patient heterogeneity of the disease renders generalizations problematic, implementation of numerous clinical instruments may be necessary. Other instruments, such as the Visual Analog Scale, are easily adapted to the clinical setting. As knowledge and treatment options within the field continue to rapidly evolve, novel means of assessment of these outcomes will be needed.

REFERENCES

1. **Pinals RS, Masi AT, Larsen RA.** Preliminary criteria for clinical remission in rheumatoid arthritis. Arthritis Rheum. 1981;24:1308-15.

2. **Katz S, Ford AB, Moskowitz RW, et al.** Studies of illness in the aged. The index of ADL: a standardized measure of biological and psychosocial function. JAMA. 1963;185:914-9.

3. **Pincus T, Summey JA, Soraci SA Jr, et al.** Assessment of patient satisfaction in activities of daily living using a modified Stanford Health Assessment Questionnaire. Arthritis Rheum. 1983;26:1346-53.

4. **Meenan RF, Mason JH, Anderson JJ, et al.** AIMS2. The content and properties of a revised and expanded Arthritis Impact Measurement Scales Health Status Questionnaire. Arthritis Rheum. 1992;35:1-10.

5. **Bellamy N, Buchanan WW, Goldsmith CH, et al.** Validation study of WOMAC: a health status instrument for measuring clinically important patient relevant outcomes to antirheumatic drug therapy in patients with osteoarthritis of the hip or knee. J Rheumatol. 1988;15:1833-40.

6. **Felson DT, Anderson JJ, Boers M, et al.** The American College of Rheumatology preliminary core set of disease activity measures for rheumatoid arthritis clinical trials. The Committee on Outcome Measures in Rheumatoid Arthritis Clinical Trials. Arthritis Rheum. 1993;36:729-40.

7. **Bombardier C, Gladman DD, Urowitz MB, et al.** Derivation of the SLEDAI: a disease activity index for lupus patients. The Committee on Prognosis Studies in SLE. Arthritis Rheum. 1992;35:630-40.

8. **Hay EM, Bacon PA, Gordon C, et al.** The BILAG index: a reliable and valid instrument for measuring clinical disease activity in systemic lupus erythematosus. Q J Med. 1993;86:447-58.

9. **Gladman D, Ginzler E, Goldsmith C, et al.** The development and initial validation of the Systemic Lupus International Collaborating Clinics/American College of Rheumatology damage index for systemic lupus erythematosus. Arthritis Rheum. 1996;39:363-9.

10. **Ware JE Jr, Sherbourne CD.** The MOS 36-item short-form health survey (SF-36). I. Conceptual framework and item selection. Med Care. 1992;30:473-83.

11. **Bergner M, Bobbitt RA, Carter WB, Gilson BS.** The Sickness Impact Profile: development and final revision of a health status measure. Med Care. 1981;19:787-805.

12. **Houssien DA, McKenna SP, Scott DL.** The Nottingham Health Profile as a measure of disease activity and outcome in rheumatoid arthritis. Br J Rheumatol. 1997; 36:69-73.

SECTION II

EROSIVE INFLAMMATORY ARTHROPATHIES

3

■ ■ ■

Rheumatoid Arthritis

Stephen A. Paget, MD

heumatoid arthritis (RA) is a chronic systemic autoimmune and inflammatory disorder of unclear etiology. It is characterized by a symmetric polyarthritis, which is often erosive, resulting in irreversible damage to the joints. Although the musculoskeletal manifestations usually dominate the clinical picture, extra-articular manifestations are also common and on rare occasions can be life-threatening. RA is the most common immune-mediated inflammatory arthropathy, with a prevalence of up to 1.5% in North America. In some Native-American populations, the prevalence may exceed 5%.

Pathogenesis

Although it is evident that dysregulation of the immune system is an important factor, and a massive amount of information has been accumulated about the immunopathogenesis of RA, a definitive cause has yet to be identified, even after nearly 50 years of directed research. Infectious organisms, particularly viruses, remain prime suspects as potential triggers in the predisposed individual. Genetic factors clearly play a role in RA, as they do in other autoimmune disorders. Both predisposition to and severity of RA appear to involve the class II histocompatibility antigens HLA-DR4 and HLA-DR1. More detailed molecular analysis has narrowed this association to a short peptide sequence present in these HLA haplotypes, which has been called the "shared epitope" (1,2).

It is conjectured that antigen-presenting cells such as macrophages, dendritic cells, and B lymphocytes process an unknown "RA antigen" and then present a component of the antigen to T lymphocytes in the context of HLA molecules bearing the "shared epitope" or another predisposing sequence. The stimulated CD4+ T lymphocyte is central to the activation of the immune system by recruiting the involvement of other immunologically active cells and by helping B lymphocytes and plasma cells produce antibodies and autoantibodies such as rheumatoid factors (RF). Complexes of autoantibodies bind complement, setting into motion pro-inflammatory processes. The expression of cytokines enable immune cells such as macrophages and lymphocytes to communicate with one another and is largely responsible for propagating or impeding downstream inflammatory and tissue-damaging processes. In RA, the net effect of cytokine expression is pro-inflammatory, resulting in the influx of inflammatory cells into the joint.

Histologically, the synovial membrane resembles an activated lymph node in which large numbers of immune cells are juxtaposed, enabling them to interact, communicate, and promote tissue damage. The inflamed synovium, known as a pannus, abuts the articular cartilage, and inflammatory cells at this interface produce enzymes that lead to cartilage erosion and destruction of the underlying bone.

The central pro-inflammatory cytokines in RA include tumor necrosis factor (TNF)-α, interleukin (IL)-1, and IL-6 (3). While natural antagonists normally maintain an inflammatory homeostasis, inappropriate or overproduction of these and other pro-inflammatory cytokines tilts the balance in the direction of inflammation in RA. These cytokines have the following actions:

- They cause the constitutional symptoms such as fatigue and weight loss that are prominent in patients with RA. They also lead to anemia and the elevations of the erythrocyte sedimentation rate (ESR), C-reactive protein (CRP), and other acute-phase reactants.

- They stimulate expression of adhesion molecules on the surface of endothelial cells. Adhesion molecules enable circulating immune cells to roll along the endothelium, adhere to its wall, and eventually integrate and extravasate between endothelial cells. Because the endothelial cells serve as the "tollbooth" through which leukocytes traverse into tissues, the eventual cellular composition and personality of the synovial disease process are defined by their state of activation.

- They stimulate chondrocytes and synovial fibroblasts to produce and secrete metalloproteinases, enzymes that can break down the chemical components of cartilage, bone, and tendons and lead to erosions and joint space narrowing.

- They can promote extra-articular disease manifestations such as rheumatoid nodules, visceral disease, osteoporosis, and even premature atherosclerosis.

The modern therapeutic approach to RA is the development of finely targeted modalities that arise from our understanding of the immunological processes described above. Traditional treatments such as methotrexate, although clearly beneficial, have broad and relatively non-specific effects upon many different cell types, affecting both pathogenic and non-patho-genic pathways. In contrast, the newer anti-cytokine treatments are aimed at the central cytokines TNF-α and IL-1, which clearly play a major role in the development and/or propagation of the inflammatory process. Con-ceptually, intervention that targets early steps in the immunopathogenic processes could reduce the likelihood of irreversible joint damage. However, it is crucial to emphasize and fully appreciate that the same pro-inflammatory elements that contribute to the pathogenesis of RA also have pleiotropic effects that protect against infections, mediate surveillance against malig-nancy, and regulate immune tolerance. Thus, as the use of newer therapies widens, vigilance for unforeseen immune-related adverse effects must be vigorously maintained.

Case Presentation

A 42-year-old previously healthy businesswoman presents with a 6-month history of progressively increasing pain, stiffness, and swelling of the small joints of her hands and feet, elbows and knees. The joint problems and severe fatigue have recently placed her job in jeopardy. She denies fever, hair loss, dry eyes, dry mouth, mucosal sores, skin rash, color change in her fingers on cold exposure, pleurisy, diarrhea, and recent tick bite. She is often awakened at night by numbness and tingling of the right thumb, index and middle fingertips. Non-prescription non-steroidal anti-inflamma-tory drugs (NSAIDs) and acetaminophen, taken in increasing doses, led to no improvement. The patient's maternal grandmother had rheumatoid arthritis.

The patient walked slowly with an antalgic gait, favoring her right leg. Although the general physical examination was normal, the musculoskeletal examination revealed diffuse and prominent abnormalities. Neck range of motion was limited on lateral flexion and extension and associated with pain. Both shoulders revealed restriction of internal rotation and abduction with some mild anterior swelling. Both elbows were limited in flexion to 85 degrees and had lateral synovitis. Both wrists revealed marked swelling, warmth, and tenderness, with limitation in range of motion in all axes. There were positive Tinel's and Phalen's signs in the right wrist, but there was no evidence of thenar atrophy.

Prominent swelling, warmth, and tenderness were found in all metacar-pophalangeal (MCP) and proximal interphalangeal (PIP) joints, and grip strength was 50% of normal. The extensor tendons of the hands revealed swelling, tenderness, and pronounced thickening. Hip flexion was limited to 90 degrees bilaterally, and there was marked pain on limited internal rota-tion. Moderate-sized knee effusions were found bilaterally, and flexion was limited to 65 degrees. Both ankles were swollen and warm with limited dor-siflexion. The dorsal aspects of both feet were quite swollen and tender, and the patient had swelling of all toes with squeeze tenderness of the forefeet.

The range of motion of the lumbar spine was normal and painless, and the sacroiliac joints were not tender.

Complete blood count demonstrated a mild anemia (hemoglobin 10.2 gm/dL) and thrombocytosis (650,000 platelets/mm^3). The ESR was high at 85 mm/h. Urinalysis and the 12-channel chemistry screening tests were normal. A serum RF test was strongly positive at a dilution of 1:2560, but a serum antinuclear antibody (ANA) test was negative. X-rays of the right hand revealed prominent soft tissue swelling and juxta-articular osteoporosis about the MCP and PIP joints, and small marginal erosions were present in the second and third MCP joints.

The diagnosis of active, moderately severe, seropositive, erosive RA was made. Carpal tunnel syndrome, probably due to RA tenosynovitis, was also diagnosed. The nature of these diagnoses and treatment options were fully discussed with the patient.

Given the marked functional limitation and early development of joint erosions in this patient, her illness was deemed to be aggressive; accordingly, an equally aggressive therapeutic regimen was chosen. A regimen of standing NSAID therapy and a 7-day rapidly tapering course of oral prednisone beginning at 20 mg was recommended to quickly control her symptoms. After it was determined that the patient had no underlying hepatic disease (e.g., chronic viral hepatitis), weekly oral methotrexate 7.5 mg and folic acid 1 mg/d were prescribed. Monthly monitoring for potential methotrexate toxicity with regular liver function tests and complete blood counts was instituted. A right volar wrist splint was crafted for use while sleeping, and a computer pad was recommended to support her hands at work.

After 6 weeks, the patient was markedly improved on NSAID therapy, and the weekly methotrexate dose had been increased to 15 mg. No adverse effects had been noted by the patient or detected by laboratory tests. The ESR fell to 45 mm/h, and the blood hemoglobin increased to 12.0 gm/dL. Mild-to-moderate puffiness in the hands and feet persisted, but the patient's grip strength and carpal tunnel syndrome symptoms improved noticeably. However, because the disease was clearly still active, the weekly dose of methotrexate was again increased.

At 3 months, the patient continued to improve functionally, and her joint examination revealed only mild puffiness of the MCP joints and anterior feet. By this time, her methotrexate dose had been increased to 22.5 mg/wk but had been switched to the subcutaneous route because of nausea.

A month later, the patient had a flare of diffuse joint inflammation and increased fatigue that was controlled with a 4-day tapering course of prednisone beginning at 20 mg on the first day and a change to another NSAID. While the patient was clearly better than when first seen, she was breaking through her drug regimen and having recurrent functional problems at home and work. The TNF-α antagonist etanercept 25 mg subcutaneously twice weekly was added to her therapeutic regimen.

Six months after her diagnosis and the onset of therapy, the patient was markedly improved, fully functional, and tolerating her drug regimen without problems. No evidence of active inflammation was found on physical examination save for some mild squeeze tenderness of the metatarsal joints.

Clinical Features

Although joint inflammation and damage generally occupy center stage in RA, constitutional symptoms and visceral disease play major supporting roles and at times can dominate the clinical picture and be life-altering or life-threatening. RA differs from patient to patient in its personality, severity, aggressiveness, pace of progression, damage potential, and capacity to limit function. Nonetheless, there are some universal constants regarding RA:

- It is a symmetrical inflammatory process that commonly involves the small joints of the hands and feet, wrists, elbows, shoulders, hips, knees, and ankles. Cervical spine disease is also often present and can severely threaten neurological structures.

- Fatigue may be prominent and is at times its most disturbing component.

- It is chronic and will eventuate in some degree of joint damage and functional limitation in all patients without proper disease-modifying treatment. Without aggressive treatment, ongoing active inflammation of joints can lead to irreparable damage and disability. Erosions will likely develop within the first 2 years of disease and progressively worsen thereafter (Figure 3-1).

- Its tempo and severity are unpredictable and may change quickly, and so close monitoring is mandated.

The clinical presentation enables the physician to solidify the diagnosis of RA, to gauge a general sense of prognosis, and to individualize optimal treatment plans accordingly.

It must be fully appreciated that the diagnosis of RA is a clinical one, based upon specific facts and symptom patterns gleaned from the history and physical examination, and supported, not defined, by laboratory tests. Inflammation of the joints is characterized by pain, redness, warmth, and swelling (i.e., *dolor, rubor, calor,* and *tumor*). Although the illness may begin in an asymmetrical or monarticular fashion, RA will eventually evolve within weeks or a few months into a symmetrical inflammatory disorder that generally involves the wrists, the MCP and PIP joints of the hands, elbows, shoulders, hips, knees, and ankles, and the small joints of the feet. Deviation from this pattern should raise the suspicion of alternative disorders. For example, a chronic asymmetrical oligoarthritis (i.e., involvement of four or fewer joints) is more consistent with a seronegative spondyloarthropathy,

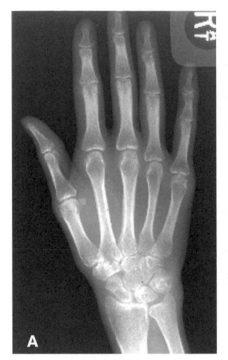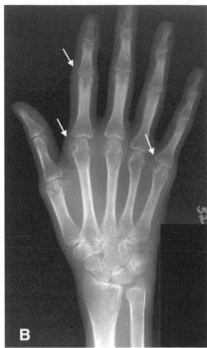

Figure 3-1 Erosive changes in rheumatoid arthritis. Panel A is a plain radiograph of the right hand and wrist of a patient newly diagnosed with RA that demonstrates juxtaarticular osteoporosis but no definitive erosive changes. In less than a year, as depicted in Panel B, clear erosions have developed at the margin of multiple joints, some of which are indicated by arrows.

such as psoriatic arthritis, the arthritis associated with inflammatory bowel disease, or reactive arthritis. The musculoskeletal symptoms associated with active RA are characteristically worse with inactivity, and therefore patients will typically complain of morning stiffness lasting at least an hour. In contrast, mechanical or degenerative joint symptoms usually improve with rest, and any complaints of stiffness last no more than several minutes.

Constitutional symptoms such as fatigue and weight loss may sometimes be the most debilitating component of RA. The patient may become exhausted by the afternoon yet otherwise appear well. These cytokine-related symptoms are similar to, but more chronic than, those of a short-lived viral illness. Interestingly, RA is generally not associated with fever. If fever is a prominent clinical manifestation, alternative diagnoses such as viral arthritis, systemic infections, or systemic lupus erythematosus should be entertained.

Tendinitis or tenosynovitis can be quite prominent and presents as diffuse swelling of the dorsae of the hands and feet. Carpal tunnel syndrome may result from pressure on the median nerve by its accompanying swollen flexor tendons, manifesting in paresthesias, pain, or motor dysfunction in the radial aspect of the hand. Similarly, cubital tunnel syndrome or tarsal tunnel syndrome can occur as the result of compression of the ulnar nerve at the elbow or of the posterior tibial nerve at the ankle, respectively.

Prominence of the ulnar styloid, ulnar deviation, interosseous muscle atrophy, swan-neck, and boutonniere deformities are signs of chronic and more severe RA and reflect greater aggressiveness of disease (Figure 3-2). Similarly, cervical spine involvement also reflects increased severity but adds a dangerous facet. If extensive, cervical instability can lead to permanent neurological deficits, myelopathy, or even death. Neurosurgical consultation is indicated at the earliest evidence of cervical spine instability (Figure 3-3).

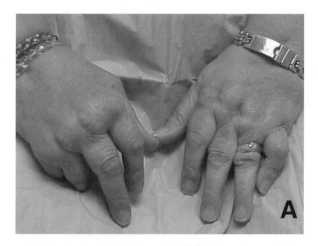

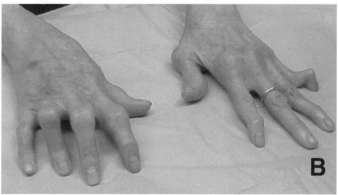

Figure 3-2   Hand changes in two patients with rheumatoid arthritis. Panel A demonstrates active synovitis of multiple metacarpophalangeal and proximal interphalangeal (PIP) joints and the boutonniere deformity [hyperflexion of the PIP joint and hyperextension of the distal interphalangeal (DIP) joint] in the left fifth digit. Panel B shows interosseous atrophy and the swan-neck deformity (hyperextension of the PIP joint and hyperflexion of the DIP joint), notably in the left fifth digit.

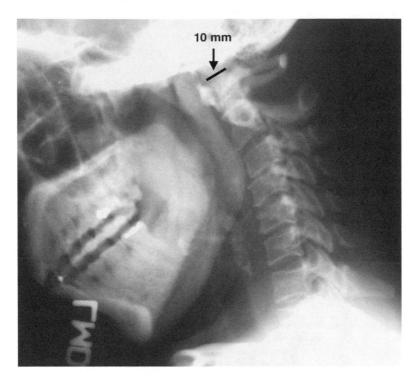

Figure 3-3   Atlantoaxial subluxation in rheumatoid arthritis. The posterior aspect of the body of the atlas (C1) is typically separated from the anterior aspect of the dens of the axis (C2) by 2-3 mm. The two vertebra are held tightly together by the transverse ligament of the atlas. In RA, the transverse ligament can become eroded by inflammation, resulting in atlantoaxial subluxation and cervical instability. In this lateral view of the flexed cervical spine of a patient with severe RA, the atlantoaxial separation is 10 mm (black bar), prompting neurosurgical intervention to fuse and stabilize the cervical spine.

Extra-articular manifestations of RA occur in a small but important subset of RA patients with the greatest likelihood for the development of rapidly progressive joint damage and functional limitation and the eventual need for joint replacement surgery. Ten percent of patients develop rheumatoid nodules at points of pressure, most particularly at the extensor surfaces of the forearms (Figure 3-4). Other extra-articular manifestations include: pleuritis and pericarditis; peripheral neuropathy; dry eyes and mouth (Sjögren's or sicca syndrome); scleritis; Felty's syndrome with spleno-megaly, neutropenia, and recurrent infections; and a rare but potentially organ-threatening and life-threatening polyarteritis nodosa-like systemic vasculitis called RA vasculitis or malignant RA. Nearly all of these patients have high serum titers of RF and rheumatoid nodules.

The average age at the onset of RA is approximately 50. Under 60 years of age, the female to male ratio is 3:1. Over age 60, accounting for one-third of all patients, the gender ratio is more even. Elderly-onset RA (onset

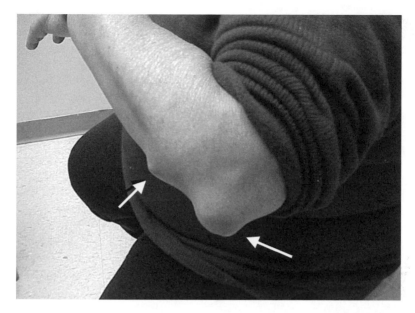

Figure 3-4 Rheumatoid nodules (*arrows*) on the extensor surface and within the olecranon bursa of the left forearm and elbow of a patient with severe rheumatoid arthritis.

after 60 years of age) may present in a somewhat atypical fashion with the co-existence of both peripheral joint and proximal muscle pain and stiffness, features reminiscent of polymyalgia rheumatica. Also, RF is often negative in these cases, and some experts believe that this subset of RA is the same illness as polymyalgia rheumatica and is appropriately treated with a gradual taper of low-dose systemic corticosteroids.

Diagnosis

Laboratory data and radiology can be used to confirm the diagnosis of rheumatoid arthritis and to monitor the course of the illness and its response to treatment.

Laboratory Testing

Anemia and thrombocytosis on complete blood counts reflect active inflammation and will improve as systemic inflammation is decreased with therapy. The white blood cell count is usually normal or mildly elevated in RA. Leukocytopenia should bring up the specter of Felty's syndrome, SLE, drug toxicity, or a bone marrow disorder such as leukemia or lymphoma.

The ESR and CRP are reasonably good reflections of the state of inflammation and are helpful in defining a response to treatment in some patients.

However, these are extremely non-specific tests, and elevations in either can occur in the settings of infections, malignancy, allergy, and tissue injury. It should be emphasized that the ESR and CRP are only general markers of disease and may not always correlate with the clinical picture. The clinician should take care to "treat the patient and not the test."

A chemistry panel including electrolytes and measures of hepatic and renal function should always be obtained. These screening tests are important in identifying co-morbidites that could alter the choice of medications (e.g. diabetes and corticosteroids; renal or hepatic dysfunction and NSAIDs or methotrexate) and for preventing and monitoring adverse effects from therapies. They occasionally may also be helpful diagnostically in distinguishing conditions that can sometimes masquerade as RA, such as gout (e.g., elevated uric acid), hepatitis C infection (e.g., elevated liver transaminases), or SLE (e.g., elevated creatinine due to nephritis). Likewise, the urinalysis can suggest lupus nephritis (e.g., proteinuria or active sediment) or drug toxicities (e.g., proteinuria in gold therapy). By itself, however, RA rarely affects the kidney, save for secondary amyloidosis in a rare patient with severe long-standing RA.

RF is an immunoglobulin that recognizes the Fc portion of IgG. IgM RF is found in the serum of 80% of patients with RA, and it is the RF that is tested for in most laboratories. If positive, a titer or level will usually be reported; a high RF titer increases the likelihood that the test is truly positive. Approximately 20% of RA patients are RF-negative, and so a negative test should not be interpreted to exclude RA as a diagnosis. Also, RF is not specific to RA and can be positive in many disorders such as SLE, scleroderma, viral hepatitis, mixed cryoglobulinemia, sarcoidosis, tuberculosis, and bacterial endocarditis, and is often present at low levels in the healthy elderly. In RA, once positive, there is generally no need to repeat the test.

Antinuclear antibody (ANA), like RF, is a screening test and thus is sensitive but not specific to RA. The ANA test is positive in almost all SLE patients but can also be positive in many disorders, including RA and scleroderma, in the setting of certain medications, in the healthy elderly, and even in healthy relatives of patients with SLE. Like RF, higher titers of ANA are more likely to be truly positive tests. There are also distinctive ANA staining patterns that can be diagnostically useful: a diffuse or homogeneous pattern is non-specific; a peripheral or rim pattern is fairly specific for SLE; a speckled pattern can be seen in SLE, Sjögren's syndrome, and scleroderma. If the ANA is positive, antibodies to double-stranded DNA (anti-dsDNA) can help assess the likelihood of SLE because it is the most specific test for lupus. Because some patients with RA do have a positive ANA but a negative RF, the anti-dsDNA antibodies can sometimes help differentiate RA from SLE. When positive, the ANA staining pattern in RA is usually homogenous and nonspecific.

In contrast to RF and ANA, circulating antibodies to citrullinated proteins (anti-CCP) show specificity for RA. Because anti-CCP antibodies

appear to predict worse outcomes in RA, they are increasingly being used
for diagnostic and prognostic purposes.

Radiological Studies

Because the presence of erosions in the wrist, MCP, or PIP joints of an RA
patient is important in defining the severity and aggressiveness of that individual's disorder and in determining therapeutic approach, a baseline X-ray
of the most-involved hand and wrist is appropriate (see Fig. 3-1). This can
be repeated in 6 months to 1 year to determine whether the disease has
progressed. Magnetic resonance imaging of the joint can reveal erosions
earlier than plain X-rays but is not routinely performed as a screening test
because of cost.

Differential Diagnosis

RA is a symmetrical polyarthritis involving the small joints of the hands and
feet (particularly the MCP and PIP joints and the analogous joints in the
feet but characteristically not the distal interphalangeal [DIP] joints), wrists,
elbows, shoulders, hips, knees, and ankles. With radiographic presence of
erosions and a positive RF, diagnoses other than RA are unlikely.

SLE, however, also commonly presents with a symmetrical polyarthritis
involving the very same joints as RA, but it is "the company that the joint
inflammation keeps" that usually differentiates SLE from RA. The absence
of characteristic skin rashes, mucosal ulcers, nephritis, cytopenias, and specific serologic tests effectively excludes SLE. Joint erosions are *not* classically seen in SLE, although a "Rhupus" overlap syndrome characterized by
joint erosions and positive lupus serologies (e.g., anti-dsDNA antibodies) is
occasionally observed.

Similarly, other types of connective tissue disorders such as scleroderma
and vasculitides such as polyarteritis nodosa (PAN) can present with a polyarthritis, but they commonly have or will develop their signature disease
manifestations such as Raynaud's phenomenon, tight skin, and esophageal
dysmotility with scleroderma, and fever, mononeuritis multiplex, and skin
lesions with PAN.

As discussed above, polymyalgia rheumatica can be difficult to differentiate from elderly-onset RA because the latter can have prominent proximal joint symptoms and a negative RF test. However, this subset of RA
patients will have prominent peripheral joint involvement, RA can be erosive, and RA is not associated with giant cell arteritis. Practically speaking,
however, both disorders will respond to low-dose prednisone.

The seronegative spondyloarthropathies such as psoriatic arthritis, reactive arthritis, or the arthritis associated with inflammatory bowel disease
share a particular presentation: asymmetrical large lower extremity joint

inflammation. Psoriatic arthritis can frequently involve the small joints of the hands, but it is usually in an asymmetrical fashion and can be differentiated from RA by the prominent involvement of DIP joints. Also, patients commonly have swollen and red sausage-shaped digits (dactylitis), nearly pathognomonic of psoriatic arthritis and other spondyloarthropathies. Because both RA and psoriasis are relatively common disorders, they can co-exist, and at times it is difficult to differentiate RA with concomitant psoriasis from psoriatic arthritis. However, because the therapies overlap significantly, this is usually not a major therapeutic problem. The co-existence of these joint presentations with enthesitis (prominent inflammation at the sites of tendon and ligament insertions), morning low back stiffness, and uveitis complete the diagnostic picture for the spondyloarthropathies.

Polyarticular gout or pseudogout can masquerade as RA. Also adding to the diagnostic conundrum are tophi that can resemble rheumatoid nodules. The diagnosis of these disorders is usually based upon their lack of truly symmetrical joint involvement, a history of acute episodes of monarticular inflammation, an elevated serum uric acid level, and a family history of gout. Also, gouty tophi have a whitish base when the skin is pulled tautly over them. Finally, the finding of characteristic crystals in synovial fluid or from tophi on polarizing microscopy makes the definitive diagnosis.

Viral arthritides can often present in a symmetrical RA-like pattern. Notable examples are rubella or rubella vaccine-induced arthritis, hepatitis B in the arthritis-dermatitis syndrome, hepatitis C as part of RF-positive mixed cryoglobulinemia, and parvovirus B19 polyarthritis. The joint symptoms of all of these disorders are self-limited, usually lasting from days to a few months. Thorough questioning will generally reveal a recent exposure history. Bacterial joint infections are usually monarticular, although disseminated gonococcal disease may be characterized by a migratory polyarthritis. Lyme disease in its early phase can be manifested by polyarthralgias without evidence of frank joint swelling. A waxing and waning monoarticular inflammatory arthritis typically involving a knee is characteristic of late, tertiary Lyme disease.

Patients with fibromyalgia will have prominent tenderness and pain in periarticular and musculotendinous structures but will not exhibit clinical or laboratory evidence of inflammation within the joint. However, it should be kept in mind that patients may have concomitant RA and fibromyalgia.

Prognosis

As with most diseases, there is an element of biological pre-determinism in RA. It is chronic and potentially destructive to joints in all patients, but the aggressiveness of RA ranges from mild to severe (Table 3-1). Fortunately, it is only rarely threatening to visceral organs or to life. Nevertheless, without aggressive treatment, significant functional impairment can result; after 10

Table 3-1   Mild, Moderate, and Severe Rheumatoid Arthritis

Mild disease
- Fewer than 10 actively inflamed joints
- No impairment of daily activities
- No radiological evidence of erosions or joint space narrowing
- No joint deformities
- No extra-articular manifestations

Moderate disease
- 10-15 actively inflamed joints
- Symptomatic fatigue or some limitations of daily activities
- Radiological evidence of erosions or joint space narrowing
- Mild/moderate joint deformities
- Mild extra-articular manifestations (e.g., anemia of chronic disease, cutaneous nodules)

Severe disease
- More than 15 actively inflamed joints
- Significant impairment of daily activities
- Significant joint destruction and/or need for surgery
- Serious extra-articular manifestations (e.g., vasculitis)

years of disease, in 50% of patients erosions will progressively worsen to the extent that the patient must stop working.

Certain clinical features are associated with increased severity of disease and overall poor prognosis:

- a large number of involved joints and a high degree of inflammation present in each;
- significant functional limitation and inability to work or perform activities of daily living;
- prominent constitutional complaints such as fatigue or weight loss;
- severe joint damage as defined by deformities, the presence of radiological erosions or joint space narrowing, or the need for joint surgery;
- laboratory evidence of systemic inflammation (anemia, thrombocytosis, elevated ESR, or CRP);
- the presence of extra-articular disease manifestations such as rheumatoid nodules, serositis, and vasculitis;
- high serum levels of RF and anti-CCP antibodies;
- a strong family history of severe RA.

Stratification of patients into categories of mild, moderate, and severe disease by employing the above data helps the physician and patient meet disease aggressiveness with appropriate treatment aggressiveness. Disease tempo and severity, however, are unpredictable, and close monitoring for changes is therefore necessary. With disease-modifying treatment, RA is less likely to progress, and its natural history can be significantly altered in a positive manner.

RA is not only a life-altering disorder with regard to function and work status but is also life-shortening. On average, both male and female patients with RA live 5 years less than age- and sex-matched controls (4). Cardiovascular disease is the most common cause of mortality, followed by infections and lymphoproliferative diseases. Aggressive treatment of RA with drugs such as methotrexate has been shown to reverse this trend towards early mortality.

Management

RA is a fairly common condition in the primary care setting, and many primary care physicians feel comfortable treating RA patients. However, because RA can be indolently progressive and because new treatment options are continually being developed, a consultation with a rheumatologist should not be delayed if the patient does not respond to treatment as expected. Like the goal of cancer treatment, the goal in managing RA is to achieve "no evidence of disease," because RA, at any level of severity, is an aggressive illness that adversely alters and shortens the patient's life. Without appropriate suppression, active inflammation of the joints eventuates in irreparable damage (5).

Whatever therapeutic decision is made initially, defined clinical outcomes and expectations are needed to assess response to therapy. Close clinical monitoring is mandatory in order to establish responsiveness to a given drug regimen and to assess the need to add to or change the armamentarium. A 70%-80% or better clinical improvement, synthesizing data from the physician's assessment, the patient's assessment, fatigue and functional scales, and laboratory tests, should be the target. Treatment approaches that are clearly ineffective should not be belabored. Optimal doses of disease-modifying anti-rheumatic drugs (DMARDs) to achieve a therapeutic response should be reached as quickly as possible. Once chosen, the regimen should be constantly reassessed and appropriate changes made as necessary to achieve desired outcomes. Short courses of corticosteroids in patients with moderate or severe RA may help enhance the efficacy of the DMARDs.

Treatment decisions are based upon a composite of the following: disease activity and severity; the patient's prior treatments for RA and response and side effects; co-morbidities; family input; patient choice of route of administration; side-effect profile; cost and logistical issues; and informed communication with the physician about recommendations.

Treatment regimens often contain combinations of the following:

- An NSAID
- Short courses of systemic corticosteroids
- One or more DMARDs
- Surgery
- Physical and occupational therapy with orthotic devices and splints as needed
- Ergonomic adjustment of the workplace or home
- Management of physical and emotional stresses

Non-Steroidal Anti-Inflammatory Drugs

There are over two dozen NSAIDs (prescription and non-prescription) currently available in the United States. These medications suppress inflammation but do not affect the natural history of RA (i.e., they are not disease-modifying). Nevertheless, they are helpful at any time during the disease course for symptomatic relief of joint complaints due to ongoing inflammation or structural damage from past disease. In an otherwise healthy person with no co-morbidities and specifically no history of peptic ulcer disease or gastrointestinal intolerance to NSAIDs or of significant renal insufficiency, any NSAID can be chosen. It may take up to 3 weeks before a beneficial effect is observed but no more than a few days after discontinuation for the beneficial effects to cease.

Patients vary greatly with regard to favorable response or adverse effects to specific drugs. It is common to try several different NSAIDs before settling on a preferred agent. In older patients or in those who have had some gastrointestinal intolerance to traditional NSAIDs, concomitant use of proton pump inhibitors or using cyclooxygenase-2-selective NSAIDs instead will lower but do not completely eliminate gastrointestinal toxicity (6,7). In general, older patients tolerate NSAIDs less well than younger patients; this is particularly true in individuals with cardiovascular, gastrointestinal, bleeding, or renal problems. A more complete discussion of these medications is presented in Chapter 29.

Corticosteroids

An overriding principle of corticosteroid therapy is that the shortest course in the lowest dose that controls severe, function-limiting RA is the optimal regimen. In moderate and severe disease, short 4-day courses of daily prednisone beginning at 20 mg will re-set the inflammatory thermostat and allow other drugs to work faster and better. This is particularly useful in the window period that is normally required before a favorable therapeutic effect of DMARD therapy is realized. Mini-pulses of intravenous methylprednisolone

(Solumedrol) (250 mg-1000 mg IV qd × 1-3 days) can be used for severe disease that is refractory to more conventional regimens or in patients with visceral disease or RA vasculitis. An average of prednisone 5 mg daily or less (or equivalent dosages of other corticosteroids) is generally regarded as safe and acceptable but is certainly not without potential adverse effects, especially with long-term use. As with all RA treatments, the risk-benefit analysis must be discussed in full with the patient.

Intra-articular corticosteroid injections (e.g., methylprednisolone [Depo-Medrol] 10-80 mg depending on the joint) are often helpful in suppressing the inflammation in single joints that are especially symptomatic. There may also be additional benefit for other joints as the injected corticosteroid is systemically absorbed. However, when a single joint is disproportionately inflamed, a possible superimposed infection should always be suspected and excluded.

Disease-Modifying Anti-Rheumatic Drugs (DMARDs)

Therapy with DMARDs should be considered for *all* patients with RA (8). These drugs are termed "disease-modifying" because in therapeutic trials the drug in question has been shown to decrease the development of joint erosions and joint space narrowing. As a general rule, DMARDs may take weeks to months before a positive symptomatic effect is observed, and the patient should be made aware of this in order to maintain realistic expectations and overall compliance. DMARDs may be used singly or in combination, instituted either all at once or in a stepwise additive fashion according to the severity of the disease. Combination therapy may target different points in pathogenesis, thereby lowering dosages of individual drugs required.

Table 3-2 lists drugs and their typical maintenance dosages that clearly fit the DMARD category and describe some of their proposed mechanisms of action. A fuller discussion of important DMARDs is presented in Chapter 31. Table 3-3 delineates some commonly employed DMARD regimens.

Methotrexate and TNF-α Inhibitors
Because of their exceptional roles in the current treatment of RA, methotrexate and the inhibitors of TNF-α deserve special mention here. Over the past three decades, methotrexate has proven to be an effective, safe, well-tolerated, and versatile agent in the management of RA and is arguably the gold standard to which other DMARDs are compared (9). It can be administered singly as a weekly oral, subcutaneous, or intramuscular dose or as the conerstone of a combination regimen. A typical initial dose is 7.5 mg per week, which can be steadily increased by 2.5-5.0 mg increments. In general, 15-25 mg per week may be needed to observe a clinical response, which may require several weeks to occur. Minor adverse effects include gastrointestinal intolerance, oral ulcers, and rashes, many of which can be

Table 3-2   Disease-Modifying Anti-Rheumatic Drugs

Drug	Maintenance Dosage	Mechanism of Action
Sulfasalazine (Azulfidine)	1000-1500 mg PO bid	Folic acid antagonist that blocks the pro-inflammatory effects of adenosine
Methotrexate (Rheumatrex, Trexall)	7.5-25 mg PO/SQ qwk	Folic acid antagonist that has immunosuppressive and anti-inflammatory properties
Leflunomide (Arava)	100 mg PO qd for 3 d followed by 10-20 mg PO qd	Pyrimidine synthesis inhibitor that interferes with DNA synthesis and is immunosuppressive
Parenteral gold salts (Myochrysine)	25-50 mg IM every week to every month	Actions unclear but possibly interferes with macrophage activation
Azathioprine (Imuran)	2 mg/kg body weight PO daily in divided doses	Purine analogue that interferes with DNA synthesis and is immunosuppressive
Cyclosporin A (Sandimmune, Neoral)	2-5 mg/kg body weight PO qd	Inhibitor of T cell activation and IL-2 activity
Etanercept (Enbrel)	25 mg SQ twice weekly	Fusion protein that binds TNF-α
Infliximab (Remicade)	3-10 mg/kg body weight IV at weeks 0, 2, 6, then every 8 weeks thereafter	Chimeric monoclonal antibody against TNF-α
Adalimumab (Humira)	40 mg SQ every 1-2 weeks	Recombinant human monoclonal against TNF-α
Anakinra (Kineret)	100 mg SQ qd	IL-1 receptor antagonist that competitively inhibits binding of IL-1 to its receptors

prevented by the concomitant administration of folic acid 1 mg daily. More serious toxicities include myelosuppression and hepatotoxicity, and so complete blood counts and serum biochemical/liver function tests need to be monitored every 4 to 6 weeks.

Three agents that inhibit the activity of TNF-α have been approved for the treatment of RA: etanercept (Enbrel), infliximab (Remicade), and adalimumab (Humira) (10-12). Despite being available for less than 10 years, these drugs have already proven to be potent and effective medications. Because they are all proteins, parenteral administration is necessary, which may be problematic for some patients, and they are very expensive. However, they are clearly effective for symptomatic relief of RA and prevention

---

Table 3-3   Optimal Choice of DMARDs Based on Disease Severity

Management of mild RA
Fewer than 10 joints actively inflamed, daily activities not impaired, and no joint deformities, erosions, or extra-articular manifestions. Consider the following single-drug regimens:

- Hydroxychloroquine
- Sulfasalazine
- Methotrexate
- Intramuscular gold salts
- Minocycline

Management of moderately severe RA
10-15 actively inflamed joints, moderately severe fatigue that limits activities of daily living or work, joint deformities or erosions, and mild extra-articular manifestions such as rheumatoid nodules. Consider the following regimens:

- Methotrexate
- Methotrexate plus hydroxychloroquine
- Methotrexate plus hydroxychloroquine plus sulfasalazine
- Intramuscular gold salts
- Leflunomide
- Azathioprine
- Etanercept
- Infliximab
- Adalimumab

Management of severe or refractory RA
20-30 actively inflamed joints with associated joint deformities, erosions, and joint space narrowing despite above listed treatment; activites markedly limited by joint symptoms and fatigue; extra-articular manifestations often present; high serum titer of RF and significant anemia of chronic disease. Consider the following regimens:

- Methotrexate plus leflunomide
- Methotrexate plus etanercept
- Methotrexate plus infliximab
- Methotrexate plus adalimumab
- Methotrexate plus anakinra
- Leflunomide plus anakinra
- Methotrexate plus cyclosporin

---

of joint damage. They appear to have a more rapid response rate than traditional DMARDs; some patients report benefit after one dose. Increased risks for infection have arisen as the greatest concern in the use of the TNF-α inhibitors.

Hydroxychloroquine and Minocycline

The anti-malarial drug hydroxychloroquine (Plaquenil) (200 mg PO bid) and the antibiotic minocycline (100 mg PO bid) are not universally regarded as true DMARDs but are quite safe and have a positive clinical impact on mild RA, above and beyond NSAIDs and prednisone (13,14). Thus, they are employed by some rheumatologists in patients with mild disease or in combination with more established DMARDs. The mechanism of action for hydroxychloroquine is unknown but may interfere with the inflammatory cascade by inhibiting antigen processing and presentation. Minocycline probably acts via the inhibition of metalloproteinase enzymes rather than through its antibacterial actions.

Surgical Options

The overwhelming trend towards early use of more effective DMARDs has resulted in better preservation of joint structure and function in patients with RA. Unfortunately, there are still patients whose disease is inadequately controlled. In many of these cases, surgical options can offer significant benefit. Procedures generally fall into four categories: synovectomy/tenosynovectomy, tendon repair/realignment, arthroplasty (joint replacement), and arthrodesis (fusion).

In general, the main goals of surgery in RA are to alleviate pain, preserve function, and restore function. Intervention purely for cosmetic reasons is discouraged because loss of function may be a significant risk of surgery. Spine fusion for treatment of cervical instability is the procedure accompanied by the greatest sense of urgency and is an example of surgery that can prevent loss of function and possibly death. Arthroplasties are demonstrating increasing longevity and can dramatically improve quality of life, particularly in patients with hip or knee disease. Shoulders and elbows are also amenable to arthroplasty, but severe wrist or ankle involvement is usually addressed with arthrodesis.

When surgery is contemplated, an orthopedic surgeon with extensive specific knowledge of RA and its physiology should be consulted to determine which option is appropriate for the situation at hand.

Non-Pharmacological Therapy and Rehabilitation

A variety of non-pharmacological and rehabilitative approaches can enhance the benefit of medical and surgical therapies. Major aims include pain control, preservation of function, joint protection, and psychological well-being. Many modalities are available to offer palliation, including heat, ultrasonography, massage for reduction of stiffness and spasm, cold for reduction of inflammation, and electrical nerve stimulation for chronic pain management. A balanced program of rest, range-of-motion exercises, and muscle strengthening are essential for preserving overall joint function. Under the guidance of trained physical and occupational therapists, patients with RA can also better protect their joints from mechanical injury by learning to more safely perform daily tasks and to use splints and assistive and ergonomic devices.

Finally, psychological therapy and counseling can often help patients, who are frequently young, to live and cope with a chronic and physically demanding disease in a healthy and adaptive manner.

REFERENCES

1. **Fries JF, Wolfe F, Apple R, et al.** HLA-DRB1 genotype associations in 793 white patients from a rheumatoid arthritis inception cohort: frequency, severity, and treatment bias. Arthritis Rheum. 2002;46:2320-9.

2. **Gorman JD, Criswell LA.** The shared epitope and severity of rheumatoid arthritis. Rheum Dis Clin North Am. 2002;28:59-78.

3. **Choy EH, Panayi GS.** Cytokine pathways and joint inflammation in rheumatoid arthritis. N Engl J Med. 2001;344:907-16.

4. **Pincus T, Sokka T, Wolfe F.** Premature mortality in patients with rheumatoid arthritis: evolving concepts. Arthritis Rheum. 2001;44:1234-6.

5. **Emery P.** Evidence supporting the benefit of early intervention in rheumatoid arthritis. J Rheumatol. 2002; 29(Suppl 66):3-6.

6. **Silverstein FE, Faich G, Goldstein JL, et al.** Gastrointestinal toxicity with celecoxib vs nonsteroidal anti-inflammatory drugs for osteoarthritis and rheumatoid arthritis: the CLASS study: a randomized controlled trial. JAMA 2000;284:1247-55.

7. **Bombardier C, Laine L, Reicin A, et al.** Comparison of upper gastrointestinal toxicity of rofecoxib and naproxen in patients with rheumatoid arthritis. VIGOR Study Group. N Engl J Med. 2000;343:1520-8.

8. **Wolfe F, Cush JJ, O'Dell JR, et al.** Consensus recommendations for the assessment and treatment of rheumatoid arthritis. J Rheumatol. 2001;28:1423-30.

9. **Williams HJ, Willkens RF, Samuelson CO Jr, et al.** Comparison of low-dose oral pulse methotrexate and placebo in the treatment of rheumatoid arthritis: a controlled clinical trial. Arthritis Rheum. 1985;28:721-30.

10. **Moreland LW, Schiff MH, Baumgartner SW, et al.** Etanercept therapy in rheumatoid arthritis: a randomized, controlled trial. Ann Intern Med. 1999;130:478-86.

11. **Maini RN, Breedvald FC, Kalden JR, et al.** Therapeutic efficacy of multiple intravenous infusions of anti-tumor necrosis factor alpha monoclonal antibody combined with low-dose weekly methotrexate in rheumatoid arthritis. Arthritis Rheum. 1998;41:1552-63.

12. **Weinblatt ME, Keystone EC, Furst DE, et al.** Adalimumab, a fully human anti-tumor necrosis factor alpha monoclonal antibody, for the treatment of rheumatoid arthritis in patients taking concomitant methotrexate: the ARMADA trial. Arthritis Rheum. 2003;48:35-45.

13. **Clark P, Casas E, Tugwell P, et al.** Hydroxychloroquine compared with placebo in rheumatoid arthritis: a randomized controlled trial. Ann Intern Med. 1993;119: 1067-71.

14. **O'Dell JR, Blakely KW, Mallek JA, et al.** Treatment of early seropositive rheumatoid arthritis: a two-year, double-blind comparison of minocycline and hydroxychloroquine. Arthritis Rheum. 2001;44:2235-41.

4

■ ■ ■

Spondyloarthropathies

Yusuf Yazici, MD

Allan Gibofsky, MD, JD

The spondyloarthropathies are a group of systemic inflammatory disorders that are pathophysiologically related and have overlapping clinical features. Included are ankylosing spondylitis (AS), psoriatic arthritis (PsA), reactive arthritis (ReA), and arthritis associated with inflammatory bowel disease (IBD). In many cases, particularly early in the course of illness, a definitive diagnosis may not be possible, and patients may be putatively given a diagnosis of an undifferentiated spondyloarthropathy. Moreover, because onset is typically quite insidious, many cases go unrecognized, and so the prevalence of spondyloarthropathies is probably much greater than has been appreciated and may be as high as 1% of the general population.

The most widely accepted classification criteria have been established by the European Spondyloarthropathy Study Group (Table 4-1) (1). Musculoskeletal involvement in the spondyloarthropathies can involve the axial skeleton (the spine and sacroiliac joints), the peripheral joints, and the entheses (the sites of bony insertions of tendons and ligaments such as the Achilles' tendon or plantar fascia). The pattern of joint inflammation (i.e., number, symmetry, and location) and extra-articular manifestations are important for determining the specific type of spondyloarthropathy. It must be emphasized that spondyloarthropathies represent a broad spectrum of conditions, and patients should be treated on a case-by-case basis even if they do not fulfill diagnostic criteria for a specific condition.

Pathogenesis

Both men and women can be affected by spondyloarthropathies, although there is clearly a male predominance. Familial aggregation frequently

Table 4-1   Classification Criteria for Inflammatory Spondyloarthropathy

Inflammatory spinal pain* or peripheral synovitis (either asymmetrical or predominantly in the lower limbs) AND one or more of the following:

- Positive family history of spondylo-arthropathy
- Psoriasis
- Radiographically or pathologically documented inflammatory bowel disease (IBD)

- Urethritis, cervicitis, or acute diarrhea presenting 1 month before arthritis
- Buttock pain alternating between right and left gluteal areas
- Enthesopathy
- Sacroiliitis

*Inflammatory spinal pain is defined by the presence of at least four of the following: 1) at least 3 months in duration, 2) onset before age 45, 3) insidious onset, 4) improvement with activity, and 5) morning spinal stiffness.
From Dougados M, van der Linden S, Juhlin R, et al. The European Spondylarthropathy Study Group preliminary criteria for the classification of spondylarthropathy. Arthritis Rheum. 1991;24:1218-27; with permission.

Table 4-2   Frequency of HLA-B27 in Whites with Spondyloarthropathies and Associated Conditions

Disease	Prevalence of HLA-B27 (%)
Ankylosing spondylitis	90
Reactive arthritis	40-80
Juvenile spondyloarthropathy	70
Spondyloarthritis associated with inflammatory bowel disease	35-75
Psoriatic arthritis	40-50
Undifferentiated spondyloarthropathy	70
Idiopathic acute anterior uveitis/iritis	50
Aortic incompetence with heart block associated with spondyloarthropathy	80

Modified from Khan MA. Update on spondyloarthropathies. Ann Intern Med. 2002;136:896-907; with permission.

occurs, and spondyloarthropathies classically begin in the late teens and early adulthood.

Although the pathogenesis of spondyloarthropathies is not completely understood, it has long been known that there is a marked association with the HLA-B27 haplotype, with AS demonstrating the strongest association (Table 4-2). ReA, juvenile spondyloarthropathy, and spondyloarthropathy associated with IBD also show strong associations. Spondyloarthropathies have also been linked to HLA class I antigens that have cross-reactivity with HLA-B27, but because HLA-B27 is present in 8% of healthy whites, it is clear that other factors also contribute to the development of disease. In ReA, in which the disease is typically preceded by a gastrointestinal or genitourinary infection, contributing factors are self-evident. However, in the other spondyloarthropathies, the nature of secondary triggers remains the subject of conjecture.

Case Presentation

A 47-year-old man with a 20-year history of ulcerative proctitis is seen for chronic back pain and new-onset right knee pain and swelling. During the past 5 years, he has developed progressive loss of mobility throughout his spine and severe low back morning stiffness. He has had anterior chest pains when he coughs or sneezes. Last week, he developed swelling and profound stiffness in his right knee. Sporadic doses of ibuprofen have not been helpful. Despite these symptoms, he has continued to engage in his usual activities and has not sought medical attention for these problems until now.

In the distant past, his colitis was treated successfully with oral sulfasalazine and up until a year ago was well controlled with only corticosteroid and mesalamine enemas as necessary during flares. However, during the past year, colitis flares have become more frequent. Recurrent episodes of iritis have become part of his disease, requiring intermittent treatment with corticosteroid eyedrops.

Notably, multiple male members of his family have IBD although not with articular or ophthalmological manifestations. The patient has had many years of recurrent aphthous ulcers but denies skin rashes, genital lesions, sexually transmitted diseases, and urethritis.

Pertinent positive findings on his physical examination include mild tenderness of costochondral and sacroiliac joints; moderate-to-severe loss of range of motion of the neck in all planes with almost no lateral flexion; inability to simultaneously press his occiput, back, and heel against a wall; and almost no lateral flexion of the lumbosacral spine. His chest excursion was less than 2 cm; he had a 5-cm Schober's test; and he was unable to bend over to touch the floor with his fingertips. The right knee was mildly warm, erythematous, and tender, with a moderately large effusion.

Complete blood count and serum biochemistries were normal. X-rays of the sacroiliac joints demonstrated mild sclerosis bilaterally, and the diagnosis of a spondyloarthropathy (IBD–associated arthritis) was made.

The patient was given ibuprofen 600 mg every 6 hours, which relieved his articular symptoms, but when he tried to discontinue the drug, he developed recurrent knee pain. Sulfasalazine 500 mg twice daily was initiated and increased to 1500 mg twice daily over several weeks, after which the patient was able to discontinue his standing anti-inflammatory medication. His gastrointestinal and ocular complaints also improved. Once he became less symptomatic, physical therapy was initiated to improve range of motion of the spine.

Clinical Features

Although there is great overlap and variability in the clinical presentation of the spondyloarthropathies, some general characteristics of individual conditions are listed in Table 4-3.

Ankylosing Spondylitis

AS is a chronic, systemic inflammatory arthritis of the axial skeleton, potentially affecting the entire spine and sacroiliac joints; symmetrical sacroiliitis is the hallmark of the disease. The shoulders and the hips are also frequently affected, but involvement of the other smaller peripheral joints is uncommon. Costochondritis and thoracic spine disease can result in clinically relevant restrictive lung disease.

AS is more common in males. It usually presents initially in adolescence or early adulthood as back pain and stiffness with prolonged inactivity. It is very rare for AS to start after age 45, although in many cases, the condition is frequently not recognized until later in life because of the subtlety of clinical manifestations. The prevalence of AS is approximately 0.1% to 0.2%.

Back pain is an exceedingly common problem in the general population (a full discussion is given in Chapter 27). Accordingly, as outlined by the classification criteria for spondyloarthropathies, specific clinical features can help to differentiate AS from other causes of back pain:

Table 4-3   General Characteristics of Spondyloarthropathies

Feature	AS	PsA	ReA	IBD
Peripheral arthritis	Uncommon	Common	Common	Common
Joint distribution	Axial, hips, shoulders	Any joint	Lower limbs	Lower limbs
Dactylitis	Uncommon	Common	Common	Uncommon
Sacroiliitis	90%	40%	80%	20%
Skin disease	Rare	Psoriasis	Circinate balanitis, keratoderma blennorrhagicum	Pyoderma gangrenosum, erythema nodosum
Mucous membrane	Uncommon	Uncommon	Common	Uncommon
Conjunctivitis	Rare	Occasional	Common	Rare
Uveitis	Occasional	Occasional	Common	Occasional
Urethritis	Rare	Occasional	Common	Rare
Aortic regurgitation	Occasional	Rare	Occasional	Occasional

AS = ankylosing spondylitis; PsA = psoriatic arthritis; ReA = reactive arthritis; IBD = inflammatory bowel disease.
From Gladman DD. Psoriatic arthritis. Rheum Dis Clin North Am. 1998;24:829-44; with permission.

- Onset before age 45
- Insidious presentation
- Persistence of symptoms for at least 3 months
- Prominent morning stiffness
- Improvement with exercise

The pain is often described as dull in character but can be quite severe. It is felt as a deep discomfort, typically localized to the sacroiliac region initially, but later can spread to other areas of the back with subsequent involvement of the entire spine. Enthesopathic changes result in discomfort or tightness in other areas such as the Achilles' tendon or the plantar fascia. With advancing disease, spinal ankylosis may develop, with flattening of the spine and development of a thoracic kyphosis.

Some patients may have constitutional symptoms such as malaise, loss of appetite, weight loss, and low-grade fever, but these are non-specific and generally quite mild. A more specific and important extra-articular manifestation of AS is acute anterior uveitis, which occurs at some point in 25%-40% of patients and is more common in HLA-B27-positive patients. A painful and inflamed eye demands an ophthalmological slit-lamp evaluation. The uveitis is usually unilateral but can be bilateral and often recurs. Visual disturbances may not always be present initially.

Dyspnea is a common complaint and is most often due to rigidity of the chest wall and/or costochondritis. However, a significant minority of patients may have cardiac or pulmonary involvement. In up to 1% of patients with AS, aortitis with dilatation of the aortic valve ring and aortic insufficiency is present (2). Cardiac conduction abnormalities and myocardial disease can also occur. In addition, 1% of patients develop progressive fibrosis of the upper lung lobes. Spinal osteoporosis can be a late complication of AS due to immobility and ongoing inflammatory cytokine activity and increases the risk of spinal fractures.

Psoriatic Arthritis

In the United States, psoriasis affects 1%-3% of whites but is less common in other ethnic groups such as blacks and Native Americans (<0.3%). The overall prevalence of psoriasis in the United States is about 1%-2%, and men and women are affected equally. More than 10% of patients with psoriasis have an associated inflammatory arthritis. The arthritis may start before the appearance of psoriasis but most commonly occurs simultaneously to or after the onset of the skin disease. Population studies point to a 50-fold increased risk of PsA in first-degree relatives of patients with the disease, and like the other spondyloarthropathies, there is an association with HLA-B27.

There is great variability in the presentation of PsA, spanning monoarthritis, asymmetrical oligoarthritis/polyarthritis, symmetrical polyarthritis resembling rheumatoid arthritis (RA), and spondylitis with or without peripheral joint involvement. The severity of the skin disease tends to be but is not always correlated with the severity of the arthritis. Onset of disease is typically before age 45.

Although the variability in clinical presentations has led to several classification schemes for PsA, patients may be divided conceptually into three general groups: 1) asymmetrical monoarthritis or oligoarthritis (40%-60% of patients); 2) symmetrical polyarthritis similar to RA (30%-50% of patients); and 3) predominant axial disease (5%-10% of patients). In addition, a rare but aggressive form of PsA called arthritis mutilans can be seen, which can lead to "telescoping" of the involved digits.

The classical presentation of PsA is an asymmetrical oligoarthritis involving a large joint (such as a knee or ankle), one or two interphalangeal joints, or dactylitis (i.e., "sausage" digit) resulting from concomitant tenosynovitis and arthritis of a digit (Figure 4-1). The RA-like symmetrical polyarthritis of PsA involves the small joints of the hands and feet, wrists, ankles, knees, and elbows. Distal interphalangeal joint involvement is almost always associated with psoriatic nail changes and helps distinguish PsA from RA; pitting (small punctate depressions) of the nail plate is a characteristic physical finding in PsA. Moreover, there is a greater propensity for bony ankylosis of interphalangeal joints than in RA.

The evolution of mild psoriasis to a widespread erythrodermic pattern with associated exacerbation of arthritis should raise the suspicion of an underlying human immunodeficiency virus (HIV) infection in high-risk patients (3). Recognition of concurrent HIV infection with psoriasis and PsA is important because immunosuppressive agents, which may otherwise be potential therapeutic options, may be contraindicated in this setting.

Inflammatory Bowel Disease

In one series, more than a third of patients with IBD, Crohn's disease, or ulcerative colitis had inflammatory arthritis, and most fulfilled the classification criteria for spondyloarthropathy (4). An additional 18% of patients in this study showed radiographic evidence of asymptomatic sacroiliitis.

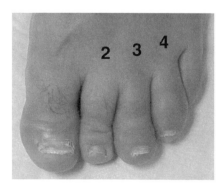

Figure 4-1 Dactylitis ("sausage" digits) of the third and fourth toes of the left foot in a patient with psoriatic arthritis, resulting from concomitant tenosynovitis and arthritis of a digit. Notice that the second toe is unaffected.

Conversely, it is interesting to note that many patients with spondylo-arthropathies have histologic evidence of microscopic colitis despite having no clinical bowel disease. The average onset of IBD-associated arthritis is approximately 30 years.

IBD-associated arthritis is usually self-limited and non-deforming and may precede the onset of bowel involvement. The arthritis may be migratory, is less often additive, and is usually asymmetrical in pattern. The peripheral arthritis tends to be more symptomatic, and its severity correlates more closely with bowel disease activity than does axial disease. Interestingly, surgical colectomy in ulcerative colitis results in permanent remission of arthritis. Cutaneous complications of IBD such as erythema nodosum and pyoderma gangrenosum often occur at the same time with arthritis. Acute anterior uveitis can also be seen in 2%-9% of patients.

Reactive Arthritis

ReA is an aseptic inflammatory arthritis that occurs 2 to 3 weeks after a gas-trointestinal or a genitourinary infection. Organisms that are commonly impli-cated include gram-negative enterobacteria (*Shigella, Salmonella, Yersinia, Campylobacter,* and other species) and *Chlamydia trachomatis.* ReA is typ-ically acute, asymmetrical, and oligoarticular. Dactylitis and enthesopathies (e.g., plantar fasciitis or Achilles' tendinitis) are commonly observed. In ad-dition, ReA is frequently associated with extra-articular manifestations, such as eye inflammation (acute uveitis or conjunctivitis), urethritis, and muco-cutaneous lesions. The triad of reactive non-gonococcal inflammatory arthritis, uveitis, and urethritis has been historically known as Reiter's syn-drome, but this term has fallen out of favor.

In most individuals, the frank arthritis usually lasts several months, al-though mild musculoskeletal problems may persist for up to a year or more. Recurrent attacks can occur, and about 15%-33% of patients even-tually develop chronic arthritis. Most of these patients have a family history of spondyloarthropathy or are positive for HLA-B27. Joints of the lower ex-tremity (knees, ankles, and small joints of the feet) are most commonly in-volved. Enthesitis usually manifests as heel or sole pain, although other sites such as the ischial tuberosities, the iliac crests, and the ribs can also often be involved. Low back pain is common and seen in half of the patients.

Some dermatological manifestations of ReA are quite distinct. Kerato-derma blennorrhagicum is a papulosquamous skin rash that most com-monly occurs on the soles and palms but can affect any part of the skin. Lesions start as raised papular lesions and later can become hyperkeratotic and scaly and indistinguishable from psoriatic skin lesions. It is histologi-cally identical to pustular psoriasis. Nails can show thickening, opacification, and crumbling, but nail pitting as seen in PsA is not characteristic of ReA. Circinate balanitis is a plaque-like rash seen on the glans penis and is also associated with ReA.

Diagnosis

Spondyloarthropathies are clinical diagnoses based on characteristic histories and physical findings. Various physical signs may be characteristic for axial skeletal involvement. Cervical spine disease may result in a fixed-forward stoop of the neck (Figure 4-2). This can be demonstrated by a positive occiput-to-wall test in which the patient is unable to push his occiput to the wall while simultaneously pressing his back and heel against the wall. The flexibility of the lumbosacral spine can be assessed with the Schober's test in which the lumbosacral junction and a point 10 cm above it along the spine are marked while the patient is standing upright. The patient is then asked to flex forward maximally. The test is considered positive if the resulting distance between the two marked points is less than 15 cm. Costovertebral involvement can be assessed by noting decreased maximal chest expansion, which is measured at the fourth intercostal space in males and under the breasts in females. Less than 5 cm of chest expansion with inspiration is considered reduced.

Several maneuvers can be used to assess sacroiliitis. Sacroiliac tenderness can be elicited by direct pressure from behind over the sacroiliac joints. Alternatively, with the patient supine, pressing and forcing the anterior superior iliac spines apart laterally can cause sacroiliac pain. Finally, again with the patient supine, sacroiliac discomfort may be elicited by forced flexion of one hip towards the contralateral shoulder during hyperextension of the contralateral hip.

When present, laboratory abnormalities like elevated erythrocyte sedimentation rates (ESR) and serum levels of C-reactive protein are non-specific but reflect the generalized systemic inflammatory condition. Rheumatoid factor positivity is not associated with the spondyloarthropathies. Although spondyloarthropathies are associated with HLA-B27, routine testing for HLA-B27 is not recommended because the diagnosis is typically defined by

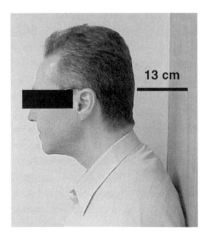

13 cm

Figure 4-2   Severe cervical spine involvement in a patient with spondyloarthropathy resulting in a fixed forward stoop of the neck. This patient is unable to extend his neck to simultaneously press his occiput and back against the wall, leaving a gap of 13 cm.

the clinical presentation, and 8% of the unaffected white population carry this haplotype.

Radiographical changes usually are not present early, but when the disease has been ongoing, radiographs can be diagnostic. Plain anteroposterior radiography of the pelvis can show sacroiliitis, which is a radiological hallmark of spondyloarthropathies (Figure 4-3). Sclerotic changes in the subchondral bone are late findings that reflect prolonged joint inflammation.

Peripheral joint involvement in PsA is characterized by concomitant erosive joint disease and periarticular bony proliferation. Fusiform soft tissue swelling, marked joint space loss, and periostitis are stereotypical findings on hand and feet X-rays. In severe cases, the joint space may appear to be widened due to aggressive resorption of the bone on both sides of the joint. The distal ends of phalanges may be eroded down to sharp points, resulting in "pencil-in-cup" deformities. Magnetic resonance imaging with gadolinium enhancement is more sensitive in detecting early joint changes but is not a cost-effective means of diagnosis.

Prognosis

Although the spectrum of disease in spondyloarthropathies is wide, several factors, when seen within the first 2 years of illness, appear to be predictors of more severe illness: hip joint involvement, an elevated ESR, poor response to non-steroidal anti-inflammatory drugs, limited mobility of the lumbar spine, dactylitis, oligoarthritis, and juvenile onset of disease (younger than

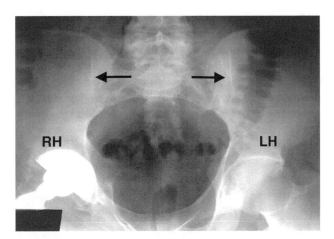

Figure 4-3   Hip and pelvis X-rays of a 35-year-old man with ankylosing spondylitis. Complete fusion of the both sacroiliac joints (*arrows*) has left only sclerotic lines with no remaining joint space. Severe right hip (RH) involvement has already resulted in the implantation of a total hip prosthesis. Left hip (LH) disease is also severe and is characterized by concentric narrowing of the joint space.

16 years) (5). Factors associated with a greater frequency of radiological changes may include male gender, family history of spondyloarthropathy, and chronic gastrointestinal lesions such as fistulae.

The disease course of AS is highly variable and can range from asymptomatic sacroiliitis to global fusion of the spine. It is difficult to predict at the outset which patients will develop more severe disease. Many patients can remain active with few limitations, but a significant number will develop permanent disabilities. In one long-term study of 100 patients, more than half were still employed full time after a mean disease duration of 16 years. Most of the loss of function occurred within the first decade of disease and was associated with the presence of shoulder or hip joint involvement and early radiographic changes in the spine.

Psoriatic arthritis can result in the same degree of joint damage and functional disability as rheumatoid arthritis and is no longer viewed as a mild condition. The severity of the arthritis tends to parallel the severity of the skin disease, and the presence of extra-articular features (e.g., uveitis) is associated with worse outcomes. In some series, joint erosions occur in up to 71% of patients with PsA. Accordingly, earlier and more aggressive therapies have become more commonplace in the management of PsA, but whether this leads to long-term benefits in outcomes remains unproven.

Peripheral arthritis and axial arthropathy in IBD tend to run independent courses. Peripheral involvement (excluding the hip) is usually non-erosive and non-deforming and often parallels the bowel disease. An extreme example of this is the observation that a complete colectomy in ulcerative colitis will induce a permanent remission of peripheral arthritis. In contrast, patients with spondylitis are prone to destructive hip disease and an erosive coxopathy that evolves separately from gut inflammation.

Post-infectious ReA is generally less severe than the other spondyloarthropathies and commonly self-limited. The initial arthritic episode may last several months, although in some cases, the inflammatory arthritis can last over a year. Mild joint discomfort and enthesopathic pain are common after resolution of the frank arthritis. Only a minority of patients (15%-33%) develop chronic peripheral joint or spine disease, but of these many can develop marked and debilitating oligoarthritis.

Management

The importance of the primary care provider is in the early recognition of spondyloarthropathies, prompting a timely rheumatology referral in order to effect rapid control of disease and to prevent permanent disability.

Physical Modalities

Patients with spondyloarthropathies require a multidisciplinary approach to treatment with a particular emphasis on a life-long program of exercise, physical activity, and life-style modification. Exercise to maintain spinal mobility helps prevent potentially disabling deformities. Swimming is usually considered to be the best kind of exercise for patients with spondylitis. Patients should sleep with a straight back and avoid being curled up on one side. Ergonomic workplace and home modifications can facilitate daily activities.

Non-Steroidal Anti-Inflammatory Drugs

The medical treatment for spondyloarthropathies generally begins with NSAIDs. Although indomethacin has been historically considered to be more effective, there is actually no definitive evidence that any specific NSAID offers more benefit than any other. Anti-inflammatory dosages (e.g., naproxen sodium, 550 mg PO bid), which are typically higher than analgesic dosages (e.g., naproxen sodium 220 mg PO bid), are often required, but most patients experience significant improvement in joint inflammation and control of pain and stiffness and are able to continue their usual activities and have an improved ability to participate in physical therapy. Many individuals with mild forms of spondyloarthropathy require only NSAIDs and a good physical exercise regimen. As discussed in Chapter 29, however, prolonged use of NSAIDs are associated with increased risks for clinically relevant toxicities such as gastrointestinal events, platelet dysfunction, and renal effects. Selective inhibitors of cyclooxygenase-2 may have fewer effects on the gastric mucosa and platelets, but they are still potentially nephrotoxic.

Corticosteroids

Intraarticular corticosteroids (e.g., Depo-Medrol 10-80 mg, depending on the size of the joint) are often very useful in treating individually inflamed joints or entheses. When necessary, injections of certain less accessible joints (e.g., sacroiliac joints or hips) can be done under fluoroscopy or ultrasonography for increased accuracy. The response to corticosteroid injections can last up to several months. Systemic corticosteroids (e.g., prednisone 10-20 mg PO qd) have also been used, particularly when many joints are affected, but there are no good controlled studies evaluating the long-term benefits and risks. In general, because clinical response is less uniform, systemic corticosteroids are less commonly used for spondyloarthropathies than for RA. They should be avoided for prolonged treatment in patients with PsA in particular because discontinuation of the corticosteroids may lead to severe flares of the skin disease. Chronic systemic corticosteroids carry significant additional risks for worsening osteoporosis and subsequent insufficiency fractures.

Disease-Modifying Anti-Rheumatic Drugs

Many of the agents used for long-term treatment of rheumatoid arthritis and prevention of irreversible joint damage have been employed for the spondyloarthropathies. Of these, sulfasalazine and methotrexate have enjoyed the widest experience. However, although peripheral joint arthritis often responds to these agents, spine involvement has not been shown to be particularly affected. Sulfasalazine has been a consistent mainstay for the treatment of mild to moderately severe spondyloarthropathies. In placebo-controlled, double-blind studies of patients with AS, PsA, and ReA, oral sulfasalazine (1.0-1.5 g twice daily) has generally shown moderate effectiveness in improving patient and physician global assessments of disease activity and reducing serological markers of inflammation (e.g., ESR) (6,7). Patients with PsA appear to respond better than patients with either AS or ReA, and peripheral disease is more responsive than axial disease. However, definitive evidence documenting retardation of radiological progression of disease is lacking.

Methotrexate (7.5-25 mg weekly administered orally or parenterally) has also been used in the treatment of spondyloarthropathies, particularly in PsA, in which both skin disease and peripheral arthritis show consistent response (8). However, significant concern over methotrexate-induced hepatotoxicity in PsA remains, and some experts continue to advocate baseline and serial liver biopsies (after each 1.5 g cumulative dose of methotrexate or after every 3-4 years of therapy) as part of routine monitoring for adverse drug effects. In AS, despite early enthusiasm, a recent randomized, placebo-controlled, double-blind study of methotrexate in severe AS showed no significant benefit compared with placebo, even in patients with peripheral arthritis (9).

TNF-α Inhibitors

For a significant number of patients with spondyloarthropathies, traditional DMARDs fail to provide significant improvement. However, recent excitement has been generated by the use of inhibitors of tumor necrosis factor (TNF)-α, a pro-inflammatory cytokine central to the perpetuation of the inflammatory process.

A randomized, placebo-controlled, double-blind trial evaluating the use of the TNF-α inhibitor etanercept (25 mg subcutaneously twice weekly) in PsA has demonstrated significant improvement in joint symptoms and skin lesions and reduced methotrexate and corticosteroid requirements in subjects given the active drug (10). Moreover, evidence also indicates that etanercept slows the progression of joint erosions. Etanercept has now been approved by the FDA for the treatment of PsA.

Infliximab, another TNF-α inhibitor, was initially developed for the treatment of Crohn's disease, and early reports indicated that associated peripheral joint disease appeared to improve with treatment. More recently, intermittent intravenous infliximab (5 mg/kg) has been evaluated in randomized, placebo-controlled, double-blind trials in the treatment of active spondyloarthropathies (primarily AS and PsA) (11). Patients treated with infliximab show clinical improvement as early as 2 weeks after the start of therapy and continue to show response after 3 months. Longer studies have also shown retardation of radiographic joint damage. Given the marginal benefit of sulfasalazine and methotrexate in patients with AS, anti-TNF-α agents may emerge as first-line therapy in the near future.

Antibiotics

Although prolonged tetracycline therapy in *Chlamydia*-induced ReA showed some promise in at least one early study, antibiotics have not been shown to be generally helpful for most cases of spondyloarthropathies (12).

REFERENCES

1. **Dougados M, van der Linden S, Juhlin R, et al.** The European Spondyl-arthropathy Study Group preliminary criteria for the classification of spondylarthropathy. Arthritis Rheum. 1991;24:1218-27.

2. **Roldan CA, Chavez J, Wiest PW, et al.** Aortic root disease and valve disease associated with ankylosing spondylitis. J Am Coll Cardiol. 1998;32:1397-404.

3. **Njobvu P, McGill P.** Psoriatic arthritis and human immunodeficiency virus infection in Zambia. J Rheumatol. 2000;27:1699-702.

4. **de Vlam K, Mielants H, Cuvelier C, et al.** Spondyloarthropathy is underestimated in inflammatory bowel disease: prevalence and HLA association. J Rheumatol. 2000;27:2860-5.

5. **Amor B, Santos RS, Nahal R, et al.** Predictive factors for the long-term outcome of spondyloarthropathies. J Rheumatol. 1994;21:1883-7.

6. **Dougados M, van der Linden S, Leirisalo-Repo M, et al.** Sulfasalazine in the treatment of spondyloarthropathy: a randomized, multicenter, double-blind, placebo-controlled study. Arthritis Rheum. 1995;38:618-27.

7. **Kirwan J, Edwards A, Huitfeldt B, et al.** The course of established ankylosing spondylitis and the effects of sulphasalazine over 3 years. Br J Rheumatol. 1993;32:729-33.

8. **Espinoza LR, Zakraoui L, Espinoza CG, et al.** Psoriatic arthritis: clinical response and side effects to methotrexate therapy. J Rheumatol. 1992;19:872-7.

9. **Altan L, Bingol U, Karakoc Y, et al.** Clinical investigation of methotrexate in the treatment of ankylosing spondylitis. Scand J Rheumatol. 2001;30:255-9.

10. **Mease PJ, Goffe BS, Metz J, et al.** Etanercept in the treatment of psoriatic arthritis and psoriasis: a randomised trial. Lancet. 2000;356:385-90.

11. **Van den Bosch F, Kruithof E, Baeten D, et al.** Randomized double-blind comparison of chimeric monoclonal antibody to tumor necrosis factor alpha (infliximab) versus placebo in active spondyloarthropathy. Arthritis Rheum. 2002;46:755-65.

12. **Lauhio A, Leirisalo-Repo M, Lahdevirta J, et al.** Double-blind, placebo-controlled study of three-month treatment with lymecycline in reactive arthritis, with special reference to *Chlamydia* arthritis. Arthritis Rheum. 1991;34:6-14.

5

■ ■ ■

Adult-Onset Still's Disease

Helen E. Bateman, MD

A dult-onset Still's disease (also referred to as adult-onset systemic juvenile rheumatoid arthritis) is a rare systemic inflammatory disorder of unknown etiology, characterized by a quotidian fever, evanescent rash, and polyarthralgias/polyarthritis. Initially described by G. F. Still in 1897, it is seen worldwide. Onset is usually between the ages of 16 and 35 with approximately equal occurrence in males and females. Waxing and waning systemic inflammatory features, with or without chronic arthritis, dominate the clinical course. Although adult-onset Still's disease is rare (incidence fewer than 2 per 100,000), it accounts for up to 15% of eventual diagnoses in patients with fever of unknown origin (1). Therefore, the primary care physician should consider this diagnosis when faced with an unexplained febrile illness and obtain a rheumatology consultation if the index of suspicion is high.

Pathogenesis

No specific etiologic triggers have been definitively identified, although viral agents have been widely suspected as potential culprits. Proinflammatory cytokines, such as tumor necrosis factor-alpha (TNF-α), interleukin-1 (IL-1), and especially interleukin-6 (IL-6), have been implicated in the pathogenesis of the inflammatory state.

Case Presentation

A 30-year-old female presented with spiking fevers and symmetric polyarthritis involving the proximal interphalangeal joints, metacarpophalangeal joints, wrists, and knees. The patient also complained of an evanescent rash associated with the fever and pleuritic chest pain. Diffuse lymphadenopathy

62

and hepatosplenomegaly were observed on physical examination. Leukocytosis (white blood cell count $22.0 \times 10^9/dL$), thrombocytosis (platelets
$532 \times 10^9/dL$), and anemia (hemoglobin 10.3 g/dL) were present, and
pleuropericarditis was suggested on chest radiography and echocardiography. Serum tests for antinuclear antibodies and rheumatoid factor were negative. Based on the clinical picture, including fever, polyarthritis, serositis,
evanescent rash, and leukocytosis, the diagnosis of adult-onset Still's disease
was made.

Treatment with NSAIDs and corticosteroids (prednisone 10-15 mg daily)
was begun, and yet the patient continued to have frequent disease flares.
Oral gold therapy was of no benefit, and treatment with oral sulfasalazine 1 g
orally twice a day resulted in only modest improvement of the synovitis. As
the patient subsequently developed more frequent exacerbations requiring
increases in her corticosteroid dosage, hydroxychloroquine 200 mg twice
daily and methotrexate 15 mg weekly were added to the regimen. Despite
this combination of disease-modifying anti-rheumatic drugs (DMARDs), the
prednisone dose could only be tapered to 10 mg daily with continued smoldering synovitis. Moreover, the patient began developing intolerance to the
multiple DMARDs, which prompted their discontinuation.

Subcutaneous etanercept 25 mg twice weekly was then initiated. The
polyarthritis improved, and the disease flares became less frequent. The
prednisone was tapered to 5 mg daily without exacerbation of disease, and
although the patient continued to have joint swelling, she experienced less
pain and stiffness.

Clinical Features

The frequency of clinical manifestations of 62 patients with adult-onset
Still's disease is shown in Table 5-1 (2). Arthralgias and arthritis occurred in
100% and 94% of patients, respectively. In order of descending frequency,
the most commonly involved joints are the knees, wrists, ankles, elbows,
shoulders, and hands. In the hands, proximal interphalangeal and metacarpophalangeal joints are most likely to be affected. Hip involvement, if present, is usually severe and debilitating and often results in arthroplasty.
Fever, occurring in 96% of patients, is usually high (> 39.5°C) and spiking
in a quotidian pattern, with return to normal temperature between spikes.
Chills may also occur. The characteristic salmon pink rash, seen in 89% of
patients, can be macular or maculopapular, usually occurs with the fever,
and is often misinterpreted as a drug allergy because it may be mildly pruritic. However, the evanescent nature of the rash is almost pathognomonic
of adult-onset Still's disease. The Koebner phenomenon, which is the occurrence of the rash at sites of irritation, is sometimes present and may be
induced by the examiner by scratching the skin. Sore throat is also
common and may cause confusion with upper respiratory tract infections.

Table 5-1   Frequency of Clinical Features in Adult-Onset Still's Disease

Quotidian fever ≥ 39° C	100%		Sore throat	92%
Arthralgias	100%		Salmon-colored evanescent rash	87%
Arthritis (any joint)	94%		Weight loss > 10%	76%
Knee	51%		Lymphadenopathy	74%
Wrist	45%		Splenomegaly	34%
Ankle	34%		Pleuritis	33%
Proximal interphalangeal	29%		Hepatomegaly	27%
Elbow	27%		Pericarditis	23%
Shoulder	25%		Pneumonitis	17%
Metacarpophalangeal	22%			
Metatarsalphalangeal	11%			
Hip	7%			
Distal interphalangeal	6%			

From Pouchot J, Sampalis JS, Beaudet F, et al. Adult Still's disease: manifestations, disease course, and outcome in 62 patients. Medicine. 1991;70:118-35; with permission.

Lymphadenopathy, hepatosplenomegaly, pleuritis, and pericarditis occur with decreasing frequency.

Diagnosis

The diagnosis of adult-onset Still's disease is based solely on clinical findings and the exclusion of other infectious, rheumatological, immunological, and neoplastic disorders. Although several classification schemes for the diagnosis of adult-onset Still's disease have been developed, the relative rarity of the condition makes validation of these schemes difficult (one recently proposed set of criteria is outlined in Table 5-2) (3). Diagnosis requires a high clinical suspicion and vigilance for specific features such as the rash, which usually presents only in the evening with the fever.

Laboratory testing (Table 5-3) generally reflects non-specific inflammatory changes including leukocytosis, thrombocytosis, an elevated erythrocyte sedimentation rate and increased serum levels of ferritin and C-reactive protein. Interestingly, however, serum levels of glycosylated ferritin are actually reduced. Although the pathogenic significance of this finding is not known, decreased levels of glycosylated ferritin have been proposed as a diagnostic criterion for adult-onset Still's disease. Elevations of serum liver transaminases are usually observed. ANA and RF are usually negative. Periarticular osteopenia is an early radiographic sign. Erosions may or may not be seen. When there is joint ankylosis, it will usually manifest in the first

Table 5-2   Proposed Criteria for the Diagnosis of Adult-Onset Still's Disease*

Major (two points)	Minor (one point)
Quotidian fever > 39°C	Onset age < 35 years
Still's (evanescent) rash	Arthritis
WBC ≥ 12,000/mm³ + ESR > 40 mm/hr	Prodromal sore throat
Negative RF and ANA	RES involvement or abnormal LFT
Carpal ankylosis	Serositis
	Cervical or tarsal ankylosis

*Probable adult-onset Still's disease: 10 points with 12 weeks observation; definite adult-onset Still's disease: 10 points with 6 months observation.
WBC = white blood cell count; ESR = erythrocyte sedimentation rate; RF = rheumatoid factor; ANA = antinuclear antibodies; RES = reticuloendothelial system; LFT = liver function tests.
From Fautrel B, Zing E, Golmard JL, et al. Proposal for a new set of classification criteria for adult-onset Still disease. Medicine 2002;81:194-200; with permission.

Table 5-3   Frequency of Laboratory Abnormalities in Adult-Onset Still's Disease

Elevated erythrocyte sedimentation rate (> 30 mm/hr)	100%
White blood cell count ≥ 10,000/mm³	94%
White blood cell count ≥ 15,000/mm³	81%
Neutrophils ≥ 80%	88%
Hypoalbuminemia	85%
Elevated liver enzymes*	76%
Anemia (hemoglobin ≤ 10 g/dL)	68%
Platelets (≥ 400,000/mm³)	62%
Serum antinuclear antibodies	11%
Serum rheumatoid factor	6%

*Alanine aminotransferase, aspartate aminotransferase, or alkaline phosphatase.
From Pouchot J, Sampalis JS, Beaudet F, et al. Adult Still's disease: manifestations, disease course, and outcome in 62 patients. Medicine. 1991;70:118-35; with permission.

few years of disease, often involving the cervical spine, interphalangeal joints, wrists, and ankles.

Differential Diagnosis

Differential diagnoses (Table 5-4) include bacterial and viral infections such as endocarditis, tuberculosis, viral hepatitis, Epstein-Barr virus, parvovirus, and rubella. Other connective tissue diseases also need to be considered. For

Table 5-4   Differential Diagnosis of Adult-Onset Still's Disease

Differential Diagnosis	Characteristic Clinical Features	Suggested Investigations and Lab/Radiologic Findings
Bacterial		
Endocarditis	Heart murmur	Blood cultures
Tuberculosis	Cough, hemoptysis, night sweats	PPD
Viral		
Hepatitis B & C	Jaundice, abdominal pain	Serologic testing, viral PCR
Human immuno-deficiency virus	Lymphadenopathy, fever, weight loss	Serologic testing
Epstein-Barr virus	Lymphadenopathy, splenomegaly, sore throat	Serologic testing, atypical lymphocytes on peripheral smear
Parvovirus B19	Rash, arthritis	Serologic testing
Drug reaction	Urticaria, pruritus	Skin biopsy
Cancer		
Leukemia	Nocturnal joint pain	Blasts on peripheral smear, periostitis on X-ray
Lymphoma	Lymphadenopathy, hepatosplenomegaly	Lymph node biopsy
Connective tissue disease		
SLE	Malar rash, fever, photosensitivity, renal disease, cytopenias	ANA, anti-ds-DNA and anti-Smith antibodies, complete blood counts, urine studies
Sjögren's syndrome	Dry eyes & mouth	ANA, anti-Ro/La antibodies
Sarcoidosis	Lupus pernio rash, dyspnea, cough	ACE level, hilar adenopathy on chest X-ray
Vasculitis		
Hypersensitivity	Palpable purpura	Skin biopsy
Wegener's granulomatosis	Hemoptysis, sinusitis, otitis, renal disease	c-ANCA
Churg-Strauss	Asthma	Eosinophilia

PPD = purified protein derivative; PCR = polymerase chain reaction, SLE = systemic lupus erythematosis; ANA = anti-nuclear antibody; ds-DNA = double stranded-DNA antibody; ACE = angiotensin converting enzyme; ANCA = anti-neutrophilic cytoplasmic antibody.

example, systemic lupus erythematosus may commonly present with fever, polyarthritis, and pleuritic chest pain, but it will be associated with a positive antinuclear antibody test and cytopenias. Rheumatoid arthritis (RA) presents as a symmetric polyarthritis, but fever and rash are not typical. Vasculitides and granulomatous diseases such as sarcoidosis can also mimic adult-onset Still's disease. Finally, leukemia and lymphomas must also be excluded, especially in cases associated with marked leukocytosis or cytopenias.

Prognosis

There are four subsets of adult-onset Still's disease based on clinical course: monocyclic systemic disease, polycyclic systemic disease, chronic articular monocyclic systemic disease, and chronic articular polycyclic systemic disease. Which subset of the disease is diagnosed affects prognosis.

Fewer than 20% of patients will have a self-limited monocyclic pattern of systemic disease (e.g., fever, rash, serositis, organomegaly), which is defined by the presence of one episode, which may last for 4-12 months, followed by clinical and laboratory remission. The majority of patients demonstrate a polycyclic systemic pattern defined by two or more episodes, again separated by sustained clinical and laboratory remissions. In both of these groups, the articular involvement is usually mild and parallels the systemic symptoms. However, in approximately 25% of patients with polycyclic systemic disease, a chronic articular disease that can be destructive and debilitating will develop.

Disease is usually considered to be chronic after 12 months of activity. The chronic articular pattern is seen in patients whose disease is dominated by chronic joint symptoms. This pattern is subdivided by the presence of co-existent monocyclic or polycyclic systemic disease. Patients with chronic articular disease have the worst outcome, with 27% progressing to functional class III with disabling arthritis in one series of patients. The presence of systemic manifestations does not necessarily contribute to poor function. HLA-DR4 positivity portends a poor prognosis with chronic arthritis. An aggressive approach to therapy with the early use of remittive or disease-modifying agents should be considered in patients with a chronic articular pattern.

Management

NSAIDs are usually the initial choice of therapy to control articular and many systemic features and are used at any point of the illness for control of fever, arthritis, or serositis. Any NSAID used at anti-inflammatory dosages (for example, indomethacin 150 mg per day) can been effective in approximately 40%-60% of patients. The risks for gastrointestinal, antiplatelet, and renal adverse effects increase with prolonged use of NSAIDs. Liver function, in particular, should be monitored very closely because the disease itself can affect the liver. Corticosteroids can been used separately or in combination with NSAIDs but should be reserved for patients with refractory disease manifested by markedly abnormal liver enzyme tests, prominent systemic features, severe serositis, or resistance to NSAIDs. Brief courses of moderate-to-high dose prednisone (40-60 mg per day) may sometimes be necessary. Minimizing the cumulative dose of corticosteroids should be a priority in order to decrease the risks of the many potential adverse effects associated with corticosteroid therapy.

When corticosteroids are inadequate for control of disease or when chronic dosage requirements are unacceptably high (e.g., more than 5-10 mg qd of prednisone), DMARDs should be considered as disease-controlling and steroid-sparing agents. Methotrexate (7.5-25 mg/week) is useful for controlling both articular and systemic symptoms and should be used early in those with severe or protracted disease (4,5). In one study of 13 patients, eight had remission of disease within 3-16 weeks, four showed no benefit, and one had to discontinue methotrexate because of severe nausea (4). Close monitoring with regular complete blood counts and liver chemistry tests is important as well as the concomitant use of folic acid 1 mg daily to minimize side effects. Other DMARDs, such as hydroxychloroquine, sulfasalazine, leflunomide, azathioprine, or cyclosporine, have also been utilized, alone or in combination, in a similar manner to the therapy for RA, particularly for patients with chronic progressive polyarthritis. However, because of the relative rarity of adult-onset Still's disease, there is a paucity of good clinical studies that assess their utility in this illness.

There is recent excitement in the use of TNF inhibitors (etanercept 25 mg subcutaneously twice a week or inflixmab infusion 3-10 mg/kg every 6-8 weeks) in the treatment of Still's disease (6-9). TNF inhibitors may be used as single agents or in combination with traditional DMARDs, especially methotrexate. They appear to be generally safe and well tolerated, but not all patients respond. Furthermore, strict vigilance for typical and atypical infections should be maintained. TNF inhibitors should be discontinued if there is evidence of severe infections.

REFERENCES

1. **Mert A, Ozaras R, Tabak F, et al.** Fever of unknown origin: a review of 20 patients with adult-onset Still's disease. Clin Rheumatol. 2003;22:89-93.
2. **Pouchot J, Sampalis JS, Beaudet F, et al.** Adult Still's disease: manifestations, disease course, and outcome in 62 patients. Medicine. 1991;70:118-35.
3. **Fautrel B, Zing E, Golmard JL, et al.** Proposal for a new set of classification criteria for adult-onset Still disease. Medicine. 2002;81:194-200.
4. **Fujii T, Akizuki M, Kameda H, et al.** Methotrexate treatment in patients with adult onset Still's disease: retrospective study of 13 Japanese cases. Ann Rheum Dis. 1997;56:144-8.
5. **Fautrel B, Borget C, Rozenberg S, et al.** Corticosteroid sparing effect of low dose methotrexate treatment in adult Still's disease. J Rheumatol. 1999;26:373-8.
6. **Cavagna L, Caporali R, Epis O, et al.** Infliximab in the treatment of adult Still's disease refractory to conventional therapy. Clin Exp Rheumatol. 2001;19:329-32.
7. **Kraetsch HG, Antoni C, Kalden JR, Manger B.** Successful treatment of a small cohort of patients with adult onset of Still's disease with infliximab: first experiences. Ann Rheum Dis. 2001;60(Suppl 3):55-7.
8. **Takei S, Groh D, Bernstein B, et al.** Safety and efficacy of high dose etanercept in treatment of juvenile rheumatoid arthritis. J Rheumatol. 2001;28:1677-80.
9. **Husni ME, Maier AL, Mease PJ, et al.** Etanercept in the treatment of adult patients with Still's disease. Arthritis Rheum. 2002;46:1171-6.

SECTION III

Collagen Vascular Diseases

6

■ ■ ■

Systemic Lupus Erythematosus

Ioannis Tassiulas, MD

Michael D. Lockshin, MD

Systemic lupus erythematosus (SLE), a chronic multisystemic connective tissue disease, is the prototypical human autoimmune disease. It is characterized by the production of numerous autoantibodies and multisystem inflammation. SLE is an extremely heterogeneous disorder, and although a number of factors are associated with more aggressive disease, its course in any individual patient is difficult to predict at the time of diagnosis. SLE predominantly affects women of childbearing age, with an overall female-to-male ratio of 7-10:1 and has an incidence of 1 in 700 among all women between the ages of 20 and 60 years and about 1 in 250 among African-American women. It should be remembered, however, that children and the elderly can also be affected.

Pathogenesis

The cause of the disease is unknown, but the interplay between genetic, hormonal, and environmental factors probably plays a significant role in the pathogenesis, severity, clinical expression, and outcome of the disease.

Immune dysfunction in SLE is multifaceted and includes the participation of pathogenic autoantibodies, defective immune complex clearance, abnormal cytokine expression, and dysfunction of cellular elements of the immune system, including lymphocytes and effector cells such as monocytes and macrophages. A general model of the pathogenesis is that SLE develops in an individual who has both inherited and acquired abnormalities of immune function. Susceptibility to SLE depends on multiple genes. For example, the relative risk of developing SLE for individuals with either the major histocompatibility class (MHC) II HLA-DR2 or HLA-DR3 haplotypes is

71

2 to 3; however, if both haplotypes are present, this risk increases to 5. Deficiencies in single genes such as the early components of complement C1q, C1r, C2, or C4 lead to SLE and SLE-like diseases but account for less than 5% of cases of SLE. Genetically defined diminished immunoglobulin receptor function leads to reduced clearance mechanisms and probably contributes to immune complex-mediated disease in SLE. Factors such as ultraviolet light, sex hormones, viruses, and certain drugs play roles both as triggers for, and as factors in, the pathogenesis of SLE.

Abnormal autoantibody production is a hallmark of SLE, and it is recognized that there are specific relationships between certain autoantibodies and clinical manifestations. Some of these relationships appear to be causal. For example, autoantibodies to specific cell types such as lymphocytes, erythrocytes, and platelets may lead to lymphocytopenia, hemolytic anemia, and thrombocytopenia, respectively. In most other instances, however, associations between autoantibodies and disease exist but causation remains less direct. Anti-phospholipid antibodies are associated with an increased risk for venous or arterial thrombosis and recurrent fetal loss. Antibodies to ribosomal P protein have been associated with depression and psychosis in SLE patients. Anti-Ro/SSA antibodies are linked to neonatal lupus and fetal heart block. Antibodies to native double-stranded (ds) DNA have a propensity for forming pathogenic immune complexes that can deposit in glomeruli and presumably foment nephritis.

Case Presentation 1

A 25-year-old white woman without significant past medical history presents for evaluation of malaise, fatigue, diffuse arthralgias that are more uncomfortable in the morning, and a sun-sensitive rash of 3 weeks duration. There is no family history for autoimmune diseases. She denies fevers, alopecia, lymphadenopathy, mucosal sores, dysphagia, pleuritic chest pain, shortness of breath, abdominal symptoms, nausea, vomiting, diarrhea, urinary frequency, dysuria, hematuria, and Raynaud's phenomenon. Physical examination reveals a fixed malar erythematous rash and symmetric synovitis of the proximal interphalangeal (PIP) joints. Minimal bilateral knee effusions are also detected. Laboratory evaluation shows a peripheral white blood cell count of $2700/mm^3$ with a normal cell differential, a hematocrit of 35%, and platelet count of $100,000/mm^3$. Measures of liver and renal function are normal, and urinalysis is negative for protein, cells, and sediment. Serological evaluation reveals an antinuclear antibody of 1:640 in a homogeneous pattern. Anti-dsDNA antibodies are not detected, and complement C3 and C4 levels are within normal limits. The diagnosis of systemic lupus erythematosus is made.

The patient is given topical low-potency corticosteroids for her rash and a non-steroidal anti-inflammatory drug (NSAID) for her musculoskeletal complaints. After a baseline ophthalmological examination, hydroxychloroquine

200 mg twice daily is initiated. After 3 months, the patient is able to discontinue the NSAID and topical steroid therapy, with only slight residual malar erythema. She continues to do well on hydroxychloroquine therapy for 2 years, with regular rheumatological and ophthalmological evaluations. She takes low doses of ibuprofen for arthralgias as needed, but there is no evidence of disease recurrence or progression to involvement of new organ systems.

Case Presentation 2

A 20-year-old African-American woman with a known history of SLE presents with a 6-week history of progressive fatigue, malar rash, epistaxis, lower extremity petechiae, bipedal edema, and a 5-kg weight gain. The patient first presented at age 17 with fever, fatigue, pleuritic chest pain, symmetric polyarthritis, mild thrombocytopenia (platelet count 100,000/mm^3), and a highly positive ANA. There was no evidence of renal disease at that time, and she was treated with an NSAID and antimalarial therapy with good response. During the next 3 years, she regularly followed up with her rheumatologist and had consistently normal laboratory tests. When she went away to college, however, she was seen less frequently.

Six weeks ago, she began feeling generally fatigued but attributed this to her workload, which she tried to lessen. Nonetheless, her symptoms persisted, and she began to notice some hyperpigmentation on her cheeks and periodic nosebleeds. She also noticed some petechiae and swelling around the ankles. In the mornings, she noticed that her face appeared swollen.

On physical examination, the patient appears uncomfortable but not toxic. Her blood pressure is 150/90 mm Hg, and she has a low-grade fever of 38.6°C. There is no periorbital edema, but a faint erythematous rash is present on her cheeks. There are no nasal or oral ulcers, but crusted blood is seen around the nares. The heart, lung, and abdominal examinations are normal. She has no active synovitis, but there are multiple petechiae and bilateral pitting edema on her legs.

The laboratory evaluation reveals a platelet count of 18,000/mm^3, and the urinalysis reveals 4+ protein and red and white cell casts. The serum albumin is 2.2 g/dL, and the serum creatinine is 1.8 mg/dL. A 24-hour urine collection reveals proteinuria of 7 g/d and a creatinine clearance of 30 mL/min. Antinuclear antibodies and anti-dsDNA antibodies are present in high titers, and complement levels C3 and C4 are markedly decreased. Prednisone 1 mg/kg daily is prescribed, which quickly increased her peripheral platelet count to 75,000/mm^3. However, no improvement in renal function is observed, and she eventually undergoes a kidney biopsy that shows diffuse proliferative glomerulonephritis with high activity and low chronicity indices.

Intravenous methylprednisolone 1 g/d for 3 days is administered, followed by intravenous cyclophosphamide 500 mg/m^2. She is given this regimen monthly for 6 months; between intravenous therapies, her prednisone is gradually weaned to 10 mg daily. By the end of 6 months, she feels well and is no longer hypertensive or edematous. Her proteinuria and creatinine clearance levels off at 400 mg/d and 70 mL/min, respectively. The urine sediment resolves, and the platelet count stabilizes at 220,000/mm^3.

Intravenous cyclophosphamide therapy is changed to every 3 months, and corticosteroid therapy is gradually discontinued. The patient continues for 2 years on intravenous cyclophosphamide every 3 months.

Clinical Features

Non-specific but prominent constitutional signs and symptoms such as fever, weight loss, malaise, and fatigue are extremely common and may be part of the initial presentation or develop at any time during the course of the illness. Raynaud's phenomenon is also very common and may precede the onset of the systemic illness by years. The diagnosis of SLE is a clinical one and depends on the recognition of specific organ system involvement, supported by laboratory test abnormalities, including serological evidence of autoimmunity.

Mucocutaneous Manifestations

Cutaneous involvement is a common manifestation of SLE. In large series, about half of the patients have skin lesions as part of their presenting symptoms, and about 80% will develop skin involvement at some time during the course of the disease. Four mucocutaneous manifestations (malar rash, discoid rash, photosensitivity, and nasal/oropharyngeal ulceration) are important enough to be included in the American College of Rheumatology classification criteria that are employed in epidemiological studies of SLE (Table 6-1). The malar or butterfly rash (Figure 6-1) is a flat or raised fixed erythematous lesion over the malar eminences usually sparing the nasolabial folds, which, although considered to be the classic inflammatory rash associated with SLE, is seen in only 15% of patients and may be confused with other conditions such as seborrheic or contact dermatitis, rosacea, dermatophyte infections, and polymorphous light eruption.

Discoid lupus is usually found on the face, scalp, ears, or arms. It begins as erythematous disc-shaped papules or plaques with moderate scaling. As the lesion ages, the scales become thick and adherent, and the follicular openings become dilated and filled with keratinous debris (follicular plugging). The late stages are characterized by pigmentary changes (hypopigmentation in the center and hyperpigmentation at the active inflammatory border), atrophy, scarring, and permanent baldness (Figure 6-2). The differential diagnosis of discoid lupus includes psoriasis and fungal infections. Immunohistochemistry of inflammatory and discoid skin lesions reveals deposition of IgG molecules at the dermal-epidermal junction (i.e., the classic

Table 6-1   American College of Rheumatology Criteria for Systemic Lupus Erythematosus

Criterion	Definition
1. Malar rash	Fixed malar erythema, flat or raised, tending to spare the nasolabial folds
2. Discoid rash	Erythematous raised patches with adherent keratotic scaling and follicular plugging; atrophic scarring may occur in older lesions
3. Photosensitivity	Skin rash as a result of unusual reaction to sunlight, by patient history or physician observation
4. Mucosal ulcers	Oral or nasopharyngeal ulceration, usually painless, observed by a physician
5. Arthritis	Nonerosive arthritis involving two or more peripheral joints, characterized by tenderness, swelling, or effusion
6. Serositis	a) Pleuritis (convincing history of pleuritic pain or rub heard by a physician or evidence of pleural effusion) *or* b) Pericarditis (documented by electrocardiography or rub or evidence of pericardial effusion)
7. Renal disorder	a) Persistent proteinuria > 0.5 g/day or >3+ *or* b) Cellular casts of any type
8. Neurological disorder	a) Seizures (in the absence of other causes) *or* b) Psychosis (in the absence of other causes)
9. Hematological disorder	a) Hemolytic anemia (with reticulocytosis) *or* b) Leukopenia (<4,000/mm^3 on two or more occasions) *or* c) Lymphopenia (<1,500/mm^3 on two or more occasions) *or* d) Thrombocytopenia (<100,000/ mm^3 in the absence of offending drugs)

10. Immunological disorder	a) Anti-dsDNA antibodies *or*
	 b) Anti-Sm antibodies *or*
	 c) Positive finding of anti-phospholipid antibodies based on
	    1) an abnormal serum level of IgG or IgM anti-cardiolipin antibody, *or*
	    2) a positive test result for lupus anticoagulant using a standard method, *or*
	    3) a false positive serologic test for syphilis known to be positive for ≥6 months and confirmed by a *Treponema pallidum* immobilization or FTA absorption test

11. Antinuclear antibody	An abnormal titer of antinuclear antibody by immuno-fluorescence or an equivalent assay and in the absence of drugs known to be associated with "drug-induced lupus" syndrome

From Tan EM, Cohen AS, Fries JF, et al. The 1982 revised criteria for the classification of systemic lupus erythematosus (SLE). Arthritis Rheum. 1982;25:1271-7.

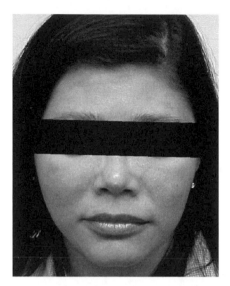

Figure 6-1   The malar or butterfly rash is a flat or raised fixed erythematous lesion over the malar eminences usually sparing the nasolabial folds. (Courtesy of Dr. D. Erkan.)

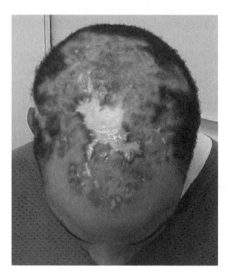

Figure 6-2   Late stages of discoid lupus with pigmentary changes (hypopigmentation in the center and hyperpigmentation at the active inflammatory border), atrophy, scarring, and permanent baldness.

lupus band test). It should be noted that only 10% of patients with discoid lupus skin lesions eventually develop systemic disease.

Mucous membrane lesions include nasal, oropharyngeal, and genital ulcers that are usually painless. Nasal septal ulcers may result in perforations. Many SLE patients have heightened skin sensitivity to sunlight (photosensitivity), which can lead to an inflammatory rash on exposed areas and may also exacerbate systemic disease activity.

Subacute cutaneous lupus erythematosus (SCLE) usually occurs as an isolated and distinct entity. SCLE can present either as a papulosquamous lesion or as an annular/polycyclic erythematous lesion. It is a photosensitive rash that, unlike discoid lupus, rarely scars. Histopathologically, SCLE is characterized by epidermal IgG deposits distinct from the classic lupus band pattern at the dermal-epidermal junction observed in acute and discoid lupus dermatitis.

Musculoskeletal Manifestations

Arthralgias and arthritis are the most common presenting manifestations of systemic lupus erythematosus, typically involving the small joints of the hands, wrists, and knees in a symmetric distribution reminiscent of rheumatoid arthritis (RA). Synovial effusions tend to be small, but soft-tissue swelling is common. Unlike classical RA, however, the arthritis of SLE is non-erosive. However, it is recognized that a small subgroup of patients with "Rhupus" do present with overlapping features of RA and SLE and can develop erosive joint disease.

Jaccoud's arthropathy is a subluxation of the hand that occurs in about 10% of patients with SLE. It resembles the ulnar deviation of RA but is reducible early in its course. Later, contractures and muscle atrophy may result in fixed deformities. Similar changes can develop in the feet.

Frank inflammatory myositis presenting as proximal muscle weakness may be seen. However, the histological features of myositis in SLE are not as striking as those found in idiopathic polymyositis/dermatomyositis, and other causes of myopathy, including drug effects (e.g., from corticosteroids and lipid-lowering agents) and hypothyroidism, need to be considered. Secondary fibromyalgia is not uncommon in patients with SLE and must be considered in patients presenting with generalized pains associated with multiple tender points.

Cardiovascular Manifestations

Valvular heart disease is an important cardiac manifestation of SLE. The spectrum of lupus-related valvular abnormalities ranges from valvular thickening and nonbacterial vegetations (predominantly on the atrial side of the mitral valve or on the vessel side of the aortic valve) to hemodynamically compromising regurgitation and/or stenosis that may require valve replacement. An increased risk of infectious endocarditis has been reported in retrospective studies of patients with SLE. Because most SLE patients with valvular disease have no symptoms referable to abnormal valves, a careful cardiovascular examination is essential to screen for significant regurgitant or stenotic lesions that may require further investigation with echocardiography.

Premature atherosclerosis and coronary artery disease are emerging as significant causes of morbidity and mortality in patients with SLE (1). The pathogenesis of accelerated atherosclerosis is multifactorial. Traditional cardiovascular risk factors such as hypertension, obesity, diabetes, and hyperlipidemia are observed with a high frequency in SLE patients, predominately as the result of chronic corticosteroid therapy. Complications from specific organ involvement (such as nephritis leading to hypertension and hyperlipidemia) may also accelerate the atherosclerotic process. Other factors such as circulating immune complexes, anti-endothelial cell antibodies, and antiphospholipid antibodies may promote vascular inflammation and/or hypercoagulability.

Pericarditis is relatively common, presenting with typical sharp precordial chest pain, a pericardial rub, and/or electrocardiographic changes. However, pericarditis is often clinically silent and detected incidentally by echocardiography or computed tomography. Constrictive pericarditis is unusual. Myocarditis may be suspected in patients who present with conduction defects, arrhythmias, or unexplained cardiomyopathy.

Pulmonary Manifestations

Pulmonary involvement in SLE is common and clinically diverse. Pleuritis is the most common pulmonary manifestation in SLE with pleuritic pain occurring in 70% and pleural effusions in up to 50% of patients. Infection and pulmonary embolism should always be considered in the differential diagnosis. Another common pulmonary finding is the "shrinking lung" syndrome, in which the lung volume appears reduced on plain chest X-rays, probably as the result of diaphragmatic weakness.

Active inflammatory disease of the lung parenchyma occurs in different forms. Acute pneumonitis and diffuse alveolar hemorrhage are uncommon but life-threatening syndromes that result from acute injury to the alveolar-capillary unit. Acute pneumonitis is characterized by the abrupt onset of fever, hypoxemia, and patchy alveolar infiltrates on chest radiography, and must be differentiated from an acute infectious process. The diffuse alveolar hemorrhage syndrome has a similar presentation except that it is associated with a drop in hemoglobin levels caused by bleeding within the lung (2). Acute reversible hypoxemia is an acute or subacute syndrome characterized by unexplained hypoxia and normal chest X-rays (3). The exact pathogenesis of this syndrome is unclear, but one hypothesis focuses on leukocyte aggregation in the pulmonary vasculature.

Chronic interstitial lung disease may develop as a consequence of acute pneumonitis or as an independent manifestation of SLE. It presents as progressive dyspnea on exertion, nonproductive cough, and bibasilar rales. Radiographic findings of interstitial lung disease may be more striking than symptoms. It is crucial to differentiate between active inflammatory lung disease and chronic fibrotic disease because only the former is treatable with anti-inflammatory and immunosuppressive therapy. High-resolution CT is a helpful non-invasive means of demonstrating the ground-glass appearance of active inflammation and distinguishing it from the honeycombing pattern of irreversible fibrosis.

Pulmonary hypertension is increasingly recognized as a long-term complication of SLE and is associated with the presence of Raynaud's phenomenon. The prognosis is poor, and a steady decline in pulmonary function, despite treatment, is typical. Serological tests show a high incidence of anti-ribonucleoprotein antibodies, rheumatoid factor, and anti-phospholipid antibodies in these patients.

Neuropsychiatric Manifestations

While seizures and psychosis are among the diagnostic criteria for SLE, the spectrum of neuropsychiatric manifestions is vast. Primary involvement of the nervous system usually occurs in the setting of other signs of active systemic disease. Neuropsychiatric lupus is defined primarily on clinical grounds and can result from direct nervous system involvement by the disease process or as a secondary complication of dysfunction in other organ systems (e.g., metabolic abnormalities due to uremia or accelerated hypertension), infections, and/or toxicities of medications.

Limited cognitive impairment has been reported in 20% to 70% of lupus patients without a history of neuropsychiatric lupus when examined using formal neuropsychological testing. Organic brain syndrome is usually characterized by apathy, impairment of memory and concentration, and loss of orientation, intellect, or judgment. Slow but progressive deterioration may occur in a few patients, sometimes resulting in severely debilitating dementia.

Intractable headaches resembling migraines are common and often do not respond adequately to narcotic analgesics. Aseptic meningitis and pseudotumor cerebri are rare but important conditions that may reflect disease activity or reactions to medications such NSAIDs and corticosteroids, respectively.

The most common ophthalmological abnormality is retinopathy, which presents as disc vasculitis, cotton-wool spots, or occasionally with normal funduscopic findings but with leakage of fluorescein on angiography. The funduscopic examination should be part of the routine evaluation of the patient with SLE.

Peripheral neuropathy may present as a mononeuritis multiplex, or as a motor, sensory, or mixed motor/sensory polyneuropathy. Transverse myelitis presenting with lower extremity paralysis, sensory deficits, and loss of sphincter control is a rare but important syndrome because appropriate and timed treatment can prevent devastating sequelae.

The predominant histopathological abnormalities in central nervous system involvement are multiple cortical microinfarctions associated with microvascular injury (4). Frank central nervous system vasculitis is rare. It is uncommon that SLE presents initially with neuropsychiatric disease, but SLE should always be in the differential diagnosis of neuropsychiatric symptoms, especially when they occur in young patients.

Autoantibodies that have been associated with neuropsychiatric manifestations in SLE include anti-neuronal antibodies, anti-ribosomal P protein antibodies, and a subset of anti-dsDNA antibodies that cross-react with certain glutamate receptor subtypes. Anti-phospholipid antibodies have also been associated with specific neuropsychiatric features, including cerebrovascular accidents, multi-infarction dementia, seizures, intracranial arterial and venous thrombosis, chorea, and acute transverse myelitis (5).

Gastrointestinal Manifestations

Non-specific gastrointestinal symptoms such as abdominal discomfort, anorexia, nausea, vomiting, and diarrhea are common. Lupus peritonitis is the result of small vessel involvement in the bowel serosa or retroperitoneum, but other potential etiologies such as infection, pancreatitis, mesenteric vasculitis, perforation, and inflammatory bowel disease should always be considered in the differential diagnosis.

Patients with mesenteric vasculitis may present with insidious lower abdominal pain that may wax and wane over a period of several weeks or months, occult or frank blood in the stool, and thickening of the bowel wall on CT. Arteriography rarely reveals obvious vasculitic changes, although poor blood flow may be seen. Bacterial peritonitis most often occurs in patients with nephrotic syndrome but may occur even in the absence of ascites. Hepatosplenomegaly may be found in the setting of active disease.

Renal Manifestations

Renal involvement is one of the more important complications of SLE because of its frequency and insidiousness and because of its potential to profoundly affect the overall morbidity and the quality of life of the patient. Like other manifestations of SLE, renal disease can be highly variable in presentation, ranging from mild asymptomatic proteinuria to rapidly progressive glomerulonephritis resulting in renal failure within weeks. Kidney involvement eventually occurs in up to half of patients with SLE. Diffuse proliferative glomerulonephritis is the most common form of renal disease and is the one associated with the worst prognosis.

Early kidney disease is often asymptomatic, subtle, and easily overlooked by the clinician. One of the earliest and most subtle symptoms is nocturia, which represents tubular dysfunction and impairment of urinary concentrating ability. Foamy urine suggests substantial proteinuria. However, only a few patients report these symptoms of early kidney involvement, and consequently lupus nephritis is frequently a "silent" complication of SLE. Unexplained accelerated hypertension can be seen but is also asymptomatic. Signs of uremia such constitutional symptoms, pleuropericarditis, and anemia occur late in the course of kidney disease but may still be mistaken for non-renal involvement of SLE.

Because early detection and treatment can significantly improve outcome, regular screening for renal disease is mandatory. Effective early detection of renal disease requires regular physical examinations to screen for signs of renal insufficiency like hypertension or edema and serial urinalyses that can detect active urinary sediment (i.e., red blood cells, white blood cells, and/or cellular casts in the urine) and proteinuria (6). Early morning urine samples are preferred because they are relatively concentrated and acidic. Macroscopic hematuria is rare and usually indicates either very severe renal involvement or lower urinary tract etiologies.

One presentation of lupus nephritis is the nephrotic syndrome with peripheral edema, proteinuria greater than 3.5 g/d, hypoalbuminemia, and hyperlipidemia. Hypercoagulability can occur because of the urinary loss of anti-thrombin III and other anti-coagulants. Nephrotic-range proteinuria reflects diffuse glomerular capillary involvement and is often seen in patients with diffuse proliferative, membranous, or membranoproliferative glomerulonephritis. Relatively low-grade proteinuria (1-2 g/d) may be seen with active nephritis and adverse effects of drugs like NSAIDs or may reflect chronic glomerular capillary wall injury (fixed proteinuria). Changes in serological parameters, such as increasing titers of anti-dsDNA antibodies or declining C3 or C4 complement components, are potentially important predictors of exacerbations of lupus nephritis.

Hematological Manifestations

Anemia of chronic disease and reactive lymphadenopathy are the most common hematological abnormalities in SLE but are non-specific findings. More specific to lupus are Coomb's positive hemolytic anemia with reticulocytosis, leukopenia (<4000/mm^3), lymphocytopenia (<1500/mm^3), and autoimmune thrombocytopenia. Thrombocytopenia has an incidence of 15%-60% in SLE patients and is a frequent presenting feature. It is often severe (platelet count <20 × 10^9/L) and resistant to treatment. Thrombocytopenia can also be part of the antiphospholipid syndrome. Functional asplenism caused by recurrent splenic infarcts can occur and may predispose lupus patients to infections caused by encapsulated organisms.

Antiphospholipid Antibody Syndrome

Circulating antiphospholipid antibodies can be detected in 30% to 40% of patients with SLE. Of these, roughly half will develop the antiphospholipid antibody syndrome. Antiphospholipid antibody syndrome is characterized by thromboembolic disease of arteries or veins and/or pregnancy morbidity, associated with circulating antiphospholipid antibodies, most commonly anticardiolipin antibodies, and lupus-anticoagulant. A complete discussion of antiphospholipid antibody syndrome is provided in Chapter 7.

Drug-Induced Lupus Erythematosus

Many medications are known to induce a clinical syndrome that is indistinguishable from SLE. The symptoms tend to include fever, rashes, joint and muscle pain, cytopenias, and serositis. Central nervous system and kidney disease rarely occur. Circulating antinuclear antibodies (ANA) demonstrate a diffuse pattern, and the presence of anti-histone antibodies is typical.

Common precipitants of drug-induced lupus erythematosus (DILE) are minocycline, hydralazine, and procainamide. Others include chlorpromazine, methyldopa, isoniazid, dilantin, quinidine, lithium salts, penicillamine, and sulfasalazine. It should be emphasized that patients with idiopathic SLE can be treated safely with these medications without fear of disease exacerbations. Recently, the anti-tumor necrosis factor (TNF)-α agents etanercept, infliximab, and adalimumab have also been shown to induce ANA production in some patients and have been associated with rare cases of DILE. Anti-dsDNA antibodies have also been detected in occasional patients treated with anti-TNF-α agents, but so far no cases of associated nephritis have been reported. The clinical manifestations of DILE resolve after several weeks to months after discontinuation of the offending agent, but short courses of NSAIDs or even systemic corticosteroids are sometimes required. ANA may still be detectable long after cessation of the culprit drug and resolution of symptoms and signs.

Lupus and Pregnancy

Whether pregnancy has a favorable, adverse, or indifferent effect on the course of SLE remains unresolved. Several controlled studies have been conducted but have arrived at seemingly contradictory conclusions (7). The difficulty lies in distinguishing disease flares in the pregnant SLE patient from pregnancy-related physiological or pathological changes. For example, arthralgias, non-specific facial and palmar erythema, thrombocytopenia, proteinuria, and anemia can all occur in otherwise healthy pregnant women who do not have SLE.

Diagnosing a lupus flare during pregnancy is a clinical endeavor. Laboratory testing should be used only as supportive data. The best specific indicators of active SLE during pregnancy include the presence of stereotypical rashes, mucosal ulcers, lymphadenopathy, and rising levels of anti-dsDNA antibody. Alternative pathway hypocomplementemia may also been associated with disease flares, but classical pathway hypocomplementemia is less helpful because this often occurs in pregnant lupus patients who are clinically well. Accordingly, low C3 but normal C4 levels would be consistent with SLE exacerbations.

Low platelet counts may be secondary to SLE, to preeclampsia as part of the HELLP (hemolysis, elevated liver enzymes, low platelet counts) syndrome, to the antiphospholipid antibody syndrome, or simply to pregnancy itself. In most cases thrombocytopenia is modest in severity (50-$150 \times 10^9/L$).

Patients with lupus nephritis frequently have worsening hypertension, proteinuria, and renal dysfunction during pregnancy because of pre-eclampsia and/or renal exacerbation of SLE. The presence of extrarenal disease manifestations of active SLE helps to distinguish between these two possibilities. However, even in a patient with unequivocal active lupus nephritis, superimposed preeclampsia often cannot be excluded definitively. In these cases, treatment for both SLE and preeclampsia is appropriate. Seizures due to SLE late in pregnancy may also be difficult to differentiate from eclampsia.

Special circumstances in which pregnancy in a patient with SLE is inadvisable include severe hypertension, progressive renal failure, severe thrombocytopenia, severe central nervous system disease, severe cardiopulmonary disease, and use of teratogenic drugs. There is no evidence supporting the general use of prophylactic corticosteroid treatment during pregnancy.

Neonatal Lupus Erythematosus

Neonatal lupus erythematosus is caused by autoimmunity that is passively acquired as a result of maternal autoantibodies that are transferred across the placenta (8). It occurs in up to 2% of infants whose mothers are positive for anti-Ro/SSA and/or anti-La/SSB antibodies. Major manifestations of the syndrome include a transient rash in the newborn period, complete heart block, or both. Approximately one third of SLE patients have one or both of these antibodies, but it is not currently possible to predict which children will acquire neonatal lupus. The occurrence and severity of neonatal lupus is unrelated to maternal disease activity or severity.

The most serious cardiac abnormalities are associated with anti-Ro/SSA and anti-La/SSB antibodies directed against specific 52 kD and 48 kD antigens, respectively, and occur in 1%–2% of infants of mothers with these antibodies. The administration of dexamethasone given to the mother has been reported to be beneficial in cases of in utero fetal myocarditis. Although the skin rash resolves with clearance of maternal antibodies, complete heart block is irreversible. The surviving infants require permanent pacemakers and have a high mortality rate in the first 3 years because of congenital cardiomyopathy and congestive heart failure. In utero fetal death may also occur.

Diagnosis

The diagnosis of SLE is made predominantly on clinical grounds with the support of laboratory testing. In 1982, the American Rheumatism Association (now the American College of Rheumatology) established 11 diagnostic criteria for SLE (see Table 6-1), with the aim of identifying clinical features that would optimize sensitivity and specificity for diagnosis. The presence of at least four of these criteria was required to make the diagnosis. Although these criteria (revised in 1997) were developed primarily for investigational purposes, they nonetheless offer a useful framework in the evaluation of the patient in clinical practice. However, it should be emphasized that many patients who do not strictly fulfill diagnostic criteria (especially early in their disease) may be regarded as having SLE and should be treated accordingly.

Serological Testing

ANA testing is usually the first step in the immunological support of the clinical diagnosis of SLE and other systemic autoimmune diseases. Immunofluorescence is the standard approach for detecting ANA and is useful for determining a titer and a staining pattern. Several staining patterns (homogeneous or diffuse, speckled, peripheral [rim], nucleolar, or centromere) may be seen depending on the location of the target antigens. These patterns correspond to the presence of autoantibodies against different nuclear antigens and are associated with different clinical syndromes (Table 6-2). The peripheral or rim pattern is fairly specific for SLE. The ANA assay is an ideal screening test because of its simplicity and sensitivity for SLE (greater than 95% when using human cultured cells as the substrate). The negative predictive value of ANA testing for SLE is over 97%. In contrast, the specificity of ANA for SLE is low. Many other conditions are associated with a positive ANA, including scleroderma, polymyositis, dermatomyositis, rheumatoid arthritis, autoimmune thyroiditis, autoimmune hepatitis, infections, neoplasms, and exposure to various drugs. Also, 10% to 35% of healthy individuals aged 65 and older may have low titers of circulating ANA (<1:40) (9).

Table 6-2   Antinuclear Antibody Patterns, Autoantigens, and Disease Associations

Pattern	Autoantigen	Disease
Diffuse	ssDNA, histones	SLE, drug-induced lupus, rheumatoid arthritis
Peripheral	dsDNA, laminin	SLE, chronic autoimmune hepatitis
Speckled	SSA, SSB, Sm, RNP, Scl-70	SLE, Sjögren's syndrome, systemic sclerosis, mixed connective tissue disease, overlap syndromes
Nucleolar	RNA polymerases I,II,III, PM-Scl	Systemic sclerosis, systemic sclerosis/myositis overlap
Centromere	CENP-A, CENP-B, CENP-C	CREST, primary biliary cirrhosis

Antibodies to dsDNA are found in up to 70% of SLE patients at some point during the course of their disease and are more than 95% specific for SLE, making them useful for confirming the diagnosis of SLE after a positive ANA test is obtained. A subset of anti-dsDNA antibodies has been shown to be nephritogenic, and their titer commonly correlates with the activity of kidney disease. High titers of anti-dsDNA antibodies are seen more frequently in high-grade proliferative nephritis. Anti-Sm (Smith antigen) antibodies are detected in 10%-30% of SLE patients, and their presence is highly specific for SLE.

Antinuclear, anti-dsDNA and anti-Sm antibodies are all included in the ARA criteria for lupus because of their usefulness as diagnostic tests. However, other autoantibodies have been identified that are often helpful in defining the clinical phenotype of individual patients. Anti-Ro (SS-A) and anti-La (SS-B) antibodies are detected in 10%-50% and 10%-20% of SLE patients, respectively. Their presence has been associated with the development of secondary Sjögren's syndrome, photosensitivity, central nervous system disease, neonatal lupus, and the development of congenital heart block in some of the children of mothers that carry these antibodies. They may also be present in the rare "ANA-negative" lupus patient. Anti-ribosomal P antibodies have been associated with neuropsychiatric manifestations of SLE, notably lupus psychosis. Autoantibodies to histones are commonly detected in drug-induced lupus.

Renal Biopsy

There are no definitive guidelines for kidney biopsy in lupus nephritis, although generally accepted indications for kidney biopsy include unexplained hematuria, renal insufficiency, cellular casts, and/or proteinuria >1.0-2.0 g/d. A biopsy should be recommended only if the results are anticipated to help guide management decisions. Accordingly, some patients with a stereotypical presentation of SLE with severe renal involvement (e.g., nephritic and nephrotic syndromes, azotemia, active urinary sediment, hypertension) may not need to undergo a renal biopsy before initiation of high-dose corticosteroid therapy. There is, however, a general consensus that most patients should have documentation of renal pathology before initiation of cytotoxic drug therapy.

The World Health Organization (WHO) classification of lupus nephritis is a practical and widely accepted system for categorizing renal lesions in lupus nephritis. It provides one measure of disease prognosis and can help influence treatment options (Table 6-3). The kidney biopsy can also give information regarding the degree of active inflammation and the severity of irreversible damage (10). Standard indices of activity and chronicity have been defined to aid in determining the likelihood of response to treatment (Table 6-4). Within the same WHO class, a high activity index indicates potentially treatable and reversible lesions, whereas high chronicity scores

Table 6-3   World Health Organization Classification of Lupus Nephritis

   I. Normal

  II. Mesangial nephropathy

 III. Focal and segmental proliferative glomerulonephritis

 IV. Diffuse proliferative glomerulonephritis

  V. Diffuse membranous glomerulonephritis

 VI. Advanced sclerosing glomerulonephritis

Table 6-4   Histologic Classification of Lupus Nephritis*

Activity Index Components	*Chronicity Index Components*
• Proliferative change	• Sclerotic glomeruli
• Fibrinoid necrosis or karyorrhexis**	• Fibrous crescents
• Cellular crescents**	• Tubular atrophy
• Leukocyte infiltration	• Interstitial fibrosis
• Hyaline thrombi	
• Interstitial inflammation	

* Each component is scored on a scale of 0 to 3.
** Weighted by a factor of 2.
NOTE—The maximum activity index score is 24. The maximum chronicity index score is 12. Activity index scores of 12 or higher and chronicity index scores of 4 or higher are considered to be indicators of poor renal prognosis.
From Austin HA 3rd, Muenz LR, Joyce KM, et al. Diffuse proliferative lupus nephritis: identification of specific pathologic features affecting renal outcome. Kidney Int. 1984;25:689-95; with permission.

reflect irreversible sclerosis and fibrosis. Activity features such as fibrinoid necrosis and cellular crescents and chronicity features such as tubular atrophy and interstitial fibrosis in particular have been associated with a higher risk for end-stage renal disease. It is recommended that all specimens be examined by pathologists with extensive experience in renal histopathology.

Prognosis

The prognosis of SLE has improved steadily over the past 50 years as a result of earlier diagnosis, better immunosuppressive treatments, and improved overall supportive care. However, despite improvements in short-term survival, SLE remains a potentially fatal disease. The three most common causes of death are major organ system failure due to active SLE, infections, and atherosclerotic disease. Nephritis, multisystem organ failure, and central nervous system disease are the most common causes of death in patients with active SLE. Several predictors of poor outcome in lupus nephritis have been identified in clinical studies. These include black and

Hispanic races, hypertension, smoking, poor compliance with treatment, elevated serum creatinine, proteinuria, thrombocytopenia, decreased C3 levels, and elevated anti-dsDNA levels.

Infections are an important cause of mortality in patients with SLE. Risk factors for serious bacterial infections include immunosuppressive treatment, proteinuria, renal insufficiency and active SLE. Patients with SLE are particularly susceptible to encapsulated organisms such as neisserial species, *Pneumococcus*, and nontyphoidal *Salmonella* (11-13). Patients who are treated with high doses of corticosteroids or with cytotoxic immunosupressive therapies resulting in leukopenia are also at increased risk for opportunistic infections. The most common fatal opportunistic infections are caused by *Pneumocystis carinii* and *Candida albicans.*

Given improved short-term prognoses, cardiovascular disease secondary to accelerated atherosclerosis has emerged as an important cause of long-term morbidity and mortality in patients with SLE. Premature vascular disease is the consequence of both prolonged exposure to corticosteroids and SLE-related endothelial injury.

Approximately 10%-15% of patients with lupus nephritis develop end-stage renal disease requiring dialysis. Patients with rapid deterioration of renal function are more likely to have some reversible renal dysfunction. There is a tendency for decreased clinical and serological lupus activity after the onset of end-stage renal disease.

Survival of lupus patients who have been on dialysis for 6 months or more is no different from that of non-SLE dialysis patients. After kidney transplantation, there is no difference in patient or graft survival in lupus versus non-lupus patients. Transplantation is usually recommended only after at least 3 months of dialysis to allow possible recovery from acute renal failure. Lupus nephritis can recur in transplanted allografts but is a distinctly rare event.

Management

General Principles of Therapy

The aggressiveness of therapy in SLE depends on the extent and severity of disease and is determined on a case-to-case basis. Accordingly, optimal care includes the involvement of a rheumatologist to help gauge and monitor disease activity and intervention. There are many goals in the treatment of SLE. First and foremost, organ- or life-threatening problems must be identified and addressed quickly. There should be no hesitation in treating acute inflammatory processes such as lupus nephritis with potent anti-inflammatory and/or immunosuppressive therapy. Less severe acute involvement such as mucocutaneous, musculoskeletal, or serosal inflammation should require less potent (and therefore less toxic) intervention.

Once acute disease is controlled, a plan for chronic maintenance therapy should be formulated. This may be simply regular observation in certain individuals or may require varying degrees of immunomodulatory therapy in others. The overall clinical picture should be monitored very closely and should guide the clinician in determining the appropriate level of pharmacological intervention. In many cases, the corticosteroid requirements are a useful surrogate marker for disease activity.

Another goal of management is to minimize morbidities associated with disease and toxicities associated with treatment. It is increasingly recognized that the appropriate care of the lupus patient extends into other areas of internal medicine beyond what is traditionally rheumatology. Because of both the disease process and the therapies, hypertension, atherosclerotic disease, diabetes, hyperlipidemia, peptic ulcer disease, increased risks for infection and malignancy, and many other conditions must be identified and addressed accordingly.

Finally, patient education is essential for optimal care and should not be underemphasized. The patient will best be served if his or her understanding of the illness is maximized, for only then can he or she fully appreciate the goals and benefits of specific interventions.

NSAIDs and Selective Inhibitors of Cyclooxygenase (COX)-2

NSAIDs are useful in the treatment of fevers, headaches, arthralgias/arthritis, myalgias, and serositis. Selective inhibitors of COX-2 have similar anti-inflammatory and analgesic effects but with probably fewer gastrointestinal toxicities when compared with traditional NSAIDs, a feature that may be of particular benefit in patients who are concurrently taking systemic corticosteroids. In addition, COX-2 inhibitors also lack the antiplatelet effects of traditional NSAIDs and therefore may be useful in patients with mild-to-moderate thrombocytopenia.

Because NSAIDs and COX-2 inhibitors reduce local production of prostaglandins, which are necessary for the maintenance of renal perfusion, these drugs should be avoided in patients with renal insufficiency. NSAIDs, most frequently ibuprofen, can be a rare cause of aseptic meningitis, a complication that appears to occur more commonly in patients with SLE. (Other general adverse effects of NSAIDs and COX-2 inhibitors are described in Chapter 29.)

Corticosteroids

Corticosteroids are the single most important class of medications available for the management of acute lupus. Prednisone, prednisolone, and methylprednisolone are the most widely used of these agents. The fluorinated corticosteroids dexamethasone and betamethasone are less commonly used but have a useful role in the treatment of heart block in neonatal lupus because of their ability to cross the placenta and enter the fetal circulation in significant amounts.

Severe or life-threatening manifestations of SLE require high-dose corticosteroid treatment (prednisone 1 mg/kg/d or equivalent) (14). High-dose corticosteroid therapy for 4-8 weeks followed by a slow taper has been considered as one of the standard regimens for the treatment of lupus nephritis. Most disease manifestations will respond in 1-2 weeks. If the condition responds inadequately to these dosages, or if the disease is severe and sparing long-term oral corticosteroids is particularly important, intravenous "pulse" corticosteroids (methylprednisolone 1 g/d for 3 days) may be given to more rapidly suppress systemic inflammation. "Pulses" may be repeated at monthly intervals and has been used to treat diffuse proliferative glomerulonephritis and severe or life-threatening manifestations of neuropsychiatric lupus, pneumonitis, systemic vasculitis, or thrombocytopenia.

Other less severe manifestations of SLE such as myositis, arthritis, serositis, and mild constitutional symptoms can be managed with lower dosages of daily corticosteroids (prednisone 0.125-0.5 mg/kg or equivalent). Alternate-day corticosteroid therapy may have a better safety profile compared with that of daily regimens, but it is less effective in gaining initial control of disease or in sustaining it.

An important general principle of corticosteroid therapy is that these agents should be used at the lowest effective doses and for the least amount of time. The use of corticosteroid-sparing agents should be considered when a patient's illness is refractory to, or side effects accrue because of, chronic corticosteroid therapy.

Corticosteroids are generally well tolerated during pregnancy. The use of typical doses of non-fluorinated corticosteroids is considered safe during pregnancy and breast-feeding and is not associated with congenital defects or adverse effects to the newborn. (An extensive discussion of different corticosteroid regimens and the litany of adverse effects associated with corticosteroid therapy is presented in Chapter 30.)

Antimalarial Agents

Antimalarial agents are now widely prescribed to most newly diagnosed SLE patients and can be used to reduce corticosteroid requirements. They have multiple potential benefits including anti-inflammatory properties, immunomodulatory properties, and sun-blocking effects. They may also lower serum lipids, improve glycemic control, and exert a mild anti-thrombotic effect. Hydroxychloroquine is the most widely used agent in the United States, with chloroquine and quinacrine as alternatives. The therapeutic efficacy of antimalarial drugs was demonstrated in a placebo-controlled withdrawal trial of hydroxychloroquine in which the replacement of the drug with placebo resulted in a significant increase in disease flares, some of which were serious (15). Patients most likely to benefit are those with mucocutaneous lupus, arthritis, or serositis.

Initial doses of hydroxychloroquine 200 mg twice daily or quinacrine 100 mg daily are recommended. Some clinicians give initial higher doses for brief periods, followed by a reduction in daily dosages once disease control is achieved. Responses to antimalarial drugs should be expected no sooner than 2 months and as late as 6 months after starting therapy. Because of synergistic effects, a combination of hydroxychloroquine and quinacrine has been used successfully in refractory skin disease.

Retinal damage is the most important toxicity of antimalarial agents and is related to the total dose and duration of treatment. It is rare in patients with normal renal function and when the drugs are given at recommended dosages (<6 mg/kg/d). Regular ophthalmological examinations with visual field testing can identify early retinal damage and should be performed at the initiation of therapy and every 6 to 12 months thereafter. If identified early, retinal toxicity can be reversible upon discontinuation of antimalarial therapy. Quinacrine appears to be associated with a lower risk of retinopathy but may cause yellow discoloration of the skin that resolves when the drug is discontinued.

Other significant adverse effects include skin rashes, gastrointestinal disturbances, and, rarely, peripheral neuropathies and myopathies of skeletal and cardiac muscle. Development of neuropathies or myopathies requires discontinuation of the drugs. The safety of antimalarial agents in pregnancy is not firmly established, but the largest published series of 33 mothers and 36 infants reported no developmental abnormalities or adverse pregnancy outcomes attributable to hydroxychloroquine (16).

Cyclophosphamide

Cyclophosphamide has been the best studied of the alkylating agents in SLE. It is very effective in depleting B and T lymphocytes, in modulating T cell activation responses, and in suppressing antibody production by B cells. Cyclophosphamide can be administered orally or by intravenous pulses, but the latter approach is associated with lower toxicity and is the generally preferred route of administration for the treatment of severe SLE manifestations. In the setting of diffuse proliferative glomerulonephritis, intravenous boluses of cyclophosphamide (0.5 to 1.0 g/m^2 of body surface area) are administered monthly for at least six months, after which the frequency is increased to every three months generally for at least eighteen months (17,18). Intravenous cyclophosphamide has also been reported to be effective in patients with severe neuropsychiatric SLE, interstitial lung disease, refractory autoimmune thrombocytopenia, and other severe manifestations of lupus.

There are many toxicities associated with cyclophosphamide therapy, most notably immunosuppression, carcinogenicity (bladder cancer, lymphoproliferative malignancies), hemorrhagic cystitis, infertility (for men as well as women), and teratogenicity. Patients must practice effective birth control techniques when being treated with cyclophosphamide.

Azathioprine

Azathioprine, a purine analog that inhibits DNA synthesis, is a widely used immunosuppressive and steroid-sparing agent in the management of SLE. Typical dosages range from 50 to 100 mg twice daily. Azathioprine has been extensively studied in lupus nephritis and has been shown to reduce proteinuria, improve or stabilize renal function, and reduce mortality in patients with DPGN. While severe and refractory nephritis is usually treated with cyclophosphamide, azathioprine in combination with systemic corticosteroids can also be effective in some patients with renal disease and may be the immunosuppressive therapy of choice if there is a desire for avoiding ovarian failure in women who are contemplating future pregnancies. Azathioprine is also favored in the control of cutaneous lupus, autoimmune cytopenias, serositis, and other non-life threatening manifestations that are refractory to moderate dosages of corticosteroids alone but not severe enough to warrant cyclophosphamide therapy. The major toxicities are gastrointestinal intolerance and bone marrow toxicity, both of which are generally reversible with reduction of the dose or discontinuation of the drug. Azathioprine is widely accepted as a relatively safe medication during pregnancy even though it is formally denoted as a class D drug.

Mycophenolate Mofetil

Mycophenolate mofetil is an inhibitor of inosine monophosphate dehydrogenase, an enzyme integral for guanine biosynthesis. Its role in the treatment of lupus appears to be comparable that of azathioprine. Typical dosages range from 500 to 1000 mg twice daily. In one study, mycophenolate mofetil showed comparable results to oral cyclophosphamide in achieving remission of lupus nephritis over a treatment period of 12 months in patients with DPGN (19), but subsequent reports suggest a high recurrence rate even if the drug is continued. The safety of mycophenolate mofetil in pregnancy is not known.

Methotrexate

A double-blind placebo-controlled study of weekly low-dose methotrexate (15-20 mg) has shown efficacy in the treatment of arthritis and skin manifestations in SLE and in permitting the reduction of corticosteroid requirements (20).

Cyclosporine A

Cyclosporine A inhibits the proliferation of T lymphocytes and selectively inhibits T cell-mediated immune responses. Its major indication in SLE is in

the treatment of pure membranous nephropathy with nephrotic range proteinuria. Cyclosporine A is used in combination with systemic corticosteroids. Usual dosages range from 2-5 mg/kg body weight. There is poor
correlation between blood levels of cyclosporine A and its clinical efficacy
in autoimmune diseases, and so monitoring drug levels is not generally
necessary. Major toxicities include hypertension and nephrotoxicity, and
renal function must be followed carefully. Cyclosporine A may be used
during pregnancy if necessary (21).

Intravenous Immunoglobulin (IVIG)

IVIG has been shown useful in managing severe lupus thrombocytopenia,
but the relapse rate following treatment is high. The primary role for IVIG
therapy is to control acute bleeding associated with lupus thrombocytopenia or to rapidly increase the platelet count prior to splenectomy or
other surgery. While there are many case reports and small series of IVIG
successfully used in the treatment of cytopenias, NP lupus, nephritis, and
manifestations of the antiphospholipid syndrome, there are no large controlled studies of IVIG in SLE. IVIG is very expensive and rare anaphylactic
reactions are cause for concern especially in patients who are IgA-deficient.

Dapsone

Dapsone has been used to manage refractory cutaneous manifestations of
lupus, including discoid, bullous, and subacute cutaneous lupus lesions.
Therapy usually starts with 50 mg/d with gradual increases to a maximum
dose of 150 mg/d. Glucose-6-phosphate dehydrogenase-deficiency should
be excluded before the initiation of therapy.

Thalidomide

The effectiveness of thalidomide in the treatment of inflammatory illnesses
has rekindled interest in this medication that had been previously infamous
for its causation of fetal developmental malformations. Thalidomide at
doses of 50-100 mg/d is effective in the treatment of severe refractory cutaneous lupus (22). Patients must be counseled thoroughly with regards to
the teratogenic properties of thalidomide, and a special license must be obtained before it can be dispensed. Other adverse effects include sedation
and peripheral neuropathy that may not improve upon drug cessation.
Withdrawal of the medication commonly results in disease relapses.

Plasmapheresis

The role of plasmapheresis in SLE is limited to acute life-threatening manifestations such as thrombotic thrombocytopenic purpura, catastrophic
antiphospholipid antibody syndrome, and pulmonary hemorrhage from

capillaritis and alveolitis. Controlled clinical trials have shown that plasmapheresis offers no additional benefit to standard therapy in the treatment of lupus nephritis.

New and Investigational Approaches

Pilot studies with the adenosine analogues fludarabine and cladribine as immunosuppressive agents have shown promise in lupus nephritis (23). High-dose cyclophosphamide with or without granulocyte colony stimulating factor has also been used successfully in patients with severe refractory autoimmune diseases including lupus nephritis but is controversial (24). In addition, autologous bone marrow or peripheral stem cell transplantation following high-dose cytotoxic therapy is being considered as a means of reconstituting normal bone marrow and immune function following the elimination of pathogenic lymphocytes.

In double-blind, randomized trials, prasterone (dehydroepiandrosterone [DHEA]), an adrenal androgen, has been shown to reduce corticosteroid requirements and stabilize or reduce disease activity in patients with mild-to-moderate disease (25). There appears to be dose-dependent response. Adverse effects, most commonly acne, are generally attributable to virilizing properties of the drug. There may be a particular role for this agent in the treatment of male patients with mild-to-moderate activity. It should be cautioned that although DHEA is available in health food stores as a nutritional supplement, regulation is lax, and labeling may not accurately reflect actual dosages.

LJP 394, consisting of four double-stranded oligodeoxynucleotides individually linked to a central scaffolding structure, is a novel agent that is thought to induce B cell tolerance to dsDNA (26). Early clinical data suggest that LJP 394 can reduce plasma levels of anti-dsDNA antibodies and cause possible beneficial effects in patients with lupus nephritis. Further studies are ongoing.

REFERENCES

1. **Salmon JE, Roman MJ.** Accelerated atherosclerosis in systemic lupus erythematosus: implications for patient management. Curr Opin Rheumatol. 2001;13:341-4.
2. **Green RJ, Ruoss SJ, Kraft SA, et al.** Pulmonary capillaritis and alveolar hemorrhage. Update on diagnosis and management. Chest. 1996;110:1305-16.
3. **Abramson SB, Dobro J, Eberle MA, et al.** Acute reversible hypoxemia in systemic lupus erythematosus. Ann Intern Med. 1991;114:941-7.
4. **Hanly JG, Walsh NM, Sangalang V.** Brain pathology in systemic lupus erythematosus. J Rheumatol. 1992;19:732-41.
5. **Asherson RA, Mercey D, Phillips G, et al.** Recurrent stroke and multi-infarct dementia in systemic lupus erythematosus: association with anti-phospholipid antibodies. Ann Rheum Dis. 1987;46:605-11.
6. **Austin HA.** Clinical evaluation and monitoring of lupus kidney disease. Lupus. 1998;7:618-21.

7. **Urowitz MB, Gladman DD, Farewell VT, et al.** Lupus and pregnancy studies. Arthritis Rheum. 1993;36:1392-7.

8. **Lee LA.** Neonatal lupus: clinical features, therapy, and pathogenesis. Curr Rheumatol Rep. 2001;3:391-5.

9. **Tan EM, Feltkamp TE, Smolen JS, et al.** Range of antinuclear antibodies in "healthy" individuals. Arthritis Rheum. 1997;40:1601-11.

10. **Austin HA 3rd, Muenz LR, Joyce KM, et al.** Diffuse proliferative lupus nephritis: identification of specific pathologic features affecting renal outcome. Kidney Int. 1984;25:689-95.

11. **Mitchell SR, Nguyen PQ, Katz P.** Increased risk of neisserial infections in systemic lupus erythematosus. Semin Arthritis Rheum. 1990;20:174-84.

12. **Yee AMF, Ng SC, Sobel RE, et al.** Fc gammaRIIA polymorphism as a risk factor for invasive pneumococcal infections in systemic lupus erythematosus. Arthritis Rheum. 1997;40:1180-2.

13. **Lim E, Hoh WH, Loh SF, et al.** Non-typhoidal salmonellosis in patients with systemic lupus erythematosus: a study of fifty patients and a review of the literature. Lupus. 2001;10:87-92.

14. **Kimberly RP, Lockshin MD, Sherman RL, et al.** High-dose intravenous methylprednisolone pulse therapy in systemic lupus erythematosus. Am J Med. 1981;70:817-24.

15. A randomized study of the effect of withdrawing hydroxychloroquine sulfate in systemic lupus erythematosus. The Canadian Hydroxychloroquine Study Group. N Engl J Med. 1991;324:150-4.

16. **Levy RA, Vilela VS, Cataldo MJ, et al.** Hydroxychloroquine (HCQ) in lupus pregnancy: double-blind and placebo-controlled study. Lupus. 2001;10:401-4.

17. **Austin HA 3rd, Klippel JH, Balow JE, et al.** Therapy of lupus nephritis: controlled trial of prednisone and cytotoxic drugs. N Engl J Med. 1986;314:614-9.

18. **Illei GG, Austin HA, Crane M, et al.** Combination therapy with pulse cyclophosphamide plus pulse methylprednisolone improves long-term renal outcome without adding toxicity in patients with lupus nephritis. Ann Intern Med. 2001;135:248-57.

19. **Chan TM, Li FK, Tang CS, et al.** Efficacy of mycophenolate mofetil in patients with diffuse proliferative lupus nephritis. Hong Kong-Guangzhou Nephrology Study Group. N Engl J Med. 2000;343:1156-62.

20. **Carneiro JR, Sato EI.** Double blind, randomized, placebo controlled clinical trial of methotrexate in systemic lupus erythematosus. J. Rheumatol. 1999;26:1275-9.

21. **Bar Oz B, Hackman R, Einarson T, Koren G.** Pregnancy outcome after cyclosporine therapy during pregnancy: a meta-analysis. Tranplantation. 2001;71:1051-5.

22. **Karim MY, Ruiz-Irastorza G, Khamasta MA, Hughes GR.** Update on therapy — thalidomide in the treatment of lupus. Lupus. 2001;10:188-92.

23. **Boumpas DT, Tassiulas IO, Fleischer TA, et al.** A pilot study of low-dose fludarabine in membranous nephropathy refractory to therapy. Clin Nephrol. 1999;52:67-75.

24. **Brodsky RA, Petri M, Smith BD, et al.** Immunoablative high-dose cyclophosphamide without stem-cell rescue for refractory, severe autoimmune disease. Ann Intern Med. 1998;129:1031-5.

25. **Petri MA, Lahita RG, Van Vollenhoven RF, et al.** Effects of prasterone on corticosteroid requirements of women with systemic lupus erythematosus: a double-blind, randomized, placebo-controlled trial. Arthritis Rheum. 2002;46:1820-9.

26. **Wallace DJ.** Clinical and pharmacologic experience with LJP-394. Exp Opin Invest Drugs. 2001;10:111-7.

7

■ ■ ■

Antiphospholipid Syndrome

Doruk Erkan, MD

Michael D. Lockshin, MD

Antiphospholipid syndrome (APS) is a distinct clinical syndrome associated with vascular thrombosis and/or pregnancy morbidity in the presence of circulating antiphospholipid antibodies (aPL), most commonly anticardiolipin antibodies (aCL) and lupus-anticoagulant (LAC). APS is a major cause of cardiovascular morbidity and mortality among young individuals. When the condition is seen in the absence of an associated underlying disease, it is known as *primary APS*. When diagnosed in the presence of an underlying disorder, it is known as *secondary APS*. Secondary APS is most commonly associated with systemic lupus erythematosus (SLE) but may also be seen in rheumatoid arthritis (RA), systemic sclerosis, or Behçet's disease. Today, 20 years after its original description, APS is recognized as an important and prevalent autoimmune disorder. Moreover, the spectrum of clinical manifestations continues to broaden.

The prevalence of aPL is 2%-12% in the general population and increases with age. Several large-scale studies report the prevalence of LAC and aCL in SLE patients to be between 11%-30% and 24%-86%, respectively. aPL have been found in less than 10% of patients with stroke but in approximately half of stroke patients who are less than 50 years of age. Approximately 14% of women who have suffered three or more pregnancy losses have circulating aPL.

Clinical Significance of Antiphospholipid Antibodies

The mere presence of aPL in the absence of clinical complications does not indicate APS. However, current literature suggests that asymptomatic aPL-positive individuals are at increased risk for developing thromboses, and a high serum titer of aCL is a significant predictor for thromboembolic disease. In the Physicians' Health Study, a high serum titer of aCL was found to be a risk factor for deep vein thrombosis or pulmonary embolism in otherwise healthy men, independent of age and smoking status.

In SLE patients, the presence of aPL is associated significantly with thrombotic events. Based on a retrospective study, 52% of asymptomatic aCL-positive SLE patients develop APS over a period of 10 years. In addition, at 20 years follow-up, there is a 50% chance of having had an arterial or venous thrombotic event among SLE patients with LAC. These events, which include strokes, myocardial infarctions, and thrombophlebitis, often result in serious debilitating sequelae. Thus APS is a major cause of cerebrovascular and cardiovascular morbidity and mortality in SLE.

Approximately one half of patients with APS do not have any underlying systemic disease. In primary APS, the female to male ratio is 2-3:1, whereas this ratio is 7-9:1 for secondary APS. Although it has been reported that family members of APS patients may be more likely to have circulating LAC and/or aCL, it is not clear whether this is associated with an increased propensity to developing APS.

Pathogenesis

Immunochemistry of Antiphospholipid Antibodies

aPL are a family of autoantibodies directed against antigenic sites (epitopes) on plasma proteins which are in complex with negatively charged phospholipids. The antigen to which aPL binds is not phospholipid but rather the phospholipid-binding plasma protein β_2-glycoprotein-I (β_2-GP-I), which has anticoagulant activity when circulating in the plasma. It likely becomes antigenic upon binding to negatively charged surfaces such as phospholipids. β_2-GP-I is not the only phospholipid-binding protein. Other plasma proteins with potential phospholipid-binding capacity include prothrombin, thrombomodulin, antithrombin III, protein C, protein S, and annexin V.

The term "anticardiolipin antibodies" refers to those aPL that are detected by their binding to cardiolipin-coated plates in standard enzyme-linked immunosorbent assays (ELISA). β_2-GP-I is a required cofactor for binding of autoimmune aCL to cardiolipin in the ELISA. Notably, anti-β_2-GP-I antibodies can be found in the sera of many patients with aCL and may, in fact, be more specific than aCL in predicting thrombotic complications according to some studies. Some patients may have antibodies that bind β_2-GP-I, detectable by the standard ELISA, but do *not* bind cardiolipin at all.

High titers of immunoglobulin (Ig) G aCL and, less so, IgM aCL are associated with increased risk for thromboembolic events. IgA aCL, as well as

---

Table 7-1   Conditions Associated with Antiphospholipid Antibodies

Infections: Syphilis, Lyme disease, leptospirosis, human immunodeficiency virus, hepatitis C virus, adenovirus, cytomegalovirus

Drugs: Chlorpromazine, procainamide, quinidine, quinine, phenytoin, phenothiazine, hydralazine, anti-tumor necrosis factor biological agents

Malignancy: Lymphoproliferative disorders

---

low titers of IgG aCL or IgM aCL (less than 30-40 U), are rarely associated with clinical events. (N.B. There continues to be significant controversy and lack of consensus as to what should be regarded as a high titer of aCL. From a practical standpoint, 40 U or greater are generally regarded as high titers.)

LAC prolongs phospholipid-dependent coagulation steps in vitro by interfering with binding of coagulation factors to phospholipid. The terms "anticardiolipin antibody" and "lupus-anticoagulant" are *not* synonymous. Approximately 80% of patients with LAC have aCL, but only 20% of patients positive for aCL have LAC.

Low titer aPL can be induced by certain drugs, malignancies, and infections (Table 7-1) but are rarely associated with thrombosis.

Mechanisms of Pathogenicity

The likely participants in aPL-promoted thrombosis are endothelial cells, platelets, and/or factors of the coagulation cascade. However, multiple synergistic mechanisms for thrombogenesis are likely to exist.

Endothelial cell damage or activation may occur due to aPL, the effects of coexisting anti-endothelial antibodies, or aPL-induced monocyte adhesion to endothelial cells. Platelets may be activated by the binding of aPL to platelet membrane phospholipid-bound proteins resulting in platelet adhesion and thrombosis. The possibility of an interaction between the coagulation cascade and aPL has also been explored intensively. Pathogenic antibodies may inhibit certain natural anticoagulation pathways such as the activation of the protein C and protein S systems. A role for aPL-induced complement activation in thrombosis has also been supported strongly by recent data from animal models.

It is not yet clear whether there are significant genetic risk factors for the production of aPL or the development of APS, even though multiple HLA-DR or HLA-DQ associations with aPL have been described.

Case Presentation

A 26-year-old white female with a medical history of two miscarriages at 15 and 17 weeks of gestation and frequent headaches wakes up with a painful and blue right index finger. Her review of systems is generally unremarkable. She is on no medications, is not a smoker, and has never had any thromboembolic events. The physical examination is normal except for diffuse livedo reticularis of the lower extremities, a decreased right radial artery pulse, and a cyanotic right index finger. Arteriography shows complete occlusion of the right radial artery. Echocardiography is normal.

Laboratory evaluation reveals positive tests for antinuclear antibodies (ANA; 1:160, nucleolar pattern) and a high serum titer of IgG aCL (>80 U). Serum IgM and IgA aCL levels were normal, as was evaluation for other hypercoagulable states, including tests for activated protein C resistance/factor V Leiden, protein C, protein S, antithrombin III, homocysteine, and the prothrombin 20210 mutation. A diagnosis of APS was made.

Intravenous heparin followed by warfarin to maintain an international normalized ratio (INR) between 3 and 4 resulted in gradual reperfusion in the patient's finger.

This case demonstrates the major manifestations of APS, which should always be considered in the differential diagnosis of a young patient presenting with vascular thrombotic events, especially with a history of miscarriages and livedo reticularis. Prompt recognition is essential to minimize the morbidity of APS.

Clinical Features

The major clinical manifestations of APS are venous and arterial thrombotic events and pregnancy morbidities (Table 7-2). These events can be acute and dramatic. Venous thromboses can occur anywhere within the vascular tree including thrombophlebitis of superficial veins. The most common site for venous thrombosis is deep venous thrombosis of the lower extremities. Arterial thromboses are most common within the cerebral vasculature, although peripheral, retinal, coronary, mesenteric, hepatic, splenic, renal, adrenal, and superficial arteries can also be involved. Thus APS patients may present with a wide spectrum of clinical manifestations including transient ischemic attacks, amaurosis fugax, strokes, occlusive ocular disease, coronary artery disease and myocardial infarction, mesenteric ischemia, Budd-Chiari syndrome, renal artery and vein thrombosis resulting in hypertension and renal failure, adrenal insufficiency due to hemorrhagic infarctions, and superficial arterial thrombosis.

Pregnancy losses in APS patients typically occur after 10 weeks of gestation, but early losses can also occur. APS-related pregnancy morbidity is due to abnormal placental function, probably resulting from thrombosis in the uteroplacental circulation. In addition to pregnancy losses, preeclampsia, intrauterine growth retardation, premature delivery, placental abruption, and HELLP syndrome (hemolytic anemia, elevated liver enzymes, and low platelet counts) can be associated with APS.

Table 7-2   Summary of Preliminary Criteria for Classification of Antiphospholipid Syndrome

Clinical criteria

Vascular thrombosis

- Arterial, venous, or small vessel thrombosis in any organ or tissue

Pregnancy morbidity

- One or more unexplained deaths of morphologically normal fetus at or beyond the 10th week of gestation; *or*
- One or more premature births of a morphologically normal neonate at or before the 34th week of gestation because of severe preeclampsia or eclampsia or severe placental insufficiency; *or*
- Three or more unexplained consecutive spontaneous abortions before the 10th week of gestation

Laboratory criteria

- Anticardiolipin antibody of IgG and/or IgM isotype present in blood in medium or high titer on two or more occasions at least 6 weeks apart; *or*
- Lupus anticoagulant present in plasma on two or more occasions at least 6 weeks apart

Definite APS is considered to be present if at least one of the clinical and one of the laboratory criteria are met.

Adapted from Wilson WA, Gharavi AE, Koike T. International consensus statement on preliminary classification criteria for definite antiphospholipid syndrome: report of an international workshop. Arthritis Rheum. 1999;42:1309-11; with permission.

Minor clinical manifestations of APS that were not designated as criteria are listed in Table 7-3. The pathophysiology of these manifestations is unclear but likely involve the previously discussed mechanisms.

Histologic examination of the vessels, skin, kidney, or other tissues shows thrombus formation *without* surrounding inflammation. The presence of significant inflammatory elements should suggest concomitant SLE, vasculitis, or other connective tissue disease.

Skin Manifestations

The most common skin manifestation of APS is livedo reticularis (20%-30% of patients), a lace-like pattern of superficial veins, most often found on the thighs, shins, and hands (Figure 7-1). Livedo reticularis reflects stasis of the blood in the superficial drainage system. In addition, pyoderma-like leg ulcers can be seen in APS patients.

Hematologic Manifestations

The major hematologic manifestations include thrombocytopenia and Coombs-positive hemolytic anemia. Thrombocytopenia is found in 15%-20% of patients. Platelet counts usually range between $50\text{-}100 \times 10^9/\mu L$ and are not generally associated with bleeding problems. Thrombocytopenia does

Table 7-3   Other Manifestations of Antiphospholipid Syndrome.

Skin	Livedo reticularis
	Cutaneous ulceration/gangrene
Hematologic	Thrombocytopenia
	Autoimmune hemolytic anemia
Neurologic	Transient ischemic attack
	Migraine (controversial)
	Seizures
	Cognitive dysfunction independent of cerebrovascular disease
	Multiple sclerosis-like syndrome
	Chorea
	Transverse myelitis
Cardiac	Cardiac valve disease
	Cardiomyopathy
	Accelerated atheroma
	Intracardiac thrombus
Kidney	Accelerated hypertension
	Thrombotic renal microangiopathy
Pulmonary	Pulmonary hypertension
	Diffuse alveolar hemorrhage
Other	Infertility (controversial)

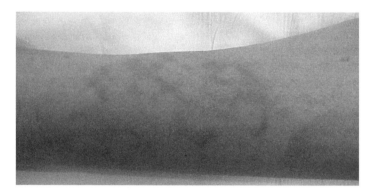

Figure 7-1   Livedo reticularis in antiphospholipid syndrome: a lace-like pattern of superficial veins.

not protect patients against thrombotic events. Although a positive direct Coombs test is not rare in APS, hemolytic anemia is actually uncommon.

Neurologic Manifestations

In addition to arterial thrombotic events, APS patients can present with psychiatric and nonthrombotic neurological features. The association between migraine and aPL is still controversial. Some patients with headache resistant to conventional treatment may experience complete or partial remission with aspirin, heparin, or warfarin anticoagulation. Seizures have been well described in primary APS patients. The etiology may be due to cerebral infarctions, but it has also been suggested that aPL may interact directly with neuronal tissue. Multi-infarct dementia can develop in APS patients as a consequence of recurrent strokes. Furthermore, cognitive dysfunction independent of cerebrovascular disease can be seen. Patients often complain of poor concentration and forgetfulness. Multiple small, hyperintense lesions can occur on brain magnetic resonance imaging (MRI) but do not appear to correlate with clinical symptoms. Other less common neurological manifestations include a multiple sclerosis-like syndrome, transverse myelitis, and chorea.

Cardiac Manifestations

Cardiac valve disease (vegetations and/or valve thickening) is present in 35%-75% of primary APS patients. Most cases are clinically asymptomatic, but roughly 5% of patients progress to cardiac failure and need valve replacement. The mitral valve is commonly affected, followed by the aortic valve. The predominant abnormality is regurgitation, and stenosis is rarely seen. Intracardiac thrombus is an uncommon manifestation of APS and can be misdiagnosed as a cardiac tumor. Diffuse cardiomyopathy is another unusual manifestation of APS. Premature coronary artery disease may occur; several investigators have suggested a role for aPL in the promotion of atherosclerosis as a result of cross-reactivity between aPL and low-density lipoprotein (LDL) particles.

Kidney Manifestations

APS patients can present with severe hypertension due to thrombosis of the renal artery or vein, which can lead to renal failure. Thrombosis of glomerular arterioles may cause non-inflammatory proteinuria.

Pulmonary Manifestations

Pulmonary hypertension can occur as a result of recurrent pulmonary emboli or small vessel thromboses in situ. Rarely, some APS patients may present with dyspnea, fever, and hemoptysis due to diffuse alveolar hemorrhage.

Other Organ Systems

Although it is controversial, aPL have been suggested as a potential etiology of presumed infertility. Increased levels of aPL occur in patients with infertility and in those who have failed in vitro fertilization. These aPL-related problems with fertility may actually reflect early spontaneous abortions. Avascular necrosis (AVN), seen in association with SLE and corticosteroid

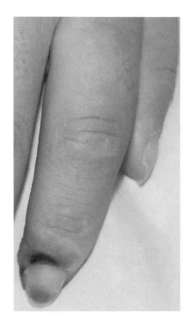

Figure 7-2 Digital ischemia and infarct in a patient with antiphospholipid syndrome. (Courtesy of Petros Efthimiou, MD.)

use, has been linked to the procoagulant effects of aPL, and AVN has been reported in non-corticosteroid-treated primary APS patients.

Catastrophic APS

Catastrophic APS is a rare but life-threatening complication of APS, which occurs in multiple organs over a period of days. Multiple thromboses of small and medium size vessels may occur despite adequate anticoagulation. Infections, pregnancy and surgical procedures have been reported as potential triggering events for catastrophic APS.

Catastrophic APS patients may present with cerebral, cardiac, hepatic, renal, adrenal, intestinal, and digital ischemia, and/or infarction (Figure 7-2). Acute adrenal failure may be the initial clinical event, one particularly challenging to recognize. Mortality of catastrophic APS is 50%, mostly due to cardiopulmonary failure.

Diagnosis

Diagnosis of APS is based on a history of a vascular or pregnancy event (see Clinical Features above) and the presence of aPL. To facilitate studies of treatment and causation, an international consensus statement on the preliminary classification criteria for APS has been developed (1). Definite APS is considered to be present if at least one of the clinical and one of the laboratory criteria given in Table 7-2 are met.

Antiphospholipid antibody testing should include assays for LAC, and IgG and IgM aCL. The LAC test is a functional assay that measures the ability of an antibody to inhibit the conversion of prothrombin to thrombin. Traditionally, the activated partial thromboplastin time (aPTT) has been the most widely used screening test for LAC. In the presence of an LAC, the aPTT is prolonged and cannot be corrected in mixing studies with normal blood; the prothrombin time (PT) is often normal or only slightly prolonged. A positive LAC test or medium-to-high serum titers IgG or IgM aCL are the laboratory criteria for APS (see Table 7-2); a false-positive test for syphilis does not fulfill the laboratory criteria. Positive tests should be verified after at least 6 weeks not only to exclude the presence of transient antibodies but also because commercial laboratories may vary greatly in their consistency of measurement.

Patients with negative IgG or IgM aCL and LAC tests should be tested for IgA aCL and anti-β_2-GP-I if they are strongly suspected of having APS.

Differential Diagnosis

Other systemic diseases (e.g., malignancy, nephrotic syndrome, polycythemia, thrombocytosis), oral contraceptive use, and congenital prothrombotic states should be considered in the differential diagnosis of APS. APS, homocystinemia, and the prothrombin 20210 mutation predispose to either arterial or venous thrombosis, whereas patients with factor V Leiden or deficiencies in protein C, protein S, or antithrombin III deficiency usually present with venous thromboses.

Conditions such as anatomic abnormalities, chronic infections of the female reproductive tract, systemic diseases, hormonal imbalances (e.g., luteal phase defect), maternal and paternal karyotype abnormalities, fetal genetic abnormalities, substance abuse, and other procoagulant states should also be considered in the differential diagnosis of recurrent pregnancy events.

As already mentioned, when LAC is present the PT is normal or only slightly prolonged; significant prolongation of PT, on the other hand, may be due to prothrombin (factor II) deficiency, hepatic insufficiency, or vitamin K deficiency. In addition, a functional prothrombin deficiency may be caused by an anti-prothrombin autoantibody, which, when present, is usually observed together with LAC. When clinically significant bleeding occurs as a result, this rare entity is called lupus anticoagulant-hypoprothrombinemia syndrome.

Prognosis and Disease Outcomes

Pulmonary hypertension, neurological involvement, myocardial ischemia, nephropathy, gangrene of extremities, and catastrophic APS are associated with a poor prognosis. In long-term follow-up, APS patients who experience major vascular events and those in whom the diagnosis and treatment are delayed are at increased risk for serious and permanent morbidity and disability. Thus the long-term functional outcome of primary APS patients is poor; at 10 years, one-third of patients will have developed permanent organ damage and one-fifth will be unable to perform activities of daily living (2).

Management

When the diagnosis of APS is entertained, a rheumatology and/or hematology consultation is indicated to help determine the appropriate intensity of anticoagulation required (4). Management options are summarized in Table 7-4.

APS with Vascular Events

Long-term anticoagulation with warfarin is the standard of care to prevent a recurrent vascular event in APS patients. The recurrence rate in untreated patients is 44%-55% following the first vascular event and approaches zero in patients treated with high-intensity warfarin therapy.

Therapeutic (as opposed to prophylactic) anticoagulation is initiated in a standard manner with either intravenous unfractionated heparin or subcutaneous low-molecular-weight heparins (LMWH). For those patients with a LAC that elevates the baseline aPTT or those who are placed initially on LMWH, peak and trough factor Xa levels can be monitored to assure appropriate anticoagulation. Initial heparin treatment is followed by long-term warfarin, usually at high intensity (INR 3.0-4.0). However, because recent studies suggest that in some individuals lower levels might be effective in preventing venous thromboembolism, some clinicians advocate an INR of 2.5-3.0 initially for treatment of a first venous thrombosis, while reserving intensive anticoagulation (INR 3.0-4.0) for those with recurrent venous thrombosis or arterial thrombosis. Low-dose aspirin (81 mg) can be added to warfarin if there is evidence of ongoing thrombosis, although this combination increases the risk of bleeding complications.

There is high risk of recurrent thrombosis especially within the 6 months following discontinuation of warfarin. Thus APS patients with vascular events should be kept on warfarin indefinitely. However, it is unclear whether patients who develop a vascular event in the presence of other hypercoagulable risk factors (e.g., abdominal or orthopedic surgery, trauma, oral contraceptive pills) should be kept on warfarin indefinitely.

APS patients are at additional risk for thrombosis when they undergo surgery. Serious perioperative thrombotic complications can occur despite appropriate prophylaxis with anticoagulants. Accordingly, perioperative

Table 7-4   Treatment Options for Antiphospholipid Syndrome

Clinical Manifestation	Treatment Options
Venous thrombosis	Warfarin (INR 2.5-3)
Arterial thrombosis	Warfarin (INR 3-4)
Recurrent thrombosis despite appropriate warfarin anticoagulation	Warfarin (INR 3-4) and LDA
Single pregnancy loss < 10 weeks	No treatment or LDA
Recurrent pregnancy loss or pregnancy loss > 10 weeks (no history of vascular thrombosis)	LDA + prophylactic-dose heparin* during pregnancy; switch to LDA postpartum 6-12 weeks
Recurrent pregnancy loss or pregnancy loss > 10 weeks (history of vascular thrombosis)	LDA + therapeutic-dose heparin** during pregnancy; switch to warfarin postpartum
Thrombocytopenia > 50,000 × 10⁹/μL	No treatment or LDA
Thrombocytopenia ≤ 50,000 × 10⁹/μL and active bleeding	Corticosteroids Intravenous immunoglobulin
Catastrophic APS	Anticoagulation Corticosteroids Intravenous immunoglobulin Plasmapheresis
Asymptomatic aPL-positive patients	No treatment, LDA, or hydroxychloroquine

INR = international normalized ratio; LDA = low-dose aspirin (81 mg).
*E.g., enoxaparin 20-40 mg daily or equivalent.
**E.g., enoxaparin 1 mg/kg twice daily or equivalent.

strategies should be clearly defined *before* any surgical procedure (3). Both pharmacological and physical anti-thrombotic interventions should be aggressively employed, and periods without anticoagulation must be minimized. Patients taking chronic warfarin therapy, for example, may require hospitalization before the day of surgery for anticoagulation with intravenous heparin up until the last possible moment. Any deviation from the expected perioperative course should be suspected as a potential APS-related event.

APS with Pregnancy Events

Aspirin plus subcutaneous (SQ) heparin is the standard prophylactic therapy during pregnancy for patients who have had previous vascular or pregnancy events. Untreated patients with high-titer aPL have about a 50%-75% chance of fetal loss, but with aspirin and SQ heparin the chance of a full-term delivery is 70%-80%. In clinical practice, low-dose aspirin alone is generally prescribed for patients with aPL but no more than a single previous first trimester loss (5). Monthly intravenous immunoglobulin (IVIG) (e.g., 2 g/kg body weight given in divided doses over 3-5 days) is a possible additional therapy for women who fail to be protected by aspirin and heparin.

Aspirin therapy is generally started before conception. Patients with a history of a thrombotic event and on warfarin are usually changed to SQ heparin before attempting to conceive in order to eliminate the risk of warfarin-induced embryopathy. LMWH is increasingly substituted for unfractionated heparin despite the lack of randomized trials for APS using LMWH in prophylactic or therapeutic dosages. Advantages of LMWH include once or twice daily dosing, decreased risks of bleeding complications and heparin-induced thrombocytopenia, and a possible lower incidence of heparin-induced osteoporosis.

The elevated estrogen level in pregnancy may contribute to the increased risk of thrombosis during gestation. Postpartum thrombosis is common in APS patients in the absence of anticoagulation. Thus APS patients with a history of vascular thrombosis should be promptly started on warfarin or continued on heparin after the delivery. In APS patients who have had only pregnancy morbidity, low-dose aspirin appears to be effective against future non-gravid vascular thrombosis.

Regardless of treatment choice, women with APS require careful observation during pregnancy and should be cared for by obstetricians experienced in high-risk pregnancies. Ultrasound evaluations to monitor fetal growth, frequent testing after 28 weeks to detect abnormal decelerations in fetal heart rate, and Doppler umbilical artery flow studies should be considered in these patients. There are no known genetic fetal abnormalities associated with aPL, and the likelihood that the child will eventually develop aPL is low.

APS with Other Manifestations

Platelet counts greater than $50 \times 10^9/\mu L$ due to APS generally require no specific therapy in patients without hemorrhagic complications. When active bleeding results from more severe thrombocytopenia, systemic corticosteroids (e.g., prednisone 1 mg/kg/d) are the first line of treatment. In life-threatening situations, intravenous methylprednisolone 1 g/d for 3 days can be given initially. IVIG (e.g., 2 g/kg body weight given in divided doses over 3-5 days) can be used as an adjunct to corticosteroids in more refractory cases (6). Platelet transfusions are usually not helpful in APS patients, because the mechanism of thrombocytopenia is thought to be due to platelet damage and may actually increase the risk of thrombosis. Besides IVIG, danazol (400-800 mg/d) or even splenectomy may be considered in corticosteroid-resistant cases (7).

Very few studies address the management of the nonthromboembolic manifestations of APS. Most of these manifestations, such as cardiac valve involvement and cognitive dysfunction, are generally managed initially with low-dose aspirin, even though no published data strongly support this approach.

Catastrophic APS

Catastrophic APS patients are usually aggressively treated with combination regimens. Plasmapheresis and/or IVIG in addition to anticoagulation and systemic corticosteroids seem to improve the outcome. Nevertheless, the survival rate is only 50%.

Asymptomatic aPL-Positive Patients

An important and poorly studied issue is the appropriate management for primary prevention of thrombosis in asymptomatic aPL-positive individuals. These patients are often identified after evaluation for an elevated aPTT detected during preoperative screening. Also, physicians have been increasingly testing their SLE patients for the presence of aPL. Asymptomatic aPL-positive patients generally receive no treatment until after they have a thrombotic event. However, there have been recent reports that advocate the prophylactic use of aspirin, despite the lack of definitive data from clinical trials. Although warfarin is superior to aspirin in the secondary prevention of thrombosis of APS patients, no data support its use in the primary prevention of thrombosis. Hydroxychloroquine (HCQ) treatment has been shown to reduce the risk of thrombosis in both SLE patients and animal models for APS (8,9). However, the number of studies evaluating HCQ is limited, and benefit may result from other effects such as controlling SLE activity and reducing hyperlipidemia.

Two ongoing clinical trials are addressing the issue of the primary prevention of asymptomatic aPL-positive patients. These trials are: placebo versus low-dose aspirin (USA – APLASA) and aspirin versus aspirin plus low-dose warfarin (UK).

In addition, education about the significance of abnormal test results and discussion of the warning signs should be included in the management plan of a patient with positive aPL but no clinical manifestations. Hypertension, hyperlipidemia, inactivity, and obesity should be aggressively addressed. Smoking should be strongly discouraged, and women should be counseled against the use of estrogen-containing oral contraceptive pills.

Summary

Although only recognized within the past 20 years as a discrete syndrome caused by aPL, APS is an important cause of thrombotic disease, especially in the young female population. In a patient presenting with arterial or venous thrombotic events, APS should be always considered.

■ ■ ■

Key Points

- Normalization of the lupus-anticoagulant test or anticardiolipin antibodies is not an indication to discontinue anticoagulation, because titers vary greatly and patients remain at risk for new thrombosis regardless of change in titer.
- Antiphospholipid antibodies (aPL) may be consumed during an acute thrombotic episode. Thus aPL should be measured again 6 weeks after an acute episode.
- Neither thrombocytopenia nor an elevated activated partial thromboplastin time (aPTT) protects against thrombosis.
- Pregnancy events are not restricted to fetal losses but include other complications such as preeclampsia.
- Prolonged aPTT and/or slightly prolonged prothrombin time (PT) when known to be due to APS do not reflect increased risk of bleeding and are *not* contraindications for surgical procedures.
- Serious perioperative clotting complications may occur in APS patients who undergo surgery.

■ ■ ■

REFERENCES

1. **Wilson WA, Gharavi AE, Koike T, et al.** International consensus statement on preliminary classification criteria for definite antiphospholipid syndrome: report of an international workshop. Arthritis Rheum. 1999;42:1309-11.
2. **Erkan D, Yazici Y, Sobel R, Lockshin MD.** Primary antiphospholipid syndrome: functional outcome after 10 years. J Rheumatol. 2000;27:2817-21.
3. **Erkan D, Leibowitz E, Berman J, Lockshin MD.** Perioperative medical management of antiphospholipid syndrome: Hospital for Special Surgery experience, review of the literature and recommendations. J Rheumatol. 2002;29:843-9.
4. **Khamashta MA, Cuadrado MJ, Mujic F, et al.** The management of thrombosis in the antiphospholipid-antibody syndrome. N Engl J Med. 1995;332:993-7.
5. **Erkan D, Merrill JT, Yazici Y, et al.** High thrombosis rate after fetal loss in antiphospholipid syndrome: effective prophylaxis with aspirin. Arthritis Rheum. 2001; 44:1466-7.
6. **Sherer Y, Levy Y, Shoenfeld Y.** Intravenous immunoglobulin therapy of antiphospholipid syndrome. Rheumatol. 2000;39:421-6.
7. **Kavanaugh A.** Danazol therapy in thrombocytopenia associated with the antiphospholipid antibody syndrome. Ann Intern Med. 1994;121:767-8.
8. **Edwards MH, Pierangeli S, Liu X, et al.** Hydroxychloroquine reverses thrombogenic properties of antiphospholipid antibodies in mice. Circulation. 1997;96:4380-4.
9. **Petri M.** Hydroxychloroquine use in the Baltimore lupus cohort: effects on lipids, glucose, and thrombosis. Lupus. 1996;5(Suppl):S16-22.

8

■ ■ ■

Sjögren's Syndrome

Athanasios G. Tzioufas, MD

Stuart S. Kassan, MD

Haralampos M. Moutsopoulos, MD

S jögren's syndrome is a slowly progressive, autoimmune disease characterized by chronic inflammation of the exocrine glands. Autoreactive lymphocytic infiltrates replace the functional epithelium, leading to decreased exocrine secretions and the clinical manifestations of keratoconjunctivitis sicca, xerostomia, xerotrachea, and vaginal dryness. Major salivary gland enlargement occurs in 60% of patients. Often there are associated extraglandular manifestations, commonly affecting the skin, lungs, kidneys, liver, peripheral nerves, or muscles. The disease can occur alone (i.e., primary Sjögren's syndrome) or in association with other autoimmune diseases such as rheumatoid arthritis (RA), systemic lupus erythematosus (SLE), systemic sclerosis, and polymyositis (i.e., secondary Sjögren's syndrome). Up to one half of patients with RA will have secondary Sjögren's syndrome. As many as 5% of patients develop B-cell lymphoid malignancies late in the course of the disease.

Primary Sjögren's syndrome can occur in all ages and in both sexes, but women between the ages of 40 and 60 years appear at highest risk. The female-to-male ratio is 9:1. The prevalence of the disease is around 3%, but this figure is probably an underestimate because many individuals with mild symptoms are unrecognized.

Pathogenesis

The minor salivary glands are the best studied organs because they are affected in almost all patients and are readily accessible. When diagnostic, minor salivary gland biopsy shows focal aggregates of at least 50 lymphocytes and plasma cells adjacent to ducts and replacing acini. Larger foci often exhibit formation of germinal centers. In addition to the lymphocytic infiltration of the affected tissues, Sjögren's syndrome is characterized by B-lymphocyte hyper-reactivity manifested as the production of a large array of organ and nonorgan specific autoantibodies. Growing evidence points to a central role of the epithelial cell in the evolution of the disease, suggesting the use of the term *autoimmune epithelitis* as an alternative to *Sjögren's syndrome* in order to reflect this pathogenetic association. Conceptually, autoimmunity is thought to be triggered by environmental factors acting on an individual with a susceptible genetic background. The autoimmune response then becomes chronic through aberrant immune regulatory mechanisms and subsequently results in organ-specific inflammation and dysfunction.

Viruses

Viruses have long been suspected as potential triggering agents in Sjögren's syndrome. Chronic viral infections are known to induce increased apoptosis (programmed cell death) of infected cells resulting in the release of intracellular antigens that may potentially initiate specific autoimmune responses. This hypothesis is supported by the observation that the epithelial cells of the exocrine glands in Sjögren's syndrome have an increased rate of apoptosis.

Patients with chronic hepatitis C virus (HCV) infection have detectable HCV RNA in their salivary glands and can develop a chronic lymphocytic sialadenitis resembling that observed in Sjögren's syndrome. Human immunodeficiency virus-1 (HIV-1) and human T-lymphotrophic virus type 1 (HTLV-1) can also infect the epithelial cells in salivary glands and cause chronic sialadenitis.

Viral infection may also contribute to the pathogenesis of lymphoma in Sjögren's syndrome through a mechanism of constant antigen-driven inflammation. Lymphomas seen in association with Sjögren's syndrome share many characteristics with those seen in chronic HCV infection, including the production of cryoglobulins and a predilection for tissue affected by autoimmune disease or by HCV infection.

Immunogenetics

Family members of patients with Sjögren's syndrome are at increased risk of also developing the disease and have a higher prevalence of circulating autoantibodies than age- and sex-matched healthy controls. Several studies have shown associations between primary Sjögren's syndrome and the major histocompatibility complex; HLA-DR3 has been reported in 50%-80% of patients with Sjögren's syndrome.

Autoantibodies

The most common serological abnormality in Sjögren's syndrome is a polyclonal hypergammaglobulinemia. Sera of patients may contain rheumatoid factor, antinuclear antibodies (usually in a speckled pattern), and autoantibodies against intracellular antigens (e.g., Ro/SSA, La/SSB), cell surface antigens (e.g., muscarinic receptors), and organ-specific antigens of salivary ductal cells, thyroid gland cells, and gastric mucosa. Anti-Ro and anti-La antibodies are detected in the serum of 45%-70% and 20%-50%, respectively, of patients with Sjögren's syndrome but are also commonly found in other autoimmune diseases, particularly SLE. The presence of anti-Ro and anti-La autoantibodies is associated with earlier onset of disease, parotid gland enlargement, infiltration of minor salivary glands, splenomegaly, lymphadenopathy, and systemic vasculitis.

Immunohistopathology

The majority of the inflammatory cells in salivary gland biopsies in Sjögren's syndrome are T cells; 20%-25% are B cells. Monocytes and macrophages make up less than 5%. Current evidence suggests that the glandular or acinar epithelial cells act as antigen-presenting cells, a role central to the induction of autoimmunity (1). The glandular and acinar epithelial cells inappropriately express HLA class II antigens in response to interferon-γ and tumor necrosis factor (TNF)-α produced locally by the activated T cell. This finding suggests that targeting these cytokines may be a possible therapeutic approach. Ductal and acinar epithelial cells may also perpetuate the autoimmune process by inappropriately secreting proinflammatory cytokines and lympho-attractant chemokines and expressing nuclear autoantigens, adhesion, and co-stimulatory molecules on their cell surface.

Case Presentation

A 64-year-old woman is seen for pancytopenia and peripheral lymphadenopathy. Ten years earlier, the patient had developed "grittiness" in her eyes and dryness in her mouth that caused discomfort while eating. She was diagnosed with primary Sjögren's syndrome on the basis of these sicca symptoms, a subsequent positive lip biopsy, and the presence of serum antinuclear, anti-Ro/SSA, and anti-La/SSB antibodies. At the time of diagnosis, she was also found to have a mild anemia (Hgb 11.5 g/dL), a positive rheumatoid factor (1:640), and mixed monoclonal cryoglobulins. She was treated with artificial tears and saliva as needed with partial relief of her symptoms. More recently, she was given a trial of oral pilocarpine that helped her xerostomia but caused her to sweat excessively.

She was in her usual state of health until 3 months ago when she developed worsening fatigue, anorexia, and a low-grade fever. On physical examination, the patient appeared pale and fatigued. A spleen tip was felt, and the liver edge was smooth and palpable 4 cm below the right costal margin. No signs of chronic liver disease were detected. The axillary lymph nodes were enlarged, smooth, and nontender. The rest of the examination was unrevealing.

Laboratory results revealed a normochromic, normocytic anemia (Hgb 8.4 g/dL), leukopenia (WBC 2600/mm^3; 53% neutrophils, 28% lymphocytes, 18.5% monocytes, 0.5% eosinophils), and a mild thrombocytopenia (105,000/mm^3). Serum levels of alkaline phosphatase, lactate dehydrogenase (LDH), and γ-glutamyl-transpeptidase (γ-GTP) were elevated.

Computed tomography of the chest, abdomen, and pelvis showed the presence of enlarged paraaortic lymph nodes and homogeneous hepatosplenomegaly. Bone marrow biopsy revealed modest infiltration with monoclonal small B-cell lymphocytes. Axillary lymph node biopsy showed destruction of the normal glandular architecture by small lymphocytes with coarsely irregular nuclei, and immunochemical staining showed κ light chain monoclonality. The histological picture was compatible with a high-grade, small cell, B-cell non-Hodgkin's lymphoma. The patient received a full course of chemotherapy with complete regression of peripheral lymphadenopathy, resolution of pancytopenia, and normalization of serum levels of alkaline phosphatase, LDH, and γ-GTP.

Clinical Features

Sjögren's disease usually runs an indolent course. Initial manifestations may be mild, and years may elapse from the initial manifestations to the full-blown development and recognition of the syndrome.

Glandular Manifestations

Diminished tear production due to lacrimal gland involvement leads to the destruction of both corneal and bulbar conjunctival epithelium and a constellation of clinical findings termed *keratoconjunctivitis sicca* (KCS). Patients usually complain of a burning, sandy, or scratchy sensation under the lids, itchiness, redness, and mild photophobia. Physical signs include dilation of the bulbar conjunctival vessels, pericorneal injection, irregularity of the corneal image, and lacrimal gland enlargement.

Xerostomia, or dry mouth, is the result of the decreased production of saliva by the salivary glands. Patients report difficulty swallowing dry food, inability to speak continuously, changes in sense of taste, a burning sensation in the mouth, an increase in dental caries, and problems in wearing complete dentures. Physical examination may show a dry erythematous sticky oral mucosa, poor dentition, scant and cloudy saliva from the major salivary glands, and atrophy of the filiform papillae on the dorsal tongue.

Parotid or major salivary gland enlargement occurs in 60% of primary Sjögren's syndrome patients. The parotid gland enlargement may be episodic or chronic, unilateral or bilateral. Dryness of the upper respiratory tract or the oropharynx causes hoarseness, recurrent bronchitis, and pneumonitis. Loss of exocrine function may also lead to loss of pancreatic function and hypochlorhydria. Patients may also experience dermal dryness and loss of vaginal secretions.

Extraglandular Manifestations

Approximately 50% of patients with the clinical picture of Sjögren's syndrome have systemic manifestations that can include general constitutional symptoms such as easy fatigability and low-grade fever, as well as specific organ involvement. There is debate whether many of these patients may actually have undifferentiated or overlap connective tissue diseases with prominent secondary Sjögren's syndrome, but this is an academic question, and patients should be treated according to their clinical problems and not according to putative diagnoses.

Extraglandular manifestations are divided into two major groups. *Periepithelial* organ involvement (e.g., arthritis, interstitial nephritis, liver involvement, obstructive bronchiolitis) is the result of lymphocytic infiltration of affected organs. These features appear early in the disease and usually have a benign course. In contrast, *extraepithelial* manifestations (e.g., palpable purpura, glomerulonephritis, peripheral neuropathy) are caused by immune complex deposition disease secondary to the ongoing B cell hyper-reactivity. These features are usually observed late in the disease and are associated with increased morbidity and risk for the development of lymphoma.

Musculoskeletal Symptoms
Musculoskeletal manifestations can include polyarthralgias, polymyalgias, morning stiffness, intermittent inflammatory synovitis, and chronic polyarthritis. Inflammatory arthritis is observed in 50% of patients but, in contrast to RA, there are usually no erosive changes. Rare cases of inflammatory myositis have been reported.

Raynaud's Phenomenon
As many as 35% of patients present with Raynaud's phenomenon that commonly precedes sicca manifestations by many years. Patients with Raynaud's phenomenon present with swollen hands but, in contrast to scleroderma, telangiectasias or digital ulcers are not typical. However, hand radiographs of these patients may show small soft tissue calcifications.

Cutaneous Involvement
Cutaneous manifestations can include purpura, annular erythema, and pernio-like lesions. Flat purpura is usually seen in patients with hypergammaglobulinemia, whereas palpable purpura is a manifestation of dermal

vasculitis. Annular erythemas have been described in patients with Sjögren's syndrome from Japan.

Respiratory Tract Disease

Manifestations from the respiratory tract and the pleura are frequent but rarely dangerous. A nonproductive cough secondary to dryness of tracheo-bronchial mucosa (xerotrachea) or dyspnea due to small airway obstruction is relatively common. High-resolution CT of the lungs often demonstrate wall thickening at the segmental bronchi, and bronchial biopsy shows peri-bronchial and/or peribronchiolar mononuclear inflammation. Interstitial lung disease in Sjögren's syndrome is less common. Pleural effusions are infrequently found in primary Sjögren's syndrome. Lymphoma should always be suspected when lung nodules or hilar or mediastinal lym-phadenopathy are present in chest radiographs.

Gastrointestinal and Hepatobiliary Features

Patients with Sjögren's syndrome often report dysphagia due to either dry-ness of the pharynx and esophagus or abnormal esophageal motility. Nausea and epigastric pain are also common clinical symptoms. Gastric mucosa biopsy specimens show chronic atrophic gastritis and lymphocytic infiltrates similar to those described in minor salivary gland biopsy. Sub-clinical pancreatic involvement is rather common, with hyperamylasemia found in approximately 25% of patients. Patients often present with hepato-megaly (25%) and antimitochondrial antibodies (AMA) (5%). Liver biopsy generally reveals mild intrahepatic bile duct inflammation.

Renal Involvement

Clinically significant renal disease is observed in approximately 5% of pa-tients with primary Sjögren's syndrome, presenting with either interstitial nephritis or glomerulonephritis. Interstitial nephritis is usually an early fea-ture and is characterized by an interstitial lymphocytic infiltration. Affected patients present with hyposthenuria and hypokalemic-hyperchloremic distal renal tubular acidosis (RTA). Distal RTA may be clinically silent, but un-treated significant RTA may lead to renal stones, nephrocalcinosis, and com-promised renal function. Glomerulonephritis is an uncommon late sequela. Membranous or membranoproliferative glomerulonephritis in Sjögren's syndrome has been described in a few patients. Cryoglobulinemia, associ-ated with hypocomplementemia, is a consistent serologic finding in these patients.

Vasculitis

Vasculitis, found in approximately 5% of Sjögren's syndrome patients, af-fects small and medium-sized vessels and presents most commonly as pal-pable purpura, recurrent urticaria, skin ulcerations, and mononeuritis multiplex. Uncommon cases of systemic vasculitis with visceral involvement affecting kidneys, lungs, gastrointestinal tract, spleen, breasts, and reproductive tract have been described.

Neurologic Involvement
Peripheral sensorimotor neuropathy can be a consequence of small vessel vasculitis. Cranial neuropathies can occur, usually affecting single nerves such as the trigeminal or the optic nerve.

Thyroid Disease
Autoimmune thyroid disease has been associated with primary Sjögren's syndrome. Twenty-five to fifty percent of patients with Sjögren's syndrome present with anti-thyroid antibodies and elevated serum levels of thyroid-stimulating hormone.

Lymphoproliferative Disease
The prevalence of non-Hodgkin's lymphoma (NHL) in primary and secondary Sjögren's syndrome is 4.3%, representing a relative risk of 44-fold compared to age-, sex-, and race-matched healthy individuals. Before the development of NHL, patients with primary Sjögren's syndrome may have monoclonal immunoglobulins or light chains in their serum and urine. Moreover, 20% of patients have mixed monoclonal cryoglobulins (type II) containing an IgM-κ monoclonal rheumatoid factor. Serial studies have shown that the presence of mixed monoclonal cryoglobulinemia correlates with lymphoma development in patients with primary Sjögren's syndrome. Persistent parotid gland enlargement, purpura, leukopenia, cryoglobulinemia, and low C4 complement levels are clinical manifestations that should raise the suspicion of lymphoma development.

Most lymphomas are extranodal and low grade and are often detected incidentally upon the evaluation of labial biopsy. The median time between the initial diagnosis of Sjögren's syndrome and the diagnosis of lymphoma is 7.5 years. Constitutional "B" symptoms (i.e., fever, fatigue, and night sweats) are usually not present at the initial diagnosis of lymphoma in Sjögren's syndrome. Poor prognostic factors include the presence of "B" symptoms, lymph node size >7 cm, and high or intermediate histologic grade.

NHL in Sjögren's syndrome is of B cell origin, and dysregulation of the p53 tumor suppressor gene has been suggested as an important contributing pathogenic factor.

Diagnosis

Diagnosis of Sjögren's syndrome is based on an internationally approved set of criteria (Table 8-1) (2). The sensitivity and specificity of the diagnostic criteria exhibited good discrimination between patients and controls. Although lip biopsy for examination of minor salivary glands is the most

---

Table 8-1   Criteria for the Classification of Sjögren's Syndrome

1. Ocular symptoms (at least one of the following): (*a*) daily, persistent and troublesome dry eyes for more than 3 months, (*b*) recurrent gritty sensation in the eyes, or (*c*) use of tear substitutes more than three times daily

2. Oral symptoms (at least one of the following): (*a*) daily feeling of dry mouth for more than 3 months, (*b*) recurrent or persistent swollen salivary glands as an adult, or (*c*) frequent requirements for liquids to aid in swallowing dry foods

3. Ocular signs (at least one of the following): (*a*) a positive Schirmer's test (<5 mm in 5 min), or (*b*) a positive Rose bengal test

4. Histopathologic features: at least one agglomeration of >50 mononuclear cells within 4 mm^3 of glandular tissue on a minor salivary gland biopsy

5. Objective testing for salivary gland function (positive test of at least one of the following): (*a*) salivary scintigraphy, (*b*) parotid sialography, or (*c*) unstimulated salivary flow (<1.5 mL in 15 min)

6. Presence of autoantibodies to Ro/SS-A, La/SS-B, or both

In the absence of any potentially associated condition, *primary Sjögren's syndrome* can be diagnosed if (*a*) four criteria are met including at least a positive biopsy or serologic test, or (*b*) if any three objective tests (i.e., criteria 3, 4, 5, or 6) are present.

In the presence of a potentially associated condition, *secondary Sjögren's syndrome* can be diagnosed if one subjective symptom (criteria 1 or 2) and any two items from criteria 3, 4, or 5 are present.

Exclusion criteria include past radiation therapy around the head and neck, hepatitis C infection, acquired immunodeficiency syndrome, pre-existing lymphoma, sarcoidosis, graft-versus-host disease, and use of anticholinergic medications.

Adapted from Vitali C, Bombardieri S, Jonsson R, et al. Classification criteria for Sjögren's syndrome: a revised version of the European criteria proposed by the American-European Consensus Group. Ann Rheum Dis. 2002;61:554-8; with permission.

---

common invasive diagnostic procedure for Sjögren's syndrome, the diagnosis is usually a clinical one based on the history and physical examination with support from laboratory data.

Serologic Testing

Anti-Ro and anti-La antibodies are included as part of the diagnostic criteria for Sjögren's syndrome and should be assessed in all patients considered for this diagnosis. Additional testing for autoantibodies (e.g., antinuclear antibodies, rheumatoid factor) can be helpful in evaluating the possible presence of underlying disorders such as SLE or RA.

Lip Biopsy

Lip biopsy confirms lymphocytic infiltration of the minor salivary glands. Focal aggregates of at least 50 lymphocytes and plasma cells and adjacent to ducts and replacing acini are seen in patients with Sjögren's syndrome. However, the lymphocytic foci are not present in all minor salivary glands, and multiple glands should be examined to secure an accurate diagnosis.

Evaluation of Xerostomia

Various tests of salivary gland function have been developed. These include direct measurement of salivary flow (sialometry), radiocontrast assessment of salivary ductal system (sialography), and functional evaluation of the rate and density of salivary gland uptake of $^{99}Tc^m$pertechnetate (scintigraphic isotope scanning). These tests are primarily used in clinical trials, rarely to confirm the diagnosis in routine clinical practice.

Evaluation of Xerophthalmia

Ocular involvement leading to keratoconjunctivitis sicca is a major glandular manifestation of Sjögren's syndrome. All tests for the evaluation of this condition are very sensitive but not specific for Sjögren's syndrome.

SCHIRMER'S TEST

The tip of a strip of filter paper 30 mm long is slipped beneath the inferior lid, with the remainder of the paper hanging out. After 5 minutes, the length of paper wetted is measured. Wetting of less than 5 mm is a strong indication of diminished tearing.

ROSE BENGAL STAINING

Rose bengal is an aniline compound that stains the devitalized or damaged epithelium of both the cornea and conjunctiva. In Sjögren's syndrome, slit-lamp examination after rose bengal staining shows a punctate pattern of filamentary keratitis.

TEAR BREAK-UP TIME

A drop of fluoroscein is instilled into the eye, and the time between the last blink and appearance of dark, nonfluorescent areas in the tear film is measured. An overly rapid break-up of the tear film indicates an abnormality of either the mucin or the lipid layer.

Differential Diagnosis

Sarcoidosis can often mimic the clinical picture of Sjögren's syndrome but can easily be diagnosed by the presence of characteristic noncaseating granulomas on salivary gland biopsy. Patients with sarcoidosis usually do not have ANA and anti-Ro and anti-La antibodies. Other conditions that can mimic the syndrome are lipoproteinemias (types II, IV, and V), chronic graft-versus-host disease, and amyloidosis. HIV, HTLV-1, and HCV may produce chronic sialadenitis and a clinical picture similar to that of primary Sjögren's syndrome and can be evaluated by appropriate serologic testing.

Table 8-2   Some Medications Associated with Sicca Symptoms

- Tricyclic antidepressants
- Antihistamines
- Narcotics
- Phenothiazines
- Anti-cholinergics (e.g., atropine)
- Sympathomimetics (e.g., epinephrine, ephedrine, pseudoephedrine)
- Dopaminergic anti-Parkinsonian medications (e.g., levodopa, carbidopa)

Patients with HIV infection can present with sicca manifestations, parotid gland enlargement, lymphadenopathy, and pulmonary involvement. Salivary gland biopsy in HIV patients reveal lymphocytic infiltrates of CD8$^+$ T cells in contrast to the predominance of CD4$^+$ T cells in Sjögren's syndrome. Patients with chronic lymphocytic sialadenitis associated with HCV infection have a higher mean age, a lower prevalence of parotid gland enlargement, and more evidence of chronic liver disease than patients with primary Sjögren's syndrome. Many commonly used medications are well known causes of sicca syndrome (Table 8-2).

Prognosis and Disease Outcomes

The glandular manifestations of Sjögren's syndrome are typically present at the time of diagnosis, and the serological profile of the patients does not tend to change substantially over time. Untreated, the consequences of diminished exocrine function can result in permanent tissue damage such as destruction of corneal and bulbar conjunctival epithelium and loss of dentition. Patients with extraglandular manifestations can be divided into two different groups with regard to the disease outcome. The presence of arthritis, Raynaud's phenomenon, interstitial nephritis, obstructive bronchiolitis, and lung and liver involvement is often associated with a generally benign course. Purpura, glomerulonephritis, hypocomplementemia, mixed monoclonal cryoglobulinemia, peripheral neuropathy, and lymphoma are poor prognostic factors. The overall mortality of patients with primary Sjögren's syndrome is increased in patients with these latter manifestations.

Management

Prevention and treatment of sicca and constitutional symptoms are among the primary objectives of management of Sjögren's syndrome. These objectives can generally be accomplished without rheumatology consultation. Because

Table 8-3   Commercially Available Preparations of Artificial Tears and Ocular Ointments

- Hydroxyethyl cellulose (Adsorbotear)

- White petrolatum (Duratears, Lacrilube)

- Polyvinyl alcohol (HypoTears, Liquifilm Forte, Tears Plus)

- Polyethylene glycol (AquaSite)

- Hydroxypropyl methylcellulose (Bion Tears, Tears Naturale)

- Methylcellulose (Murocel)

- Carboxymethylcellulose (Refresh Plus)

Sjögren's syndrome is a chronic disease with a broad clinical spectrum, patients should also be regularly followed for significant functional deterioration and evidence of disease complications such as extraglandular involvement or lymphoma; if these occur, specialty consultation is appropriate.

Treatment of Sicca Symptoms

Preventive measures for sicca manifestations is very important. Lubrication of dry eyes with artificial tear drops and ocular ointments should be done as often as necessary, even hourly if required. A variety of commercially available preparations differ primarily in viscosity and type of preservative (Table 8-3). Patients usually test several different preparations to determine which is most suitable for their individual needs. Bicarbonate-buffered electrolyte solutions, which mimic the electrolyte composition of human tears, have shown promising results. Avoidance of windy and/or low humidity indoor and outdoor environments is helpful. Cigarette smoking and drugs with anticholinergic side effects such as phenothiazines, tricyclic antidepressants, antispasmodics, and anti-Parkinsonian agents should be avoided. Oral pilocarpine 5 mg four times daily has been shown to reduce the ocular symptoms of Sjögren's syndrome without serious adverse effects (3,4). Topical administration of cyclosporine 0.05% has been shown to be moderately effective in a placebo-controlled clinical trial and is now FDA-approved for keratoconjunctivitis sicca (5). In severely dry eyes, punctal cauterization should be used. When corneal opacification or perforation occurs, corneal transplantation is recommended.

Treatment of Xerostomia

Treatment of xerostomia is difficult. No single method is consistently effective, and most efforts are aimed only at palliation. Stimulation of salivary flow by sugar-free highly flavored lozenges is helpful. Various artificial saliva preparations are available, but they tend to be not highly liked by

Table 8-4	Commercially Available Preparations of Artificial Saliva and Oral Lubricants
• Salivart	• Biotène Mouthwash
• MouthKote	• Xero-Lube
• Saliment	

patients (Table 8-4). Conscientious oral hygiene after meals is a prerequisite for prevention of dental disease. Topical treatment with stannous fluoride enhances dental mineralization and retards damage to tooth surfaces. In cases of rapidly progressive dental disease, the fluoride can be directly applied to the teeth from plastic trays that are used at night. Two muscarinic agonists, pilocarpine hydrochloride (Salagen) and cevimeline (Evoxac), have recently been approved for the treatment of symptoms of xerostomia in Sjögren's syndrome. These agents stimulate the M_1 and M_3 muscarinic receptors present on salivary glands, leading to increased secretory function (6). Increased salivary flow rate can occur within 15 minutes of oral-dose pilocarpine hydrochloride 5 mg (generally administered four times daily) and can last for at least 4 hours (3). Cevimeline (30 mg three times daily) has also been shown also to increase the salivary flow (7). Pilocarpine and cevimeline can cause transient hemodynamic changes and arrhythmias and should be used with caution in patients with cardiovascular disease. Side effects such as flushing, headache, and sweating are uncomfortable but usually mild.

Treatment of Vaginal Dryness and Dry Skin

Vaginal dryness is best treated topically with lubricant jellies. Moisturizing lotions are best for dry skin.

Drug Therapies

Hydroxychloroquine
Hydroxychloroquine 200-400 mg/day can be effective in a subgroup of patients complaining of arthritis/arthralgias, myalgias, and constitutional symptoms (8).

Methotrexate
An open trial of weekly methotrexate 0.2 mg/kg for the treatment of primary Sjögren's syndrome resulted in subjective improvement in symptoms of xerophthalmia and xerostomia, dry cough, and purpura, but there was no beneficial effect on objective measures of dry eyes and mouth (9). Some of the musculoskeletal symptoms may respond to methotrexate, but the overall role of this drug in Sjögren's syndrome remains to be determined.

Systemic Corticosteroids and Cytotoxic Agents

Severe extraepithelial disease (e.g., diffuse interstitial pneumonitis, glomer-ulonephritis, vasculitis, peripheral neuropathy) requires high-dose systemic corticosteroid therapy (starting at prednisone 0.5-1.0 mg/kg daily or equivalent) and/or immunosuppressive therapy with agents such as cyclophosphamide. The duration of corticosteroid and/or immunosuppressive therapy is dictated by the severity of the disease manifestation. Typically, corticosteroid tapers are not initiated until control of the acute problem is achieved and then are conducted gradually over weeks to months with careful monitoring for disease relapses. When immunosuppressants are required, they are usually maintained at least 6 months after a remission is obtained before they are tapered or discontinued. The impact of these agents on the natural course of Sjögren's syndrome is not well established.

TNF Inhibition

In a recent single-center, open-label pilot study, 16 patients with primary Sjögren's syndrome received three infusions of infliximab, a chimeric human-mouse anti-TNF-α monoclonal antibody, at a dose of 3 mg/kg, at 0, 2, and 6 weeks (10). There was statistically significant improvement in all clinical and functional parameters, including global assessments (patient's global assessment, patient's assessment of pain and fatigue, physician's global assessment), erythrocyte sedimentation rate, salivary flow rate, Schirmer's test, tender joint count, fatigue score, and dry eyes and dry mouth indices. However, a subsequent multi-center, randomized, double-blind, placebo-controlled study of 103 patients with primary Sjögren's syndrome did not demonstrate any efficacy for infliximab over 22 weeks (11).

Treatment of Lymphoma

Treatment of lymphoma depends on histologic type, location, and extent of disease (12,13). Low-grade lymphomas may remain localized for many years or may even undergo spontaneous remission without therapy. On the other hand, patients with high and intermediate grades have the worst prognoses. The management of lymphoma and decisions regarding chemotherapy and/or radiation therapy should be dictated by experienced oncologists.

REFERENCES

1. **Manoussakis MN, Moutsopoulos HM.** Sjögren's syndrome: current concepts. Adv Intern Med. 2001;47:191-217.
2. **Vitali C, Bombardieri S, Jonsson R, et al.** Classification criteria for Sjögren's syndrome: a revised version of the European criteria proposed by the American-European Consensus Group. Ann Rheum Dis. 2002;61:554-8.

3. **Vivino FB, Al-Hashimi I, Khan Z, et al.** Pilocarpine tablets for the treatment of dry mouth and dry eye symptoms in patients with Sjögren syndrome: a randomized placebo-controlled, fixed dose, multicenter trial. P92-01 Study Group. Arch Intern Med. 1999;159:174-81.

4. **Tsifetaki N, Kitsos G, Paschides CA, et al.** Oral pilocarpine for the treatment of ocular symptoms in patients with Sjögren's syndrome: a randomized 12 week controlled study. Ann Rheum Dis. 2003;62:1204-7.

5. **Sall K, Stevenson OD, Mandorf TK, Reis BL.** Two multicenter, randomized studies of the efficacy and safety of cyclosporine ophthalmic emulsion in moderate-to-severe dry eye disease. CsA Phase 3 Study Group. Ophthalmology. 2000;107:631-9.

6. **Fox RI, Konttinen Y, Fisher A.** Use of muscarinic agonists in the treatment of Sjögren's syndrome. Clin Immunol. 2001;101:249-63.

7. **Fife RS, Chase WF, Dore RK, et al.** Cevimeline for the treatment of xerostomia in patients with Sjögren's syndrome. Arch Intern Med. 2002;162:1293-1300.

8. **Tishler M, Yaran I Shirazi I, Yaron M.** Hydroxychloroquine treatment for primary Sjögren's syndrome: its effect on salivary and serum inflammatory markers. Ann Rheum Dis. 1999;58:253-6.

9. **Skopouli FN, Dafni U, Ioannidis JP, Moutsopoulos HM.** Clinical evolution, and morbidity and mortality of primary Sjögren's syndrome. Semin Arthritis Rheum. 2000;29:296-304.

10. **Steinfeld SD, Demols P, Salmon I, et al.** Infliximab in patients with primary Sjögren's syndrome: a pilot study. Arthritis Rheum. 2001;44:2371-5.

11. **Mariette X, Ravaud P, Steinfeld S, et al.** Inefficacy of infliximab in primary Sjögren's syndrome: results of the randomized, controlled Trial of Remicade in Primary Sjögren's Syndrome (TRIPSS). Arthritis Rheum. 2004;50:1270-6.

12. **Voulgarelis M, Moutsopoulos HM.** Malignant lymphoma in primary Sjögren's syndrome. Isr Med Assoc J. 2001;3:761-6.

13. **Moutsopoulos NM, Moutsopoulos HM.** Therapy of Sjögren's syndrome. Springer Semin Immunopathol. 2001;23:131-45.

9

Inflammatory Myopathies

Yusuf Yazici, MD

Lawrence J. Kagen, MD

The three major inflammatory myopathies seen in adults are dermatomyositis, polymyositis, and inclusion body myositis (1). Although the three conditions have in common the subacute or insidious onset of symmetrical weakness resulting from an inflammatory infiltration of the musculature, they differ in very specific clinical and pathological features (Table 9-1).

Pathogenesis

Dermatomyositis is characterized by prominent proximal muscle weakness associated with a dermatitis that can involve the face, the trunk, and the extremities. Histologically, dermatomyositis is characterized by inflammation in the muscle and skin. Muscle biopsy demonstrates an inflammatory infiltrate composed largely of B cells and CD4 lymphocytes, emanating from vessels and extending into the myofibers. Myofiber necrosis and regeneration are seen, and in chronic cases, replacement of portions of the fascicle with collagen and adipose tissue occurs. Macrophages are found at areas of myofiber necrosis, and polymorphonuclear leukocytes are also occasionally present. The vascular nature of this disorder is evidenced by the reduction in the numbers of capillaries and microvessels and by the presence of perifascicular atrophy. Immunoglobulins, complement components, and the membrane attack complex may line the capillary walls. Tumor necrosis factor (TNF-α) and monocyte-attractant proteins are produced locally and serve to attract leukocytes to the site. In the skin, CD4 lymphocytes and macrophages are found in close proximity to small vessels in the dermis, and immunoglobulins and complement components are found at the dermal-epidermal junction and in dermal microvessels.

Table 9-1   Characteristics of Inflammatory Myopathies

Disease	Gender	Age of Onset	Rash	Pattern of Weakness	Serum CPK	Histo-pathology	Response to Pharmacological Therapy?
DM	F > M	Childhood, adult	Yes	Proximal > distal	Increased	Perimysial perivascular inflammation	Yes
PM	F > M	Adult	No	Proximal > distal	Increased	Endomysial inflammation	Yes
IBM	M > F	Elderly	No	Proximal = distal	Normal or mildly increased	Endomysial inflammation, rimmed vacuoles, amyloid deposits	No

Abbreviations: CPK, creatine phosphokinase; DM, dermatomyositis; PM, polymyositis; IBM, inclusion body myositis; F, female; M, male.
Modified with permission from Amato AA, Barohn RJ. Idiopathic inflammatory myopathies. Neurol Clin. 1997;14:615-48.

Polymyositis also primarily affects the proximal musculature of both upper and lower extremities, but there is no rash. Histologically, there is endomysial infiltration by cytotoxic CD8 lymphocytes that send out processes containing the tissue-damaging enzymes perforin and granzyme directed toward the myofiber. Studies of the T cell receptor in these lymphocytes have demonstrated a reduced repertoire compared with that present in the circulation, suggesting a local expansion of certain clones of T cells, possibly as the result of antigenic stimulation.

Inclusion body myositis is so called because of intranuclear and intracytoplasmic tubulofilamentous inclusions seen on muscle biopsy. The inclusions have been found to contain beta amyloid, ubiquitin, and phosphorylated tau protein, but their pathogenetic roles remain unclear. Histologically, the inflammatory infiltrate resembles that of polymyositis with the presence of cytotoxic CD8 lymphocytes invading the endomysium. Clinically, inclusion body myositis involves not only the proximal musculature but also has a predilection for the finger and wrist flexors.

Case Presentation

A 64-year-old woman without significant medical history presented with an erythematous pruritic rash over the back of her hands and on her forehead. Over the course of a month, she began to feel generally fatigued and experienced mild proximal muscle aches. Physical examination at this time revealed a raised erythematous rash on the dorsum of her hands and on her forehead, but her general examination seemed otherwise normal. Routine laboratory studies, however, showed a mildly elevated erythrocyte sedimentation rate (ESR) of 42 mm/hr and elevated serum levels of alanine aminotransferase (ALT; 62 U/L) and aspartate aminotransferase (AST; 81 U/L). Serum tests for alkaline phosphatase, α-glutamyltranspeptidase, and bilirubin were in the normal range. Topical corticosteroids were prescribed for the rash but did not offer sustained benefit.

Over the next several weeks, her fatigue worsened, and, moreover, she found it increasingly difficult to comb her hair and rise from a chair because of weakness. The rash spread to other areas and now was present over the forehead, around the eyes, at the upper outer surfaces of the arms and thighs, in the V-area of the neck and chest, over the upper, posterior thorax, over the dorsum of the hands, and at the knees. Over flat surfaces, the rash was macular in nature. Over bony prominences at the knuckles and knees, the rash appeared heaped up, papular, and slightly scaly. There was also marked periungual erythema. Proximal muscle strength was reduced. She could walk normally without the use of aids but had difficulty in raising her arms over her head and in crossing her legs. She could not stand up from a sitting position in a regulation chair without the use of her hands, and she was unable to perform a deep knee bend or rise from a crouch without the use of her hands. She also could not raise her head up from the supine position. Facial and distal musculature was normal in strength. The rest of the physical examination was normal.

Serum creatine phosphokinase (CPK) was markedly elevated at 8,600 U/L, and an antinuclear antibody test was positive at 1:80. A muscle biopsy of the left quadriceps femoris demonstrated an inflammatory infiltrate within the muscle, with myofiber necrosis and regeneration. Computed tomography of the chest, abdomen, and pelvis was also obtained. A mass in the left ovary was found that was eventually diagnosed as an adenocarcinoma.

Clinical Features

Dermatomyositis

Dermatomyositis affects females more frequently and can occur at any age. The dermatological manifestations frequently precede the appearance of muscular disease, occasionally up to several years. Patients in this category who have not as yet developed or who do not have recognizable muscle involvement are referred to as having amyopathic dermatomyositis. Nonetheless, in many of these cases, subclinical muscle involvement manifested by borderline abnormalities in serum enzymes or electromyography findings may be present.

There are various characteristic rashes associated with dermatomyositis. On the chest, a macular erythema in a "V" distribution anteriorly and in a shawl-like distribution posteriorly may be seen and may extend over the shoulders (Figures 9-1 and 9-2). The scalp may also be involved, as may be the back of the neck below the hairline. Periorbital heliotrope or purple

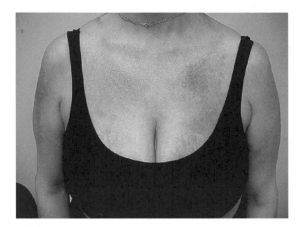

Figure 9-1   V sign and anterior chest rash. Rash of dermatomyositis over the anterior thorax and upper outer arms.

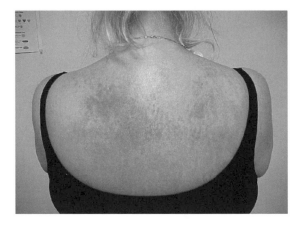

Figure 9-2   Shawl sign. Rash of dermatomyositis over the posterior thorax.

discoloration with edema may be present, along with erythema and telangectasia at the borders of the upper eyelids. Over bony prominences, particularly at the knuckles of the hands, Gottron's papules assume a papular heaped up psoriasis-like appearance (Figure 9-3). In addition to these features, severe erythema of the palms, scaling scalp plaques, hyperkeratosis of the fingers ("mechanic's hands") are also commonly encountered. Less frequently, papular or even vesicular rashes over flat skin surfaces have been observed.

Muscle involvement initially presents as weakness and mild achiness. Pain is not normally severe or debilitating and is generally responsive to simple analgesics. Weakness progresses subacutely, while myalgias decline over weeks to months. Severe pain and tenderness are rare. Muscle atrophy

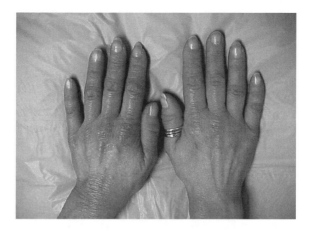

Figure 9-3 Gottron's papules. Rash of dermatomyositis on the bony prominences overlying the proximal interphalangeal and metacarpophalangeal joint areas.

is not present at the outset but may occur with repeated disease exacerbations and chronicity. Although many muscle groups may be affected, neck flexors and proximal musculature of the extremities are most prominently involved. Affected individuals have difficulty lifting their head when supine, raising their arms to comb their hair or feed themselves, and rising from seated or crouched positions. Generally, muscles supplied by the cranial nerves and distal musculature are spared. However, with severe involvement, even these areas may become affected. Falls are a major concern, not only because of resulting trauma but because patients may not be able to get up if alone or unaided.

The proximal third of the esophagus is composed of skeletal muscle and can be affected in dermatomyositis. Patients may complain of proximal dysphagia, and in severe involvement aspiration and malnutrition due to inadequate oral intake may occur.

In addition, pulmonary alveolitis and interstitial pulmonary fibrosis may occur (2). In certain patients, these may precede the appearance of muscular manifestations. Interstitial lung disease secondary to fibrosing alveolitis is seen in both dermatomyositis and polymyositis and is associated with esophageal involvement and with the presence of circulating antibodies to aminoacyl transfer RNA synthetases. In some patients, chest radiographs or pulmonary function testing can indicate the presence of interstitial lung disease even in the absence of clinically apparent signs or symptoms. In others, exertional dyspnea is an indolently progressive problem. Finally, some patients can present acutely with aggressive diffuse lung disease, with fever, nonproductive cough, and rapidly progressive respiratory compromise.

Calcinoses also can be a major problem (3). These may occur as eruptions on the surface of the skin from subcutaneous deposits, and there may be calcific investment of perimyseal tissues leading to woody thickening of the extremities with concurrent loss of mobility. Infections, usually with *Staphylococcus aureus,* may complicate calcific surface eruptions.

An underlying malignancy is seen in approximately one quarter of adult patients with dermatomyositis (4). Diagnosis of the cancer may precede or follow the diagnosis of dermatomyositis. Although there has been no statistically validated prospective verification of this frequency, several recent retrospective studies from Scandinavia, Australia, and Scotland have emphasized the risk of occult neoplasia. Many types of malignancies have been reported, including carcinomas, sarcomas, and lymphomas. In general, the most frequently observed tumors are those that are most commonly seen in the general population, although several studies have suggested an apparent increased risk of ovarian tumors. Older age at onset and male gender may be independent predictive factors for malignancy in myositis patients. Most published guidelines recommend that patients with dermatomyositis have an age-appropriate examination for occult malignancy with further evaluation of any suggestive signs or symptoms. However, many rheumatologists routinely perform imaging studies of the chest, abdomen, and pelvis in all dermatomyositis patients over 50 to screen for occult malignancies, as seen in the case study presented. Complicating or associated features such as calcinosis, pulmonary disease, and malignancies also occur in amyopathic dermatomyositis.

Polymyositis

Upper and lower extremity proximal muscle weakness also characterizes polymyositis, but there are no characteristic dermatological lesions associated with this disorder. It is more prevalent in females, and the age of onset is usually in adulthood. As in dermatomyositis, proximal esophageal dysfunction and interstitial pulmonary disease may also occur. An increased risk of associated malignancy exists for polymyositis but is much less than for dermatomyositis. The malignancies seen in polymyositis reflect those found in an age-matched population, except for a possible preponderance of ovarian cancer.

Inclusion Body Myositis

Inclusion body myositis most commonly affects elderly men. Proximal muscle weakness is present but, unlike dermatomyositis and polymyositis, also has a predilection for distal musculature, particularly the wrist and finger flexors. The disease onset is frequently insidious, and a considerable delay of months to years may elapse before recognition of the disease occurs. In many patients, weakness is initially ascribed to the effects of age, thereby delaying diagnosis and leading to irreparable myofiber loss, significant atrophy, and disability. Noteworthy is the fact that inclusion body myositis is poorly responsive to pharmacological therapies.

Diagnosis

Laboratory Testing

Myonecrosis results in the leakage of intracellular proteins and enzymes from muscle into the circulation. The most commonly measured components are myoglobin, CPK, aldolase, lactate dehydrogenase, aspartate aminotransferase, and alanine aminotransferase. These tests are not only diagnostically useful but also are a guide to the course of the disease and its response to therapy. Serum CPK is the most widely used in this regard because of its abundance in muscle. Although many autoantibodies have been found to be associated with inflammatory myositis, at this juncture they are largely of academic interest. They are generally not helpful in the management of individual patients and should not be routinely assessed. Markers of systemic inflammation such as ESR or C-reactive protein may be normal or moderately elevated but are generally not as useful for monitoring disease activity as the clinical examination or muscle enzyme tests.

Imaging Techniques

Magnetic resonance imaging (MRI) and ultrasonography (US) have become increasingly useful in the diagnosis of inflammatory myopathies. Edema seen on T2-weighted MRI sequences can demonstrate edema, a marker of active inflammation. Chronic muscle atrophy can also be visualized. In addition to its usefulness in diagnosis, MRI may be utilized in the choice of an actively inflamed muscle for biopsy.

US offers the advantages of decreased expense and greater availability. It also allows for the assessment of both upper and lower extremities at the same examination, a feature less possible with MRI. Closely spaced reflections of sound from connective tissue indicate atrophy. The power Doppler technique can reveal hyperemia, an indicator of active inflammation, and thus can also be used in the selection of muscle for biopsy.

MRI and US can both be used to assess changes in muscle and the response of muscle to therapy. However, the usefulness of both techniques is limited by the experience of the radiologist.

Electromyography

This technique provides another powerful tool for the assessment of myopathy. Myopathic changes are characterized by small, short, low amplitude potentials with irritative phenomena. Because electromyography itself may induce local areas of inflammation, muscles on only one side of the body are generally examined, leaving the contralateral side available for biopsy.

Muscle Biopsy

Muscle biopsy is the most direct and accurate means of diagnosing inflammatory myopathies. It can reveal the presence of inflammatory infiltration and myofiber necrosis, atrophy, and regeneration. In chronic cases, loss of portions of the fascicle with replacement by collagenous connective tissue and fat may be seen as well. Evidence of vasculitis, a hallmark of dermatomyositis, can also be apparent.

Biopsy may be performed by an open procedure or with a fine needle, but neither method is infallible. Multiple specimens should be taken since inflammation may be "spotty" in its localization and affected tissue may be missed with limited samples. For this reason, a negative biopsy does not exclude the diagnosis of inflammatory myopathy. In order to further improve the diagnostic yield of muscle biopsy, the clinician should carefully select a muscle that is clinically involved for sampling. Common sites include the deltoid, the biceps humeri, or a member of the quadriceps femoris group. The hamstrings musculature of the lower extremity is often spared and therefore is not generally sampled. Imaging by MRI or ultrasound or electromyography findings may also be employed in selecting the optimal muscle for biopsy.

Differential Diagnosis

Inflammatory myositis can be seen as part of other collagen vascular diseases such as systemic lupus erythematosus, scleroderma, and mixed connective tissue disease. In these conditions, however, the histological features of myositis are not as striking as those seen with polymyositis or dermatomyositis. Muscle involvement of sarcoidosis can also manifest as weakness and is typically characterized by granulomatous inflammation of muscle. In addition, Table 9-2 lists some other conditions that should be considered in the evaluation of the patient with diffuse muscle weakness.

Prognosis

The inflammatory myopathies are chronic disorders with clinical courses that have exacerbations and remissions. It is important for both the clinician and patient to realize that the course of illness may be prolonged and that it may be necessary to periodically adjust the amount and type of medication to meet the clinical needs. All of this may produce a sense of psychological strain, which can be met with patience and understanding.

Prompt recognition and treatment of myositis is essential to save myofibers and thereby maximize preservation of muscle strength. Delays in diagnosis increase the likelihood of permanent loss of strength. Severe muscle disease, cardiopulmonary complications, and the presence of an underlying malignancy are all poor prognostic features. In addition,

Table 9-2   Conditions Associated with Diffuse Muscle Weakness

Drugs and Toxins
- Corticosteroids
- Lipid-lowering agents (particularly "statins")
- Zidovudine (AZT)
- Penicillamine
- Colchicine
- Propylthiouracil
- Azathioprine
- Ethanol
- Cocaine

Endocrine Disorders
- Acromegaly
- Hypothyroidism
- Hyperthyroidism
- Addison's disease
- Cushing's disease

Electrolyte Disturbances
- Hypokalemia
- Hypocalcemia

Electrolyte Disturbances *(cont'd)*
- Hypercalcemia
- Uremia

Neurological Disorders
- Myasthenia gravis
- Eaton-Lambert syndrome
- Amyotrophic lateral sclerosis
- Guillain-Barré syndrome

Infections
- Trichinosis
- Human immunodeficiency virus
- Lyme disease

Genetic Diseases
- Muscular dystrophies
- Glycogen storage diseases
- Lipid storage diseases
- Mitochondrial myopathies

dermatomyositis patients with open ulcerated lesions on the torso appear to have poorer outcomes.

Management

The involvement of a rheumatologist is essential once a diagnosis of inflammatory myositis is made. The major aim of treatment is to reduce or halt the inflammatory process that, if left unrestrained, would lead to irreparable tissue destruction. Early intervention has been shown to improve overall outcome and preserve strength. At present, systemic corticosteroid agents, administered either orally or parenterally, are the mainstay of the therapy. Moderate-to-high doses of prednisone (30-60 mg daily) or their equivalent are typical starting oral dosages. In severe cases, intravenous boluses of methylprednisolone (500-1000 mg daily) for a brief period have also been employed initially to more rapidly bring about control of the inflammation. Careful clinical and CPK monitoring of the response to therapy is essential as corticosteroids are tapered over the course of several months. Formal muscle strength assessments using torque analysis are available at some academic centers to provide objective measures of response to therapy.

Although there are many adverse effects of corticosteroid therapy (discussed in Chapter 30), steroid myopathy is a particularly relevant issue in the context of myositis because the two conditions both cause proximal muscle weakness and may coexist. Resultant disuse and atrophy can further complicate the clinical picture. The overall recent clinical picture and pattern of strength are important in distinguishing between inflammatory myositis and steroid myopathy. Evidence of active extramuscular involvement such as skin or lung disease and rising serum levels of muscle enzymes indicate active myositis and call for more potent therapy. In contrast, progressive weakness with no concomitant change in muscle enzymes in the setting of a stable steroid dosage suggests steroid toxicity warranting reduction of dosage. At times, empiric increase or lowering of corticosteroid dosing can be diagnostic.

Because there is, as yet, no predictable or certain cure for the inflammatory myopathies, corticosteroid therapy of sufficient potency will be needed as long as required to halt disease progression. Return of strength and improvement of laboratory abnormalities towards normal usually accompany successful therapy, but complete normalization of muscle enzyme tests is not absolutely necessary before attempts at corticosteroid tapers can be made. Individual circumstances including comorbidities, response to treatment, and adverse effects of therapies all affect the decision on when medication dosages should be modified.

Intravenous gamma globulin (IVGG) therapy has become an important therapeutic adjunct to corticosteroids and may minimize the risk for steroid-related toxicities. IVGG (total 2 gm/kg body weight given in divided daily doses over 2 to 5 days) has proven effective in bringing about remissions in case-controlled studies of dermatomyositis and inclusion body myositis (5,6). The mechanism of action of IVGG remains unknown, although one effect in dermatomyositis may be the inhibition of the complement pathway. IVGG therapy is generally safe, but infusion reactions occur rarely and include fever, flushing, and hypotension. Patients with selective IgA deficiency who possess anti-IgA antibodies are not suitable candidates for IVGG.

Other immunosuppressive or cytotoxic drugs have also been shown to be of value in certain patients. General indications for the use of these agents are inadequate response to corticosteroids, the development of steroid-induced complications, recurrent relapses, severe pulmonary involvement, and rapidly progressive disease. Azathioprine, methotrexate, cyclophosphamide, and cyclosporin have been most widely utilized thus far, but large controlled studies are lacking. Newer agents including mycophenolate mofetil, leflunomide, and the B cell–directed antibody rituximab have also been used in small groups of patients.

Because of the demonstration of TNF-α at sites of muscle inflammation, there is recent interest for the use of the anti-TNF-α agents, etanercept, adalimumab, and infliximab, in the treatment of myositis. Individual case studies and small case series have shown exciting promise (7), but, thus far, data documenting overall efficacy and advantages over currently available agents are lacking.

Treatment of Cutaneous Manifestations and Calcinosis

The rash of dermatomyositis may respond to systemic therapy in parallel to the myopathy but can often run a separate and recalcitrant course. The rash typically appears before muscle weakness is appreciated and is often the last manifestation to resolve. In general, topical corticosteroids are marginally beneficial but, because of low toxicity, are worth trying. In addition to therapies used for the muscle disease, hydroxychloroquine 200 mg once or twice daily can be helpful (8). Mycophenolate mofetil has been reported to be effective in a small series of patients (9). Calcinosis is notoriously difficult to treat. Although many agents including colchicine, diltiazem, warfarin, and corticosteroids have been reported to be effective in some patients, no one agent has shown consistent benefit. Surgical excision of subcutaneous calcifications is sometimes necessary, particularly when function is threatened.

Treatment of Interstitial Lung Disease

Like the muscle disease, interstitial lung disease in the inflammatory myopathies may sometimes respond to corticosteroid therapy alone, but often require the addition of immunomodulatory medications like intravenous gammaglobulin, azathioprine, methotrexate, cyclophosphamide, or cyclosporin. No adequate clinical trials are available to render a standard or definitive approach. However, it is accepted that prompt intervention must be implemented to prevent irreversible pulmonary fibrosis (10).

Physical Therapy

The goals of physical therapy are to maintain joint mobility and to preserve and/or recover strength. During acute exacerbations of myositis, passive range of motion exercises can be instituted to prevent joint contractures without risk of incurring further injury to muscle. In general, 2 to 3 weeks after stabilization of disease, strength training can be safely initiated to prevent muscle atrophy due to disuse (11).

REFERENCES

1. **Amato AA, Barohn RJ.** Idiopathic inflammatory myopathies. Neurol Clin. 1997;15: 615-48.
2. **Hirakata M, Nagai S.** Interstitial lung disease in polymyositis and dermatomyositis. Curr Opin Rheumatol. 2000;12:501-8.
3. **Fusade T, Belanyi P, Joly P, et al.** Subcutaneous changes in dermatomyositis. Br J Dermatol. 1993;128:451-3.
4. **Yazici Y, Kagen IJ.** The association of malignancy with myositis. Curr Opin Rheumatol. 2000;12:498-500.
5. **Dalakas MC.** The molecular and cellular pathology of inflammatory muscle diseases. Curr Opin Pharmacol. 2001;1:300-6.

6. **Cherin P, Pelletier S, Teixeira A, et al.** Results and long-term followup of intravenous immunoglobulin infusions in chronic, refractory polymyositis. Arthritis Rheum. 2002;46:467-74.

7. **Hengstman GJ, van den Hoogen FH, Barrera P, et al.** Successful treatment of dermatomyositis and polymyositis with anti-tumor necrosis factor-alpha: preliminary observations. Eur Neurol. 2003;50:10-15.

8. **Wallace DJ.** The use of chloroquine and hydroxychloroquine for non-infectious conditions other than rheumatoid arthritis or lupus: a critical review. Lupus. 1996;5(Suppl 1):S59-64.

9. **Gelber AC, Nousari HC, Wigley FM.** Mycophenolate mofetil in the treatment of severe skin manifestations of dermatomyositis: a series of 4 cases. J Rheumatol. 2000;27:1542-5.

10. **Schnabel A, Reuter M, Biederer J, et al.** Interstitial lung disease in polymyositis and dermatomyositis: clinical course and response to treatment. Semin Arthritis Rheum. 2003;32:273-84.

11. **Varju C, Petho E, Kutas R, Czirjak L.** The effect of physical exercise following acute disease exacerbation in patients with dermato/polymyositis. Clin Rehabil. 2003; 7:83-7.

10

■ ■ ■

Systemic Sclerosis and Related Conditions

Sergio Schwartzman, MD

Petros Efthimiou, MD

Systemic sclerosis (SSc), also known as scleroderma, is a multisystem connective tissue disorder characterized by abnormal fibrosis and resultant dysfunction of skin, vasculature, and internal organs. Strictly speaking, two forms of SSc are recognized: diffuse scleroderma and limited scleroderma. In the diffuse form, cutaneous disease is diffuse, involving the face, neck, trunk, and both proximal and distal parts of the limbs and can be associated with severe and rapid visceral disease, notably in the lungs and kidneys. In contrast, limited scleroderma, otherwise known as the acronym CREST syndrome (calcinosis, Raynaud's phenomenon, esophageal dysmotility, sclerodactyly, telangiectasias), is characterized by thickening of the skin on the face and neck and the distal parts of the limbs only. However, significant diversity in presentation and overlap in symptoms with other rheumatological disorders can exist from patient to patient.

SSc is an uncommon illness with a yearly incidence between 3.7 and 19.1 per million and a prevalence of 30.8 to 286 patients per million. There is a clear female predominance. SSc can affect any racial group, but epidemiological studies have suggested that SSc is more common and more severe in African Americans. Disease onset most commonly occurs between 20 and 50 years of age, but SSc can occur in childhood and in the elderly.

Pathogenesis

Although various drugs and toxins have been associated with the development of scleroderma, no such exposure is identified in the majority of patients. However, in all cases, abnormal and exuberant fibrosis is the common pathway, resulting in end-organ structural damage and dysfunction. T-cells and monocytes play a critical early role in the disease process and, through the effects of various pro-fibrotic cytokines (notably interleukin-4 and transforming growth factor-β), recruit the involvement of endothelial cells and fibroblasts. Ultimately, dysregulation of genes that control collagen synthesis is induced, resulting in the overproduction of collagen.

Pathological specimens from patients with early SSc reveal increased lymphocyte and mast cell infiltration and some collagen deposition. With disease progression, continued deposition of extracellular matrix and collagen can be seen, and this eventually leads to development of tissue fibrosis. In the skin, thinning of the epidermis ensues with the loss of all skin appendages. In the vasculature, activated smooth muscle cells proliferate within the wall of affected arteries, obliterating the lumen. The resultant endothelial changes also promote platelet activation and thrombosis. Involvement of the adventitia can lead to fibrotic encasement of the vessel. Cumulatively, the multiple insults to the blood vessels contribute significantly to the vasculopathy and ischemia characteristic of severe Raynaud's phenomenon and visceral disease in SSc.

Case Presentation 1

A 28-year-old Asian female presented with a history of Raynaud's phenomenon for 8 years, mild diffuse hand swelling for the past 7 months, and the recent onset of diffuse erythema over the anterior chest and face. The patient had also noted recent mild dyspnea on exertion.

On physical examination, vital signs were normal. The patient was found to have mild skin tightening bilaterally over the hands, forearms, chest, and face. The size of her oral aperture was diminished, and there was an erythematous macular rash on her face and anterior chest wall. Chest auscultation revealed dry crackles at the left lung base. The metacarpophalangeal and proximal interphalangeal joints of the hands were diffusely swollen. Her hands were cool to touch, and there was mild cyanosis of the distal tufts of the fingers, but no digital ulcers were present.

Routine laboratory testing, including complete blood count, biochemical profile, and urinalysis, was remarkable only for a mild anemia. Further laboratory testing revealed a slightly positive anti-nuclear antibody and an erythrocyte sedimentation rate of 48 mm/h. Anti-Scl-70 (anti-topoisomerase) antibodies were later found to be present.

A plain chest radiograph was normal. However, computed tomography of the chest revealed mild interstitial changes with a ground glass appearance in the periphery of both lung fields. Pulmonary function tests demonstrated a mild restrictive ventilatory defect with a slightly reduced diffusing capacity. Echocardiography was normal.

The patient subsequently underwent bronchoscopy with broncho-alveolar lavage, which yielded an increased number of neutrophils and lymphocytes. Diffuse systemic sclerosis with inflammatory interstitial lung disease was diagnosed based on the distribution of the scleroderma and alveolitis. She was treated with high doses of systemic cortico-steroids and oral cyclophosphamide. During the next year, her pul-monary symptoms and function tests improved, and corticosteroids and cyclophosphamide were subsequently tapered successfully. The skin changes remained unaltered. She continues to be followed closely for exacerbation of pulmonary disease and new involvement of other organ systems.

Case Presentation 2

A 33-year-old African-American female was evaluated for several years of progressive hand pain and swelling. She reported Raynaud's phenomenon of her hands since age 17 that has been bothersome but was never severe enough to interfere with any of her activities. At age 25, she first developed joint pain in her hands and feet that was distinct from her Raynaud's phe-nomenon. Ibuprofen as needed offered moderate relief.

During the past year she has gradually noted puffiness in the skin of her hands and difficulty opening her mouth fully. She also reported increasing episodes of heartburn and mild difficulty swallowing. She denied any cardiopulmonary symptoms. Other than mild tightening of the skin on the dorsum of her hands and some difficulty in fully opening her mouth, her general physical examination was normal. However, two digits on her right hand became reversibly cyanotic when immersed in cold tap water. Otherwise, there was no evidence of cutaneous calcinosis or telangiectasias on her skin or mucosal surfaces.

Laboratory analysis revealed a mild normocytic anemia and a slightly ele-vated sedimentation rate. Serum anti-nuclear and anti-centromere antibod-ies were present. Videoesophagography demonstrated moderate esophageal dysmotility and reflux. Chest x-ray, pulmonary function testing, electrocar-diography, and echocardiography were all normal.

The diagnosis of limited scleroderma (CREST) was made and fully dis-cussed with the patient. She was started on an occupational therapy pro-gram. Sustained-release nifedipine and a baby aspirin were prescribed for treatment of digital ischemia due to Raynaud's phenomenon. A selective cyclooxygenase-2 inhibitor was offered for joint pains as needed. Finally, dietary modifications and a proton-pump inhibitor were recommended to reduce her gastrointestinal symptoms.

For the next 3 years, her disease remained stable, except for some mild progression of skin tightening over the dorsum of her hands. Her joint pains, Raynaud's phenomenon, and gastrointestinal complaints have been well controlled.

Clinical Features

Although diffuse and limited forms of systemic sclerosis are defined by the extent of cutaneous involvement, they also have other generally distinguishing features (Table 10-1). Diffuse scleroderma is more commonly associated with a rapidly progressive course, early and severe visceral disease (notably

Table 10-1   Scleroderma Spectrum of Disorders

Syndrome	Clinical Characteristics	Serological Findings*
Diffuse scleroderma	• Rapidly progressive facial, truncal and peripheral (proximal and distal) skin sclerosis • Onset of skin changes often within 1 year of onset of Raynaud's phenomenon • Scleroderma renal crisis • Inflammatory interstitial lung disease • 40%-60% 10-year survival	• Anti-nuclear antibody (90%) • Anti-Scl-70 antibody (40%) • Anti-centromere antibody (5%)
Limited scleroderma/ CREST	• Skin sclerosis limited to the face, neck, and distal parts of the limbs • Onset of skin changes often occurring after longstanding Raynaud's phenomenon • CREST syndrome (subcutaneous calcinosis, Raynaud's phenomenon, esophageal dysmotility, sclerodactyly, telangiectasias) • Pulmonary hypertension • >75% 10-year survival	• Anti-nuclear antibody (90%) • Anti-Scl-70 antibody (10-15%) • Anti-centromere antibody (70-90%)
Mixed connective tissue disease	• Overlap syndrome combining features of scleroderma, systemic lupus erythematosus, rheumatoid arthritis, and/or inflammatory myopathy (typically, Raynaud's phenomenon, acrosclerosis, hand edema, synovitis, and myositis) • Fibrosing alveolitis	• Anti-nuclear antibody (100%) • Anti-U1 ribonucleoprotein antibody (100%) • Rheumatoid factor (70%)
Overlap syndromes	Limited or diffuse skin sclerosis with characteristic features of at least one other autoimmune disease.	Variable

* Frequencies of positive tests are in parentheses.

renal crisis and inflammatory lung disease), the presence of anti-Scl-70 (anti-topoisomerase) antibodies, and overall worse prognosis. In contrast, limited scleroderma is characterized by the classic features of CREST syndrome: calcinosis, Raynaud's phenomenon, esophageal dysmotility, sclerodactyly, and mucocutaneous telangiectasias. Visceral disease in limited scleroderma tends to evolve slowly and to be characterized by progressive fibrosis rather than prominent inflammatory features; pulmonary hypertension and gastrointestinal motility problems are typical. However, it should be emphasized that significant variability exists, and individual patients should not be pigeon-holed diagnostically. Moreover, many patients will also simultaneously exhibit features of other defined autoimmune diseases and are commonly denoted as patients with "undifferentiated" or "overlap" syndromes. One better-defined overlap syndrome is mixed connective tissue disease, which is associated with features of scleroderma, systemic lupus erythematosus, rheumatoid arthritis, and/or inflammatory myositis, and with antibodies against U1 ribonucleoprotein.

Raynaud's Phenomenon

Raynaud's phenomenon, a hallmark feature of scleroderma, is characterized by abnormally exaggerated vasospasm of arteries, typically in response to cold or stress. It most commonly involves acral areas of the body (e.g., digits, ears, and tip of the nose), but the vasculature of internal organs can also be affected. Although classically characterized by a triphasic color change (pallor, cyanosis, and erythema) in the hands and feet, this progression is not absolutely necessary for diagnosis. It is present at some point in almost all patients with CREST syndrome and in most patients with diffuse scleroderma. With long-standing and severe ischemia, loss of tissue at the distal tufts of the digits can occur (Figure 10-1). Raynaud's phenomenon frequently precedes the overt manifestations of the fibrotic illness by many

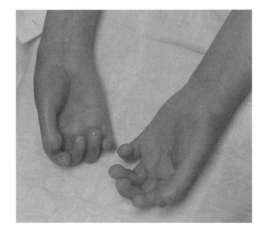

Figure 10-1 Severe sclerosis of the hands of this patient with diffuse scleroderma has caused permanent contractures of the fingers. Significant loss of tissue at the tufts of the digits due to persistent ischemia from chronic Raynaud's phenomenon is also evident.

years. Although Raynaud's phenomenon is common in the general population, initial evaluation of a patient of Raynaud's phenomenon should include the assessment of an underlying secondary cause. In early scleroderma, friction rubs can be palpated along tendons as the underlying joint is moved and indicates fibrotic changes. In addition, capillary loops at the nailfolds may reveal misshapen vessels also suggestive of early scleroderma. A more complete discussion of Raynaud's phenomenon is presented in Chapter 28.

Cutaneous Findings

Skin thickening seems to evolve through several phases. Initially, there is generalized puffiness of the involved skin. Over a period of months to years, the skin becomes taut and may ulcerate. Occasionally, when skin changes are minimal or progress slowly, the diagnosis may be delayed or confused. In some patients, after several years of progressive skin changes, the fibrotic phase ceases, and the skin may actually soften slightly. Unfortunately, this does not occur in all patients. The distribution of skin involvement is important in the classification of scleroderma. Patients with diffuse scleroderma have sclerodermatous changes in the head, neck, trunk, and the proximal and distal parts of the extremities; limited scleroderma/CREST syndrome is characterized by involvement of only the skin of the face and neck and in the extremities distal to the elbows and knees.

Two other skin findings are typical of CREST syndrome: subcutaneous calcinosis, which manifests as firm subcutaneous nodules or swelling that can frequently ulcerate, and telangiectasias, which commonly occur on the face, neck, and chest wall. Telangiectasias can also be seen on the mucosal surfaces throughout the gastrointestinal tract.

Gastrointestinal Involvement

Involvement of the gastrointestinal tract is extremely prevalent in systemic sclerosis, potentially affecting any segment. Both upper and lower tract symptoms are common in scleroderma and can frequently be attributed to impaired peristalsis due to enteric smooth muscle dysfunction. Esophageal involvement is the most common gastrointestinal manifestation, occurring in up to 80% of patients. Dysphagia, caused by involvement of the distal esophagus, can result in regurgitation and aspiration. Gastroesophageal reflux commonly causes esophagitis and gastritis and can also result in severe peptic ulcer disease. Decreased peristalsis can be manifested by delayed gastric emptying, hypomotility of the small intestine, and wide mouth diverticuli of the large bowel. Small intestine involvement may result in malabsorption and malnutrition. Large intestine disease may present as either severe diarrhea or constipation. Dysphagia or malnutrition can at times be severe enough to demand parenteral nutrition. Significant gastrointestinal bleeding may occur as the consequence of peptic ulcer disease or telangiectasias in the gastrointestinal tract.

Cardiopulmonary Manifestations

Cardiopulmonary involvement is a common cause of morbidity and death in patients with scleroderma. Chest pain, cough, dyspnea, and palpitations are frequent complaints. Raynaud's phenomenon of the coronary arteries can mimic atherosclerotic heart disease or Prinzmetal's angina. Myocardial fibrosis can result in cardiomyopathies or arrhythmias, the latter occurring in as many as 50% of patients (1,2). Involvement of the pericardium typically manifests as pericardial fibrosis, but pericardial effusions can occur and can sometimes be massive.

Although pulmonary involvement is very common, many patients are relatively asymptomatic. Patients with diffuse scleroderma may develop alveolitis and inflammatory interstitial lung disease, which can progress to pulmonary fibrosis and respiratory failure. In CREST, pulmonary hypertension due to slowly progressive fibrotic changes of the pulmonary vasculature without significant inflammatory changes is the most common pulmonary complication.

Scleroderma Renal Crisis

In this life-threatening complication of diffuse scleroderma, patients present with accelerated hypertension, renal insufficiency, and microangiopathic hemolysis. Although hypertension is characteristic, about a tenth of affected patients may actually be normotensive during scleroderma renal crisis, a finding that may delay diagnosis and treatment (3).

High plasma renin activity is characteristic, and urinary sediment usually reveals proteinuria and hematuria. If left untreated, progressive renal failure ensues, and mortality is high. Fortunately, while still a feared complication, the advent of angiotensin-converting enzyme (ACE) inhibitor therapy has vastly improved the prognosis of scleroderma renal crisis. Because of the risk of renal crisis, frequent monitoring of blood pressure and renal function is essential in all patients with diffuse scleroderma.

Musculoskeletal Findings

Myalgias and arthralgias, joint stiffness, and tendinitis with palpable friction rubs are common symptoms. Frank polyarticular arthritis can occur, particularly early in the course of illness; however, this manifestation is less common and is usually seen as part of overlap syndromes. Later in the disease, longstanding scleroderma around articulations result in chronic joint contractures (Figure 10-1).

Inflammatory myositis presenting as proximal muscle weakness and elevations in serum levels of muscle enzymes can also occur, frequently in the setting of undifferentiated or overlapping collagen vascular conditions. Subsequently, a chronic fibrotic non-inflammatory myopathy may ensue.

Diagnosis

Anemia and elevated erythrocyte sedimentation rates are common but non-specific findings that indicate a chronic inflammatory state. Serum creatinine levels and urinalyses should be performed regularly to assess for renal involvement. Muscle enzyme testing (e.g., creatine phosphokinase, aldolase, and others) should be performed in patients with evidence of muscle weakness.

Anti-nuclear antibodies are present in most patients with diffuse scleroderma, limited scleroderma (CREST), and mixed connective tissue disease. Anti-centromere antibodies occur frequently in limited scleroderma but are relatively unusual in diffuse scleroderma. Anti-Scl-70 (anti-topoisomerase) antibodies are more specific for diffuse scleroderma but are present in only 20% to 40% of patients. Anti-U1 ribonucleoprotein (RNP) antibodies are highly sensitive for mixed connective tissue disease.

Evaluation of cardiopulmonary disease may necessitate echocardiography, chest radiography, pulmonary function testing, or helical computed tomography. Pulmonary function testing and helical computed tomography are particularly helpful in identifying early pulmonary disease, in which interstitial inflammatory changes and a decreased diffusing capacity with low lung volumes are observed. Bronchoscopy with alveolar lavage is indicated for patients suspected of alveolitis in which bronchoalveolar lavage fluid analysis typically reveals increased cellularity (2 to 3 times normal), with increased numbers of activated macrophages, neutrophils, and frequently eosinophils (4).

Prognosis

The disease spectrum of systemic sclerosis ranges from relatively benign disease with limited and isolated skin thickening to severe forms with rapidly progressive and diffuse skin and visceral organ involvement. Negative prognostic factors at the time of diagnosis include diffuse skin involvement, increased skin thickness, the presence of visceral disease, elevated erythrocyte sedimentation rate, anemia, and the presence of anti-Scl-70 (anti-topoisomerase) antibodies. In most but not all studies, worse outcomes were associated with older patients.

Studies from the pre-1980 era reported overall 5-year survival rates of 34% to 73% after initial diagnosis of scleroderma. One study during this period reported 10-year survival rates of 71% and 21% for limited and diffuse SSc, respectively. However, prognosis has dramatically improved since then, notably with the advent of ACE-inhibitor therapy for the management of scleroderma renal crisis (5). A recent study reported current 10-year survival rates of 79% for CREST and 62.4% for diffuse SSc. At present, standardized mortality ratios for patients with CREST and diffuse SSc are, respectively, 2-fold and 6-fold higher than for sex- and age-matched healthy controls. (The standardized mortality ratio is the ratio between the observed rate of death in a study cohort and the expected rate of death in sex- and age-matched individuals.)

Management

Treatment of scleroderma is a major challenge to the clinician because the cause of the disease is unknown and the rarity of the disease hinders the ability to conduct large clinical trials. Moreover, great variability in clinical manifestations, severity, and disease courses, in combination with the potential for spontaneous improvement, renders outcomes data difficult to interpret. Coordinated care between the primary care physician and subspecialists (e.g., rheumatologist, nephrologist, pulmonologist, and cardiologist) is essential for optimal management.

Consistently effective treatment strategies targeting vascular abnormalities, immune dysfunction, and dysregulated collagen production are lacking. However, major advances in organ-based therapies have vastly decreased the morbidity and mortality of the disease. Examples include:

- ACE inhibitors for scleroderma renal crisis
- calcium channel blockers and other vasodilators for Raynaud's phenomenon
- proton pump inhibitors for reflux esophagitis
- parenteral prostaglandin analogues (e.g., epoprostenol and iloprost) and, more recently, oral endothelin receptor antagonists (bosentan) for pulmonary hypertension
- broad-spectrum antibiotics for small bowel bacterial overgrowth
- prokinetic agents for bowel hypomotility
- corticosteroids and immunosuppressive therapy (e.g., cyclophosphamide) for active alveolitis and other inflammatory complications

Systemic Immunomodulatory Therapies

Because there is evidence for inappropriate activation of cellular and humoral immunity in SSc, several immunomodulatory agents have been used empirically but with marginal benefit at best. Methotrexate (15-25 mg weekly) is regularly employed as a disease-modifying agent, but its use is controversial. A Dutch placebo-controlled study suggested benefit for both skin and pulmonary manifestations (6), but a larger North American study did not support this conclusion (7). Limited evidence also supports beneficial effects of cyclosporin A, tacrolimus, interferon-γ, and mycophenolate mofetil, but the roles of these agents remain to be defined. Systemic corticosteroids are generally reserved for inflammatory myositis, active alveolitis, serositis, and synovitis. Excessive corticosteroid use has been implicated in precipitating scleroderma renal crisis and should be prescribed cautiously.

Anti-Fibrotic Therapies

D-penicillamine can block cross-linking of collagen in vitro and has been used extensively in scleroderma. Multiple early studies, largely retrospective and poorly controlled, have suggested that the use of D-penicillamine in scleroderma can result in skin softening, reduced new organ involvement, lower risks of scleroderma renal crisis, and improved overall survival. However, a multicenter, double-blind, controlled study of 134 patients with early diffuse scleroderma followed for 2 years showed no statistical difference between patients treated with a standard dose of D-penicillamine (750-1000 mg/d) and those treated with 125 mg every other day, raising legitimate questions about its efficacy (8). An early uncontrolled study has suggested that oral colchicine 0.6 mg twice daily may have anti-fibrotic properties, but these findings have not been confirmed in rigorous trials. Also, despite initial enthusiasm, relaxin, a hormone known to reduce the synthesis of type I collagen by scleroderma fibroblasts, was shown to be ineffective in scleroderma in a recent large well-conducted study.

Musculoskeletal Complications

NSAIDs, selective inhibitors of COX-2, acetaminophen, and tramadol can be helpful in the treatment of musculoskeletal manifestations, with more refractory cases requiring opiate analgesics or low doses of corticosteroids (e.g., less than 10 mg/d of prednisone). Extreme care should be exercised when using NSAIDs and COX-2 inhibitors, however, because they may exacerbate renal insufficiency, raise the blood pressure, aggravate esophagitis, or cause gastrointestinal bleeding. Also, the use of opiates or tramadol may be cause for concern in patients with severe gastroparesis.

Carpal tunnel syndrome is often an early complication but generally responds to wrist splints, local corticosteroid injections, or surgical release if necessary. Physical and occupational therapy and paraffin baths are invaluable in reducing the development of soft tissue contractures and in maintaining function and should be instituted early in the course of the disease.

Scleroderma Renal Crisis

Prior to the introduction of ACE inhibitors in 1980, scleroderma renal crisis was the most dreaded complication of diffuse scleroderma, with a 1-year survival of only 18% (9). Its prognosis improved dramatically with the advent of ACE inhibitors, and 1-year survival increased to 76%. Scleroderma renal crisis occurs with a frequency of 13% within the first 3 years after the diagnosis of diffuse scleroderma. Hospitalization is warranted, optimally in a setting where the arterial pressure can be closely monitored. An intra-arterial catheter can be utilized judiciously if sclerodermatous changes of the upper extremity make use of a sphygmomanometer problematic, but care should be taken to ensure that perfusion is not endangered. ACE inhibitors are the cornerstone of therapy even if additional anti-hypertensive medications such as calcium channel blockers are also required to more completely control blood pressure. Short-term hemodialysis is occasionally required. Recovery of renal function after an acute episode may occur slowly over many months.

Pulmonary Complications

Pulmonary hypertension is one of the most insidious and dangerous complications of SSc. Most commonly, a vasculopathic condition similar to primary pulmonary hypertension is seen patients with limited SSc. In diffuse scleroderma, pulmonary hypertension can occur in the context of sustained interstitial inflammation and subsequent fibrotic changes. Therapy for pulmonary hypertension includes low-flow oxygen and anticoagulation with warfarin. ACE inhibitors and prazosin may also offer some benefit. Continuous intravenous infusions of epoprostenol, a prostacyclin analogue, have been used in patients with severe pulmonary hypertension but are a costly intervention and may be associated with many potential adverse effects (10). Bosentan (62.5-125 mg b.i.d.), a new orally active antagonist of endothelin receptors, was recently approved for the treatment of primary pulmonary hypertension or pulmonary hypertension secondary to collagen vascular diseases (11). Lung transplantation may be considered in patients who do not respond to medical therapy.

Patients with active neutrophilic alveolitis should be treated with a combination of systemic corticosteroids (initial prednisone 10-40 mg daily) and daily oral cyclophosphamide (50-150 mg/d) to prevent the development of fibrotic pulmonary disease (4,12). A low threshold should be held for initiating antibiotic therapy for possible pulmonary infections, and all patients with lung involvement should be given both influenza and pneumococcal vaccines. It should also be emphasized that esophageal dysfunction and reflux increases the risk of aspiration pneumonia in patients with SSc.

Gastrointestinal Complications

Esophageal involvement is the most common gastrointestinal complication of SSc. Behavioral modifications such as head elevation during sleep; avoidance of late evening snacks; limiting caffeine, peppermint, and alcohol intake; smoking cessation; eating small, frequent meals; and maintaining normal body mass index are simple measures to minimize symptoms.

Reflux esophagitis generally requires acid suppression, best achieved with proton pump inhibitors. Proton pump inhibitors are also useful for the treatment of esophageal strictures, NSAID-induced gastropathy, and bleeding complications from gastric vascular ectasia or "watermelon stomach." Esophageal strictures often require periodic dilatation. Pro-kinetic agents (e.g., metoclopramide, cisapride, or erythromycin) are useful in treating esophageal hypomotility. Because of the risk of cardiac arrythmias, cisapride is currently restricted for compassionate use only. Some success has been reported in the treatment of pseudoobstruction with octreotide, a somatostatin analogue. Anti-reflux surgical procedures remain controversial. Mucosal telangiectasias and "watermelon stomach" are important causes of gastrointestinal bleeding and respond to endoscopic laser photocoagulation.

Malabsorption due to small bowel hypomotility and bacterial overgrowth requires broad-spectrum antibiotics, optimally with a rotating schedule to avoid antibiotic-resistance. When suspected, small bowel malabsorption syndromes can be diagnosed by standard hydrogen breath tests. Two-week rotating courses of metronidazole, oral vancomycin, amoxicillin, tetracycline, ciprofloxacin, doxycycline, and co-trimoxazole can have a dramatic effect on symptoms and can reverse a previously positive hydrogen breath test. Oral supplementation with vitamins, minerals, trace elements, and medium chain triglycerides should be considered in mild-to-moderate cases of malabsorption; severe cases may require parenteral hyperalimentation.

Raynaud's Phenomenon

Treatment of Raynaud's phenomenon may include a combination of non-pharmacological therapies, pharmacological approaches (e.g., vasodilators and anticoagulation), and surgical interventions. A full discussion of treatment of Raynaud's phenomenon is presented in Chapter 28.

Novel Therapeutic Strategies

In the absence of clearly defined disease-modifying therapies in patients with SSc, a wide range of agents has been investigated for the treatment of skin fibrosis. Agents undergoing active investigation include minocycline, halofuginone (a plant alkaloid that is a specific inhibitor of collagen alpha1[I] synthesis), various antioxidants, oral native bovine collagen, anti-transforming growth factor-β monoclonal antibodies, anti-tumor necrosis factor-α agents, etretinate, psoralen/ultraviolet-A, and thalidomide. A phase I/II study of 41 patients with diffuse scleroderma undergoing immuno-ablation with peripheral stem cell rescue showed a favorable skin response in the majority of patients. Unfortunately, there was a 27% mortality rate during the first year after transplantation.

REFERENCES

1. **Follansbee WP, Curtiss EI, Medsger TA Jr, et al.** Myocardial function and perfusion in the CREST syndrome variant of progressive systemic sclerosis. Exercise radionuclide evaluation and comparison with diffuse scleroderma. Am J Med. 1984;77:489-96.

2. **Follansbee WP, Curtiss EI, Rahko PS, et al.** The electrocardiogram in systemic sclerosis (scleroderma). Study of 102 consecutive cases with functional correlations and review of the literature. Am J Med. 1985;79:183-92.

3. **Helfrich DJ, Banner B, Steen VD, Medsger TA Jr.** Normotensive renal failure in systemic sclerosis. Arthritis Rheum. 1989;32:1128-34.

4. **Silver RM, Mitler KS, Kinselssa MB, et al.** Evaluation and management of scleroderma lung disease using bronchoalveolar lavage. Am J Med. 1990;88:470-6.

5. **Steen VD, Medsyer TA Jr.** Case-control study of cortiocosteroids and other drugs that either precipitate or protect from the development of scleroderma renal crisis. Arthritis Rheum. 1998;41:1613-9.

6. **van den Hoogen FH, Boerbooms AM, Swaak AJ, et al.** Comparison of methotrexate with placebo in the treatment of systemic sclerosis: a 24 week randomized double-blind trial, followed by a 24 week observational trial. Br J Rheumatol. 1996;35:364-72.

7. **Pope JE, Bellamy N, Seibold JR, et al.** A randomized, controlled trial of methotrexate versus placebo in early diffuse scleroderma. Arthritis Rheum. 2001;44:1351-8.

8. **Clements PJ, Furst DE, Wong WK, et al.** High-dose versus low-dose D-penicillamine in early diffuse systemic sclerosis: analysis of a two-year, double-blind, randomized controlled clinical trial. Arthritis Rheum. 1999;42:1194-203.

9. **Lopez-Ovejero JA, Saal SD, D'Angelo WA, et al.** Reversal of vascular and renal crises of scleroderma by oral angiotensin-converting-enzyme blockade. N Engl J Med. 1979;300:1417-9.

10. **Badesch DB, Tapson VF, McGoon MD, et al.** Continuous intravenous epoprostenol for pulmonary hypertension due to the scleroderma spectrum of disease. A randomized, controlled trial. Ann Intern Med. 2000;132:425-34.

11. **Rubin LJ, Badesch DB, Barst RJ, et al.** Bosentan therapy for pulmonary arterial hypertension. N Engl J Med. 2002;346:896-903.

12. **Akesson A, Scheja A, Lundlin A, Wollheim F.** Improved pulmonary function in systemic sclerosis after treatment with cyclophosphamide. Arthritis Rheum. 1994; 37:729-35.

11

■ ■ ■

Sarcoidosis

Leah Lande, MD

Arthur M.F. Yee, MD, PhD

arcoidosis is a systemic disease of unknown etiology characterized by the presence of noncaseating granulomas in various organs. Although almost any organ system can be involved, sarcoidosis most commonly affects the lung, the lymphatic system, the skin, and the eyes. Its clinical manifestations vary widely: from self-limited asymptomatic hilar lymph node involvement to progressive multiorgan failure. Sarcoidosis commonly affects young and middle-aged adults, with the highest prevalence rates in African-Americans and whites of Irish or Scandinavian descent. In the United States, its overall prevalence is 10 to 40 per 100,000 with an African-American:white ratio of 10:1.

Pathogenesis

The cause of sarcoidosis remains unknown. The most widely accepted hypothesis is that sarcoidosis results from the exposure of genetically susceptible hosts to as yet undefined environmental or infectious agents (1). The development of disease likely requires three different events:

1. Exposure to a putative inciting antigen
2. Acquired cellular immunity directed against the antigen, mediated through activated antigen-presenting cells and antigen-specific CD4+ T lymphocytes
3. The appearance of immune effector cells and cytokines that stimulate a more generalized inflammatory response and granuloma formation.

Thus an antigen-specific, yet uncontrolled, cellular immune response occurs within target organs.

The characteristic pathological lesion of sarcoidosis is a discrete, compact, noncaseating granuloma composed of highly differentiated epithelioid cells, multinucleated giant cells, and lymphocytes. Over time, a dense band of fibroblasts, mast cells, collagen fibers, and proteoglycans begins to encase this ball-like cluster of cells. This fibrotic response can produce substantial and often irreversible organ destruction and physiological dysfunction. Granulomas can be found upon biopsy of any affected organ, and the diagnosis of sarcoidosis is established when clinicoradiological findings are supported by histological evidence of granulomas.

Granuloma formation is dependent on the pro-inflammatory cytokine tumor necrosis factor (TNF)-α. Animals deficient in TNF-α synthesis have impaired ability to form granulomas in response to bacterial antigens (2). In patients with sarcoidosis, levels of spontaneous TNF-α secretion by alveolar macrophages correlate with disease activity and may positively predict disease flares (3,4). These data suggest that TNF-α has a central role in the pathogenesis of sarcoidosis and may be an attractive target for therapeutic intervention.

Case Presentation 1

A 40-year-old asymptomatic white male without significant past medical history was noted to have bilateral hilar lymphadenopathy on a chest radiograph performed as part of a routine insurance physical examination. A thorough review of systems revealed no evidence of systemic disease, and the patient reported no complaints. Routine laboratory testing was normal. Subsequent computed tomography (CT) confirmed the findings of bilateral hilar lymphadenopathy and revealed paratracheal and subcarinal lymphadenopathy, but lung parenchyma appeared normal. Pulmonary function tests were also normal. Close observation without pharmacological intervention was recommended. At 6 months, CT of the chest was normal with complete resolution of the lymphadenopathy.

This patient has stage I sarcoidosis that was discovered incidentally. Because 60% to 80% of patients with stage I sarcoidosis will undergo spontaneous remission, it is reasonable to observe such patients presenting with stereotypical clinical and radiological features without treatment and to forego a biopsy at the initial discovery of radiological abnormalities.

Case Presentation 2

A 35-year-old previously healthy African-American female presents with a 2-month history of progressive fatigue, dry cough, anterior chest pain, and dyspnea on exertion. She had also noted polyarthralgias and swelling in her cheeks. On physical examination, she was breathing comfortably with a normal respiratory rate, although the resting room air oxygen saturation was 94%. Bilateral parotid gland swelling and cervical lymphadenopathy were noted. Lung examination revealed bibasilar rales and a few scattered expiratory wheezes. She had tenderness and warmth of her elbows and knees but no swelling or erythema. Chest radiography revealed bilateral hilar lymphadenopathy and diffuse interstitial infiltrates.

The patient's pulmonary function tests were markedly abnormal. The forced expiratory volume in one second (FEV_1) was 50% of predicted; the forced vital capacity (FVC) was 70% of predicted; the FEV_1/FVC ratio was 71% of predicted; the total lung capacity was 75% of predicted; and the diffusing capacity was 45% of predicted. Her complete blood count, serum chemistries, and electrocardiogram were normal, but the erythrocyte sedimentation rate was elevated at 60 mm/h.

During bronchoscopy, "cobblestone-like" lesions were noted on the tracheobronchial mucosa. Transbronchial biopsies showed noncaseating granulomas, and smears for fungal and mycobacterial organisms were negative.

The diagnosis of sarcoidosis was made, and the patient was given prednisone 40 mg daily. Over 6 weeks, all of her pulmonary and extra-pulmonary symptoms completely resolved and her pulmonary function test abnormalities returned to near-normal values. The prednisone dose was tapered over the next few months, and the patient was followed with serial pulmonary function tests. However, during several attempts to taper the prednisone dosage to below 15 mg daily, the patient experienced recurrence of her symptoms.

This patient has stage II sarcoidosis with prominent systemic symptoms and significant impairment of pulmonary function. A biopsy was indicated to make the diagnosis and to exclude other conditions, and treatment with corticosteroids was required because the disease was clinically active. This case also demonstrates dependence on chronic corticosteroid therapy, one of the common difficulties in treating patients with sarcoidosis. In these cases, steroid-sparing agents should be considered to minimize corticosteroid requirements and limit their attendant adverse effects.

Clinical Features

The clinical manifestations of sarcoidosis vary widely. Many asymptomatic cases are discovered incidentally after chest radiographs are obtained as part of presurgical evaluations or other screening programs. Because sarcoidosis is a multiorgan disorder with diverse manifestations, patients may present initially to clinicians of many different medical specialties. Approximately one third of patients with sarcoidosis will report nonspecific constitutional symptoms (e.g., fever, fatigue, weight loss, anorexia) that are suggestive of a systemic inflammatory illness. Patients with pulmonary involvement may report dyspnea on exertion, retrosternal chest pain, or chronic cough. Lofgren's syndrome, the triad of erythema nodosum, bilateral hilar lymphadenopathy, and inflammatory arthritis/periarthritis (characteristically in and around the ankles), may be seen in 20% to 50% of patients with acute presentations. In the United States, more than one half of patients present initially with chronic respiratory symptoms and few constitutional symptoms.

Pulmonary and Mediastinal Disease

The lungs are affected in more than 90% of patients with sarcoidosis (5). Even when extrapulmonary manifestations predominate, subclinical lung involvement is usually present. One third to one half of patients will have dyspnea, dry cough, and chest pain that is usually retrosternal. Pulmonary sarcoidosis can be staged according to chest radiographic findings:

- *Stage I*—Bilateral hilar lymphadenopathy
- *Stage II*—Bilateral hilar adenopathy accompanied by parenchymal infiltrates (Fig. 11-1)
- *Stage III*—Parenchymal infiltrates without hilar adenopathy
- *Stage IV*—Pulmonary fibrosis with evidence of honeycombing, emphysema, bullae, and hilar retraction

Pulmonary involvement of sarcoidosis is most commonly an interstitial lung disease involving the alveoli, blood vessels, and bronchioles that results in clinical findings of dry "velcro-like" rales, restricted lung volumes, and abnormalities in gas exchange (6). In addition, patients can have airway involvement, with granulomatous infiltration of the nares, larynx, trachea, and bronchi, leading to airway obstruction and occasionally bronchiectasis. In fact, up to 20% of patients may have airway hyperactivity and present with wheezing. Uncommon pulmonary manifestations include

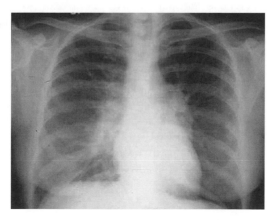

Figure 11-1   Plain chest radiograph of a patient with stage II sarcoidosis demonstrating prominent hilar lymphadenopathy and diffuse interstitial infiltrates.

pleural effusions, pneumothorax, pleural thickening and calcification, lymph node calcification, and cavity formation.

Cutaneous Manifestations

Cutaneous involvement occurs in approximately 25% of patients, and dermatologists are often the first to diagnose a new case of sarcoidosis after the biopsy of atypical skin lesions. Sarcoid skin lesions are highly heterogeneous and may include plaques, subcutaneous nodules, macules, papules, hypo- and hyper-pigmented areas, and changes in old scars or tattoos.

The two classic skin lesions of sarcoidosis are erythema nodosum and lupus pernio. Erythema nodosum is more commonly seen in white, Puerto Rican, and Mexican patients, less frequently seen in the African-American and Japanese populations. The lesions consist of raised, red, exquisitely tender subcutaneous nodules characteristically on the anterior aspects of the legs and commonly seen in the setting of Lofgren's syndrome (see Fig. 25-1 in Chapter 25). Over the course of weeks, the lesions darken and resemble deep purplish bruises. Adjacent ankle joints may be swollen and painful, and the rash is often coalescent with joint erythema. Biopsy of the nodules typically does not show granulomas. Erythema nodosum usually resolves spontaneously within several weeks to months. In some series, up to 25% of patients will develop erythema nodosum (7). Lupus pernio consists of violaceous doughy infiltration commonly involving the nose and nasal mucosa, cheeks, lips, and ears and may be associated with an increased risk for upper respiratory tract disease; skin biopsy typically reveals granulomas. With the exception of erythema nodosum, the chronic skin lesions of sarcoidosis typically do not cause pain or itch.

Musculoskeletal Manifestations

Arthralgias or inflammatory arthritis occurs in approximately 25% to 40% of patients with sarcoidosis, although almost never with deforming arthritis. The knees, ankles, elbows, wrists, and small joints of the hands and feet are most commonly affected. The arthralgias may be acute and transient, or chronic and persistent.

A myopathy that clinically resembles the proximal muscle weakness of inflammatory myositis can occur. Proximal muscle weakness can also be an adverse effect of chronic systemic corticosteroid use, which can complicate making the diagnosis. "Punched-out" bony lesions can occur, usually in association with chronic skin disease and a dactylitis-like swollen digit appearance. Diffuse granulomatous involvement of bone is rare but can lead to severe local or generalized skeletal pain.

Hematological Abnormalities

An anemia of chronic disease can be seen in approximately 10% to 20% of patients with sarcoidosis, and mild leukopenia in up to 40%. The leukopenia may represent bone marrow infiltration, be secondary to redistribution of circulating T lymphocytes to sites of active disease, or be related to hypersplenism. Thrombocytopenia can be present and occasionally severe.

Approximately one third of patients with sarcoidosis have peripheral lymphadenopathy, with the cervical, axillary, epitrochlear, and inguinal regions most frequently involved. The lymph nodes are generally easily movable and nontender. Splenomegaly may rarely occur.

Cardiac Manifestations

It is essential that all patients with suspected or proven sarcoidosis be evaluated at baseline and then periodically for cardiac involvement because it is the leading cause of death among affected individuals. Clinically evident myocardial involvement is present in only about 5% to 10% of patients, and so, in many cases, cardiac involvement may be overlooked. Up to one half of patients with cardiac sarcoidosis have evidence of rhythm, conduction, or repolarization abnormalities. Twenty-four–hour Holter monitoring is more sensitive than an electrocardiogram in the detection of ventricular tachycardia, heart block, or other conduction system abnormalities. Prophylactic implantation of cardioverter-defibrillators and/or pacemakers is indicated in patients identified as having potentially malignant arrhythmias.

Other cardiac manifestations include papillary muscle dysfunction, infiltrative cardiomyopathy, and pericarditis. Myocardial imaging with thallium-201 scanning may reveal segmental defects that correspond to either granulomatous infiltration or a fibrous scar. The finding of granulomas on endomyocardial biopsy confirms the diagnosis of cardiac sarcoidosis, but the diagnostic yield of this procedure is low due to the heterogeneous distribution of disease.

Head and Neck Manifestations

Ocular lesions occur in approximately 25% of patients with sarcoidosis. Any part of the eye or orbit may be affected, with uveitis being the most common eye lesion. Acute anterior uveitis presents with blurred vision, photophobia, and excessive lacrimation and usually clears spontaneously or after topical or locally injected corticosteroids. Chronic uveitis may lead to adhesions between the iris and the lens, glaucoma, cataracts, and blindness. Other eye lesions include conjunctival nodules, retinal vasculitis, keratoconjunctivitis sicca, lacrimal gland enlargement, and dacryocystitis.

Approximately 6% of patients will develop parotitis with painful, swollen enlargement of either one or both parotid glands; in one half of these patients, the parotitis is self-limiting.

Neurological Manifestations

Approximately 5% of patients have nervous system involvement, and virtually any part of the nervous system may be affected. The disease has a predilection for the base of the brain, and cranial nerve involvement is common, particularly seventh nerve palsies. Patients can also have peripheral neuropathy and neuromuscular involvement. Unusual combinations of neurological deficits affecting the central nervous system and/or peripheral nerves should raise the suspicion of sarcoidosis. The diagnosis of neurosarcoidosis can be supported by abnormal findings on gadolinium-enhanced magnetic resonance imaging (MRI); lymphocytosis with an increased $CD4^+/CD8^+$ ratio and elevated protein in cerebrospinal fluid (CSF) in about 80% of patients; and elevated CSF angiotensin-converting enzyme levels in about 50% of patients. However, while all of these findings are suggestive of sarcoidosis, biopsy of the affected tissue is the only definitive way to secure this diagnosis.

Hepatic Involvement

Although liver biopsy reveals granulomas in 40% to 70% of patients, clinically significant hepatic dysfunction secondary to sarcoidosis is rare. Approximately one third of patients will have asymptomatic hepatomegaly or abnormalities in hepatic enzymes. Rarely, pruritis may be a significant problem due to the accumulation of bile acids in the plasma caused by hepatic obstruction.

Gastointestinal Manifestations

Aside from liver involvement, less than 1% of patients have gastrointestinal tract disease, with the stomach being the most common site. Less frequently, esophageal, colorectal, and pancreatic involvement can occur and can mimic inflammatory bowel disease, tuberculosis, fungal infections, or pancreatic neoplasms.

Metabolic Manifestations

Patients with sarcoidosis have abnormal regulation of 1,25-dihydroxyvitamin D production by activated macrophages and granulomas, resulting in increased intestinal absorption of calcium, enhanced bone resorption, and resultant hypercalciuria with or without hypercalcemia. This increases risks for nephrocalcinosis and renal failure. Rarely, the granulomatous process may produce interstitial nephritis by direct involvement of the kidneys.

Diagnosis

The diagnosis of sarcoidosis requires a compatible clinical picture, histological demonstration of noncaseating granulomas, and exclusion of other diseases capable of producing a similar histological or clinical picture. When considering a diagnosis of sarcoidosis, it is important to rule out other types of granulomatous disease (Table 11-1), notably mycobacterial and atypical infections. The diagnostic evaluation for patients with suspected sarcoidosis should fulfill four goals:

1. To provide histological confirmation of the disease
2. To assess the extent and severity of organ involvement
3. To assess whether the disease is stable or progressive
4. To determine if therapy is indicated

The initial evaluation of a patient with suspected sarcoidosis should include a careful history including occupational, environmental, and medication exposures; a thorough physical examination; a complete blood count and biochemical panel to evaluate hepatic and renal function and serum calcium; chest radiography; and other tests specific to suspected areas of organ involvement. Other studies as dictated by the initial assessment may include electrocardiography, CT of the chest, pulmonary function testing (PFT), and an ophthalmological evaluation with slit-lamp examination.

Table 11-1   Differential Diagnosis of Granulomatous Diseases

Cause	Examples	Tests to Distinguish from Sarcoidosis
Mycobacteria	• Tuberculosis • Atypical mycobacteria	• Positive stain or culture for acid-fast bacilli
Fungi	• Histoplasmosis • Coccidioidomycosis	• History of possible exposure; positive culture or urinary histoplasmosis antigen
Bacteria	• Brucellosis • Chlamydia • Tularemia	• History of possible exposure; culture; serology
Spirochetes	• Syphilis	• Serology
Parasites	• Leishmaniasis • Toxoplasmosis	• Serology; demonstration of organism in tissue
Malignancy	• Lymphoma • Solid tumors	• Biopsy
Immune and inflammatory disorders	• Wegener's granulomatosis • Churg-Strauss syndrome • Primary biliary cirrhosis • Common variable immunodeficiency	• Wegener's granulomatosis: anti-neutrophil cytoplasmic antibody; biopsy • Churg-Strauss syndrome: peripheral eosinophilia; biopsy • Primary biliary cirrhosis: anti-mitochondrial antibodies • Common variable immuno-deficiency: quantitative serum immunoglobulins

Although serum angiotensin-converting enzyme (ACE) levels are elevated in two thirds of patients with sarcoidosis, they do not consistently correlate with disease activity and are also elevated in numerous other disorders that involve the lungs; thus routine measurement of serum ACE levels is generally not useful. The Kveim-Siltzbach test consists of the intradermal injection of homogenates of spleen or lymph node cells from an individual with known sarcoidosis, followed by biopsy of the injected area, which should show a granulomatous reaction in patients with sarcoidosis. This test is neither widely available nor well standardized and has the potential for transmission of infectious agents. It is largely of historical interest and is rarely used even at specialized centers. Table 11-2 outlines a reasonable organ-based approach to baseline and serial noninvasive testing for disease assessment and monitoring.

Clinical and radiological features alone may be diagnostic in 98% of patients with stage I and 89% of patients with stage II pulmonary disease; in many cases, tissue biopsy may not be necessary if the disease is not clinically active. Similarly, patients presenting with Lofgren's syndrome will not generally require a tissue diagnosis. However, when there is sufficient question as to diagnosis or when pharmacological intervention is being considered for symptoms, a biopsy should be taken from the most readily accessible organ by the least invasive method. The most common means are skin, peripheral lymph node, and transbronchial lung biopsies. When necessary, hilar lymph node biopsies can generally be obtained through transbronchial needle aspiration or mediastinoscopy. Transbronchial lung biopsies have a diagnostic yield of up to 90% in patients with radiographic abnormalities and of 50% to 80% in patients without radiographic evidence of parenchymal disease. Examination of bronchoalveolar lavage (BAL) fluid can also have diagnostic utility. BAL fluid lymphocytosis is a common finding and, according to some authorities, a ratio of CD4/CD8 cells in BAL fluid of greater than 3.5 has a sensitivity of 53% and a specificity of 94% for sarcoidosis.

Table 11-2   Organ-Specific Tests for Monitoring Sarcoidosis

Organ	Test
Lungs	Chest radiography, computed tomography, pulmonary function tests
Heart	Electrocardiography, thallium scintigraphy, echocardiography
Skin	Physical examination
Central nervous system	Physical examination, magnetic resonance imaging
Liver	Liver function tests
Kidneys	Serum calcium and creatinine, urinalysis, urine calcium
Eyes	Slit-lamp examination

Pulmonary function tests should be performed on all patients at baseline and then periodically to follow for changes in lung function, even for patients without radiographic evidence of lung involvement. The most sensitive parameters for detecting functional impairment are the diffusing capacity and the forced vital capacity. Both restrictive and obstructive pulmonary function abnormalities may be found.

CT of the chest may also be a helpful tool in evaluating patients with suspected pulmonary sarcoidosis, particularly in the presence of pulmonary function abnormalities. The classic findings on CT scan are diffuse small nodules that follow the bronchovascular bundle or subpleural distribution, thickened interlobular septae, architectural distortion, and masses. Less common findings are honeycombing, cyst formation, bronchiectasis, and alveolar consolidation. In the setting of stage IV disease, cavities and bullae may become infected or chronically colonized with opportunistic pathogens such as *Aspergillus* and *Pseudomonas aeruginosa*.

When an extent of disease evaluation is indicated, total-body gallium-67 scanning has proven to be helpful in delineating specific areas of organ involvement and assessing disease activity.

Prognosis and Disease Outcomes

It is not well understood why some patients with sarcoidosis have very mild, self-limited disease, whereas others have severe, progressive, and relapsing disease. The radiographic staging of pulmonary sarcoidosis has prognostic significance: stage I disease spontaneously remits in 60% to 80% of patients; stage II remits in 50% to 60%; and stage III remits in less than 30%. More than 85% of spontaneous remissions occur within 2 years of presentation. Failure to regress spontaneously within 2 years predicts a chronic or persistent course. Features associated with a poorer prognosis include black race, onset of disease after age 40, symptoms lasting for more than 6 months, the absence of erythema nodosum, splenomegaly, involvement of more than three organ systems, and stage III or IV pulmonary disease. The Lofgren's syndrome variant of sarcoidosis is associated with a good overall prognosis.

Management

Appropriate management of sarcoidosis depends on the individual case. The key role of the primary care physician is to coordinate care. Because the lungs become involved in almost all patients, a pulmonologist should be consulted upon diagnosis. Other specialists should be called upon depending on which organ systems become affected.

Because of the potential for spontaneous improvement, close observation is often a reasonable initial course of action in cases with no evidence of active disease. Accordingly, patients with stage I pulmonary disease almost never require treatment. Lofgren's syndrome can usually be managed with relatively brief courses of nonsteroidal anti-inflammatory drugs or low-dose systemic corticosteroids for symptomatic relief of the joint and skin problems. However, most physicians feel that patients with significant pulmonary symptoms or with progressive loss of lung function should be treated. The mainstay of treatment for sarcoidosis is systemic corticosteroids, which usually results in rapid relief of respiratory symptoms and improvement in chest X-ray findings and pulmonary function tests. However, after discontinuation of treatment, symptoms and lung function abnormalities often recur (8). Therapy is also clearly indicated for cardiac disease, neurological disease, ocular disease not responding to topical therapy, and severe hypercalcemia. There have been no placebo-controlled clinical trials evaluating the long-term outcome of patients treated with corticosteroids.

The optimal dose and duration of therapy with corticosteroids have not been studied in a randomized, prospective controlled trial. For pulmonary sarcoidosis, initial therapy is usually 20 to 40 mg of prednisone (or equivalent) daily. Higher doses (1 mg/kg/d) are often necessary for cardiac or neurosarcoidosis. Patients should be evaluated monthly to assess response to therapy. If there is no improvement by 3 months, response is unlikely and alternative agents should be considered. Nonresponders should also be evaluated for the presence of irreversible fibrotic disease, in which case continued treatment may incur unnecessary risks associated with medication without prospect for significant benefit. Among those patients who do respond to systemic corticosteroids, the dose should be slowly tapered over 6 months to the minimal effective dose, ideally to less than prednisone 10 mg/d, and then continued for a minimum of 1 year before further dose reduction. Up to 25% of patients with stage II or III disease will relapse once therapy is tapered or discontinued; thus dependence on chronic corticosteroid therapy and its attendant toxicities may evolve into serious complications. Moreover, although close monitoring of symptoms and pulmonary function is required at all times, particular vigilance is necessary during corticosteroid dose reduction or cessation of therapy. Topical and injectable steroids are often adequate for the treatment of skin papules and plaques, as well as for most cases of anterior uveitis.

Several alternative therapies have been used for patients with disease refractory to corticosteroids, in those experiencing steroid-related toxicities, and in cases of severe pulmonary, cardiac, or neurological involvement, in which the mortality risk is significant. Among these are methotrexate (7.5-25 mg/wk) (9), azathioprine (50-200 mg/d in divided doses) (10), and oral or intravenous cyclophosphamide (11,12), but the potential toxicities of many of these agents may limit their use. None of these therapies has ever been proven to prolong survival, and most of the data are in the form of case reports and uncontrolled studies. Therefore, a careful benefit-versus-risk analysis must be made before recommending their use. Hydroxychloroquine

(200-400 mg/d) has been used to treat hypercalcemia and the skin manifestations of sarcoidosis (13).

Because TNF-α has been strongly implicated in promoting the granulomatous inflammatory process in sarcoidosis, recently developed specific antagonists of TNF-α have been considered to be novel therapeutic options. Infliximab (5 mg/kg IV) is a chimeric IgG monoclonal antibody directed against human TNF-α; etanercept (25 mg twice weekly) is a soluble TNF-α receptor fused to the Fc fragment of a human IgG. Both of these agents inhibit the activity of TNF-α, and in case reports and small series both have shown promise in bringing about subjective and objective improvement in varied clinical manifestations of steroid-refractory sarcoidosis (14-16). One open-label uncontrolled study, however, did not find a benefit from etanercept therapy for stage II and III pulmonary sarcoidosis (17). Thalidomide (50-200 mg/d), which also has anti-TNF-α properties, has also been shown to be effective, particularly in the treatment of cutaneous manifestations in uncontrolled case series (18). Appropriately strict precautions are absolutely necessary given its notorious teratogenicity.

REFERENCES

1. **Hunninghake GW, Crystal RG.** Pulmonary sarcoidosis: a disorder mediated by excess helper T lymphocyte activity at sites of disease activity. N Engl J Med. 1981;305:429-34.

2. **Marino MW, Dunn A, Grail D, et al.** Characterization of tumor necrosis factor-deficient mice. Proc Natl Acad Sci USA. 1997;94:8093-8.

3. **Baughman RP, Strohofer SA, Buchsbaum J, Lower EE.** Release of tumor necrosis factor by alveolar macrophages of patients with sarcoidosis. J Lab Clin Med. 1990;115:36-42.

4. **Ziegenhagen MW, Benner UK, Zissel G, et al.** Sarcoidosis: TNF-alpha release from alveolar macrophages and serum level of sIL-2R are prognostic markers. Am J Respir Crit Care Med. 1997;156:1586-92.

5. **Lynch JP 3rd, Sharma OP, Baughman RP.** Extrapulmonary sarcoidosis. Semin Respir Infect. 1998;13:229-54.

6. **Keogh BA, Hunninghake GW, Line BR, Crystal RG.** The alveolitis of pulmonary sarcoidosis: evaluation of natural history and alveolitis-dependent changes in lung function. Am Rev Respir Dis. 1983;128:256-65.

7. **Diab SM, Karnik AM, Ouda BA, et al.** Sarcoidosis in Arabs: the clinical profile of 20 patients and review of the literature. Sarcoidosis. 1991;8:56-62.

8. **Gottlieb JE, Israel HL, Steiner RM, et al.** Outcome in sarcoidosis: the relationship of relapse to corticosteroid therapy. Chest. 1997;111:623-31.

9. **Lower EE, Baughman RP.** Prolonged use of methotrexate for sarcoidosis. Arch Intern Med. 1995;155:846-51.

10. **Muller-Quernheim J, Kienstat K, Held M, et al.** Treatment of chronic sarcoidosis with an azathioprine/prednisolone regimen. Eur Respir J. 1999;14:1117-22.

11. **Demeter SL.** Myocardial sarcoidosis unresponsive to steroids: treatment with cyclophosphamide. Chest. 1988;94:202-3.

12

■ ■ ■

Polyarteritis Nodosa, Microscopic Polyangiitis, and Mixed Cryoglobulinemia

Kristina B. Belostocki, MD

Stephen A. Paget, MD

The vasculitides affecting small and medium-sized vessels can involve many organ systems, resulting in diverse signs and symptoms and frequently leading to diagnostic confusion (Table 12-1). Polyarteritis nodosa characteristically affects medium-sized arteries, whereas microscopic polyangiitis and mixed cryoglobulinemia tend to involve smaller blood vessels (arterioles, capillaries, and venules). However, significant overlap can occur in the size of the vessels and clinical manifestations. Correct and timely diagnosis and prompt initiation of appropriate therapy are essential for achieving optimal outcomes.

Polyarteritis Nodosa

Polyarteritis nodosa (PAN) is an immune complex-mediated necrotizing vasculitis affecting medium-sized arteries, typically sparing arterioles, venules, and capillaries. It is commonly characterized by peripheral nervous system, skin, muscle, and gastrointestinal tract involvement, but it is *not* associated with glomerulonephritis or lung disease. The annual incidence of PAN ranges from 2 to 9 cases per million and predominantly affects individuals between 40 and 60 years of age. It is twice as common in men as in women. In the recent past, PAN was associated with hepatitis B virus (HBV) infection in up to one third of cases, but this association has declined to approximately 10%, probably due to the improved quality of the blood supply as well as vaccination against the virus.

Table 12-1   Clinical Features of Polyarteritis Nodosa, Microscopic Polyangiitis, and Mixed Cryoglobulinemia

Disease	Vessel Involvement	Prominent Organ Involvement	Renal Disease	Pulmonary Disease	Immune Complex Mediated	Disease Associations
Polyarteritis	Medium-sized arteries	Peripheral nerve, skin, muscle, gastro-intestinal tract, kidney	Medium-sized artery disease, hyper-tension	None	Yes	Hepatitis B
Microscopic poly-angiitis	Arterioles, capillaries, venules; less commonly medium-sized arteries	Kidney, lungs, skin, peripheral nerve	Glomerulo-nephritis	Pulmonary capillaritis	Uncom-mon	None
Mixed cryoglob-ulinemia	Arterioles, capillaries, venules; not infrequently, medium-sized arteries	Skin, joint, kidney, gastro-intestinal tract	Glomerulo-nephritis	Rarely	Yes	Hepatitis C

Pathogenesis

The immunopathogenesis of PAN is incompletely understood, although immune complex-induced activation of the complement cascade appears to play a role, particularly in PAN associated with active HBV infection. Hepatitis B surface antigen (HBsAg) is probably the triggering mechanism, and the mean time from infection with HBV to development of PAN is generally less than one year.

Case Presentation 1

A previously healthy 45-year-old Caucasian male presents with a 3-week history of fevers to 39°C, fatigue, malaise, and polyarthralgias. Over the past week, he has noted a nonpruritic rash on the lower parts of both legs and progressive pain and weakness of his left foot. Three days previously he developed postprandial periumbilical abdominal pain. On examination, he appeared to be moderately uncomfortable, with a temperature of

38.8°C and a pulse of 115. His abdomen was diffusely tender but without guarding or rebound. Livedo reticularis and palpable purpura were present over the lower extremities, and a left foot drop was present. Laboratory evaluation was significant for a normochromic anemia, thrombocytosis, and an erythrocyte sedimentation rate of 95 mm/h. Serum chemistries, urinalysis, and abdominal X-rays were normal. Blood cultures, serum cryoglobulins, and serologies for antinuclear antibodies (ANA), anti-neutrophil cytoplasmic antibodies (ANCA), and hepatitis B and C viruses were all negative.

Skin biopsy confirmed the presence of a nongranulomatous necrotizing vasculitis. Abdominal angiography revealed microaneurysms and stenoses within medium-sized arteries in the mesentery. Electromyography and nerve conduction velocity studies were consistent with the presence of a mononeuritis multiplex of the left peroneal nerve. The diagnosis of polyarteritis nodosa was made.

Because of visceral end-organ involvement in the form of mesenteric vasculitis, intravenous methylprednisolone (1 g/d for 3 days) was administered, followed by daily oral prednisone (1 mg/kg). Monthly intravenous cyclophosphamide was also initiated. After 3 months of high-dose corticosteroids, the severe manifestations of his disease were felt to be under sufficient control, and the daily corticosteroids were slowly tapered over the next year. Monthly intravenous cyclophosphamide was also continued over this time, after which the patient did well without permanent sequelae from his disease or therapy and without relapse of the vasculitis.

This patient has polyarteritis nodosa with visceral end-organ involvement, mandating an aggressive course of therapy with a combination of systemic high-dose corticosteroids and cyclophosphamide.

Clinical Features

The initial signs and symptoms of PAN may be nonspecific, frequently causing diagnostic ambiguity and delaying diagnosis. Constitutional symptoms such as malaise, fever, and weight loss are common. More specific findings are peripheral neuropathy, manifestations of gastrointestinal ischemia, and vasculitic skin lesions. Patients can appear acutely ill, but in others the illness is insidious.

The nervous system is often involved in PAN. Peripheral neuropathy is one of the most common manifestations, occurring in as many as 70% of patients, and is a result of inflammation of the vasa nervorum. This may present as a painful mononeuritis multiplex, an ischemic neuropathy involving large mixed motor and sensory nerves, or multiple mononeuropathies. The peroneal, ulnar, median, and sural nerves are those most commonly affected. Motor and sensory involvement is asymmetric, tends to be more distal than proximal, and predominantly affects the lower extremities, leading to a toe or foot drop and/or painful dysesthesias. Cranial nerve palsies and hand drop have also been described but are less common. Central nervous system involvement is rare but can result from vasculitis of a cerebral artery, leading to stroke and motor or sensory deficits. Ocular involvement can take the form of retinal vasculitis, retinal detachment, or cotton-wool spots.

Cutaneous involvement occurs in 27% to 60% of patients and usually takes the form of purpura or livedo reticularis. Small, tender, subcutaneous nodules and nailfold infarcts due to vasculitis can also occur. Ischemia due to vasculitis in small vessels may lead to distal gangrene. Isolated cutaneous PAN may represent 10% of cases. In these patients, the lower extremities frequently develop palpable purpura and painful nodules surrounded by livedo reticularis and necrotic lesions. Isolated cutaneous PAN may regress spontaneously or progress to systemic PAN at any juncture. A search for visceral involvement at the onset of disease and continued vigilance over time are essential.

Musculoskeletal involvement in the form of myalgias and arthralgias is reported in 30% to 73% of patients. Asymmetrical arthritis of the lower extremity large joints can occur early in the course of the disease.

Renal involvement due to vasculitis of medium-sized renal and intrarenal arteries is commonly seen in PAN, but glomerulonephritis is *not* a feature. Multiple renal infarcts can, rarely, lead to renal failure. Renal angiography reveals multiple microaneurysms, which can rupture and lead to intrarenal or perirenal hematomas. Hypertension due to renal artery involvement is seen in one third of patients. Peri-ureteral vasculitis and secondary fibrosis causing ureteral stenosis can lead to anuria and renal failure.

Involvement of the gastrointestinal tract can be severe, presenting as abdominal pain, gastrointestinal bleeding, or bowel perforation. Bowel ischemia can cause intractable abdominal pain and weight loss and may be confused clinically with inflammatory bowel disease. Small bowel involvement is most common, but the stomach and colon can also be affected. Hepatic infarctions and hematomas can also occur. PAN may affect the gallbladder or appendix, presenting as acalculous cholecystitis or appendicitis.

Cardiac manifestations are due to vasculitis of the coronary arteries or to severe or malignant hypertension. Resultant cardiomyopathy is present in 25% of cases, and congestive heart failure commonly ensues. Despite coronary artery vasculitis, classical angina is rare and coronary angiography is usually normal.

Orchitis is present in 36% of men with HBV-related PAN but is less common in PAN without HBV.

Notably, *classic PAN does not involve the lungs,* and the diagnosis of microscopic polyangiitis should be considered if nongranulomatous vasculitis of small-to-medium sized vessels is identified in the lung.

The clinical manifestations of non-HBV-related PAN are similar to those observed in HBV-related PAN, although malignant hypertension, renal infarction, and orchiepididymitis are more frequently associated with HBV infection. Identifying cases that are HBV-related is important because therapeutic approaches can often differ.

Diagnosis

Most laboratory abnormalities found in PAN are nonspecific. Most patients exhibit evidence of systemic inflammation reflected as an elevated erythrocyte sedimentation rate (ESR) and C-reactive protein (CRP) levels, normochromic anemia, leukocytosis, and thrombocytosis. Hypocomplementemia and low titer rheumatoid factor may also be found. Anti-neutrophil cytoplasmic antibodies (ANCA) occur in less than 20% of patients with PAN. Given the association of HBV infection in approximately 10% of cases, HBV serological testing (including HBsAg, HBsAb, HBeAg, HBeAb, and HBcAb) should be obtained for all patients.

Although the diagnosis of PAN can be and is often made on clinical grounds solely, confirmation by tissue biopsy is nonetheless desirable and useful, especially when cytotoxic therapy is being considered. The site of biopsy is determined by the clinical picture, and the skin, skeletal muscle, sural nerve, and kidney are typical sites for sampling. Unfortunately, the yield of biopsy is not assured, even if guided by clinical signs or symptoms. For example, among patients with neuropathic symptoms and abnormal electrophysiological studies, a diagnostic nerve biopsy is found in only 45%. However, a simultaneous muscle biopsy can enhance the yield substantially. If the clinical presentation does not identify an accessible tissue for examination, a "blind" biopsy of clinically unaffected muscle (i.e., no muscle weakness or muscle enzyme abnormalities) may reveal vasculitis in 30% to 50% of cases.

Histological examination reveals a nongranulomatous, focal, segmental, sectoral, necrotizing vasculitis of medium-sized arteries that can lead to aneurysmal bulging of the arterial wall. There is a predilection for sites of bifurcation. Veins and venules are not involved. Neutrophilic infiltrates predominate early in the disease, whereas mononuclear cells characterize latter stages of the inflammatory process. Due to the segmental nature of this vasculitis, examination of multiple cuts of biopsy specimens may be required for improved sensitivity.

Abdominal angiography should be obtained when pathological evidence of vasculitis is lacking despite high clinical suspicion for PAN. However, caution must be exercised with the use of intravenous contrast dye in patients with evidence of renal insufficiency. Abdominal angiography can reveal microaneurysms and stenoses in medium-sized arteries in the liver, kidneys, and mesentery. These abnormalities, however, are not specific to PAN and may be seen in many other conditions (e.g., atrial myxoma, neurofibromatosis, Ehlers-Danlos syndrome, systemic lupus erythematosus [SLE], Wegener's granulomatosis, endocarditis) and thus need to be put in the context of the entire clinical picture. Angiography can be useful in identifying a subset of patients with more severe end-organ involvement and who may benefit from early aggressive intervention (1).

Prognosis and Disease Outcomes

The prognosis of PAN has improved with the use of corticosteroids and immunosuppressive drugs. Untreated PAN has an extremely poor prognosis, with a 5-year survival rate of only 10%. However, with the advent of systemic corticosteroid therapy and cytotoxic agents, the 5-year survival rate has increased to over 70%. Age greater than 50 years and cardiac, gastrointestinal, or renal involvement are associated with increased mortality (2). Infectious complications, particularly during courses of profound immunosuppression, add significantly to overall morbidity.

Chronic problems resulting from PAN or its therapy can include sensorimotor deficits from peripheral neuropathy, renal insufficiency, hypertension, or osteoporosis. The relapse rate is low: approximately 19% in patients with non-HBV-related PAN and 8% in HBV-related PAN (3). Unlike Wegener's granulomatosis, SLE, and Churg-Strauss syndrome, PAN tends to be characterized by discrete episodes rather than by a chronically progressive course.

Management

Without prompt intervention, PAN may result in severe complications such as renal failure, permanent neurological deficits, bowel perforation, or even death. The goals of management are to quickly identify the extent and severity of disease, to rapidly control inflammatory processes with systemic corticosteroids, and to choose an immunosuppressive agent of appropriate potency to induce disease remission and enable tapering and discontinuation of corticosteroid therapy. In practice, a major management challenge for the clinician is to balance the therapeutic benefits and the potentially severe toxicities of pharmacological agents.

Pharmacological Therapy

The initial management of PAN *not* associated with HBV infection often includes high-dose oral corticosteroids with or without intravenous "pulse" corticosteroid therapy. Due to its rapid onset of action, intravenous methylprednisolone (1 g/d for 3 days) can be given at the initiation of therapy for severe systemic vasculitis with life-threatening organ involvement. Maintenance oral corticosteroids (1 mg/kg prednisone or equivalent daily) are then initiated and slowly tapered after disease control is achieved, typically after 2 months. For less severe, non-life-threatening organ involvement, the oral regimen alone, initially in divided doses, can be given and then consolidated to single daily dose when a therapeutic response is attained.

Cyclophosphamide is commonly used in conjunction with corticosteroids for severe or unresponsive cases with visceral end-organ involvement (e.g., mesenteric vasculitis, cardiac disease, nervous system involvement) or as a steroid-sparing agent to avoid or minimize toxicities of long-term corticosteroid use. Intravenous cyclophosphamide (0.5-1.0 g/m^2) is administered monthly, with doses adjusted as needed to maintain a peripheral leukocyte count of no less than 3000/mm^3 and a neutrophil count of no less than 1500/mm^3 at 10 to 14 days after infusion. Daily oral cyclophosphamide is another option but, while clinically effective in the treatment of PAN, it has a low therapeutic/toxicity index and is associated with a high incidence of adverse effects including hemorrhagic cystitis, bladder fibrosis, bone marrow suppression, ovarian failure, bladder cancer, and hematological malignancy. Cyclophosphamide therapy is generally maintained for at least a year after a remission is achieved, while systemic corticosteroid therapy is slowly tapered. In order to limit potential toxicities of cyclophosphamide therapy, an alternative approach is to induce initial control of disease activity with cyclophosphamide and then, once the symptoms are under control (generally after at least 3 months), an alternative, less toxic, immunosuppressant such as methotrexate or azathioprine can often be effectively and safely substituted.

In HBV-related PAN, the prolonged use of immunosuppressive agents may allow the virus to persist, which can lead to chronic hepatitis, cirrhosis, and hepatocellular carcinoma. Although corticosteroids may be initially used in high doses within the first two weeks to promptly gain control over severe vasculitic manifestations, a quick discontinuation of corticosteroids and a switch to maintenance therapy with antiviral agents such as vidarabine or interferon-α is recommended (4), preferably in consultation with a hepatologist. Plasma exchanges have also been used to remove immune complexes and control manifestations of PAN, while avoiding the potential complications of immunosuppressive therapy, particularly with regard to enhancement of viral replication.

Disease Monitoring
Patients should be monitored at least monthly during the first year of therapy to assess for clinical response, toxicities related to medications, and evidence of disease relapse. Close clinical observation for relapse/reactivation of disease is critical during the tapering of immunosuppressive drugs. In addition to thorough clinical evaluations, complete blood counts, acute phase reactants (ESR and CRP), electrolytes, renal and hepatic profiles, and urinalyses should be assessed. Once patients achieve remission and the course of cyclophosphamide is completed, they may be evaluated less frequently (e.g., every 2-3 months). Given the association of cyclophosphamide with transitional cell carcinoma of the bladder, cystoscopy should be performed in all patients with unexplained hematuria in the setting of prior exposure to cyclophosphamide. The development of bladder cancer may occur even ten years after cyclophosphamide therapy, and so long-term bladder surveillance with regular urinalyses with microscopy is necessary.

Microscopic Polyangiitis

Microscopic polyangiitis (MPA) is a nongranulomatous necrotizing vasculitis affecting small-to-medium-sized blood vessels (arterioles, capillaries, and venules). Unlike PAN, MPA frequently presents with glomerulonephritis and pulmonary capillaritis and is commonly associated with circulating anti-neutrophil cytoplasmic antibodies (ANCA), typically in the perinuclear pattern (pANCA). MPA is more common than PAN, with an annual incidence ranging from 3.3 cases per million in the United Kingdom to 24 cases per million in Kuwait. Men are twice as likely to be affected as women, and the average age of onset is 50 years.

Pathology reveals a focal segmental necrotizing nongranulomatous small vessel vasculitis *without* prominent immune complex deposition. Medium-sized blood vessels are rarely involved. Kidney involvement is prominent in MPA, with segmental thrombosis, necrotizing glomerulonephritis, glomerular crescents, tubular damage, and interstitial infiltrates seen on renal biopsy. Active lesions may coexist with healed lesions.

Case Presentation 2

A previously healthy 52-year-old Caucasian male presents with a 3-month history of fevers to 39°C, fatigue, and malaise. He has also noted a cough productive of bloody sputum with accompanying dyspnea progressing over the previous three days. On examination, he appeared to be moderately uncomfortable, with a temperature of 38.8°C and a resting room air oxygen saturation of 93%. Auscultation of the lungs revealed scattered crackles bilaterally without wheezing. The remainder of his physical examination was unremarkable.

Laboratory evaluation was significant for a normochromic anemia, thrombocytosis, and erythrocyte sedimentation rate of 95 mm/h. Urinalysis revealed proteinuria and hematuria, and serum chemistries were notable for a creatinine of 1.6. Bilateral patchy alveolar infiltrates were found on chest X-ray. ANCA serology was positive in a perinuclear pattern. Renal biopsy demonstrated focal segmental necrotizing small vessel vasculitis, and the diagnosis of microscopic polyangiitis was made.

The patient was treated initially with intravenous methylprednisolone (1 g/d for 3 days) in conjunction with monthly intravenous cyclophosphamide. Maintenance oral corticosteroids (e.g., prednisone 1 mg/kg) were also initiated and slowly tapered when disease activity was brought under control. Cyclophosphamide was given monthly over the next year, during which time the patient achieved a sustained remission. Cyclophosphamide dosing was then tapered to every 3 months over the next year. During this time, the patient felt clinically well but was noted to have a recurrence of microscopic hematuria on routine follow-up urinalysis. Cystoscopy revealed hemorrhagic cystitis due to cyclophosphamide bladder toxicity.

This patient has microscopic polyangiitis with both pulmonary and renal involvement, which requires aggressive therapy with a combination of systemic corticosteroids and cyclophosphamide. Unlike PAN, relapse is common upon discontinuation of treatment or during the period of corticosteroid taper, and the hematuria noted upon follow-up evaluation may have been indicative of either disease relapse or an adverse treatment effect.

Clinical Features

The clinical onset of MPA is often insidious, with nonspecific symptoms such as fatigue, malaise, fever, myalgias, and arthralgias often preceding the diagnosis of vasculitis by months or longer.

Renal involvement, classically in the form of a rapidly progressive glomerulonephritis (RPGN), is seen in 90% of MPA cases. The urinalysis may show proteinuria, hematuria, and/or leukocyturia, and histopathology characteristically reveals a focal segmental necrotizing small vessel vasculitis.

In contrast to PAN, MPA frequently involves the lungs and is the most common cause of pulmonary-renal syndrome. (Other notable causes include SLE, Churg-Strauss syndrome, Wegener's granulomatosis, and Goodpasture's syndrome.) Pulmonary involvement occurs in approximately 50% of cases. Pulmonary capillaritis may lead to potentially life-threatening alveolar hemorrhage and hemoptysis in up to 29% of cases. Plain radiographs reveal alveolar shadowing in the absence of pulmonary edema or infection. Pulmonary small vessel vasculitis may also present clinically as an interstitial pneumonitis.

Palpable purpura is the most common cutaneous manifestation. Gastrointestinal symptoms include abdominal pain, hematemesis, and melena. Neurological manifestations are reported in about 30% of patients and include both peripheral and central nervous system involvement. Ear, nose, and throat involvement occurs in one third of patients and may include sore throat, oral ulcers, epistaxis, or sinusitis.

Diagnosis

More than 80% of patients with MPA are ANCA-positive, most often in a perinuclear pattern. Unlike PAN, MPA is not associated with HBV infection, and complement levels are usually normal. Evidence of renal involvement in the form of an elevated serum creatinine, microscopic hematuria, and proteinuria is common. Anemia and nonspecific markers of inflammation are also common.

Because MPA is characterized by small vessel disease, visceral angiography reveals microaneurysms in only a very small percentage of MPA patients; if microaneurysms are present, alternative diagnoses such as PAN should be strongly considered. Biopsy of clinically affected sites is recommended for diagnosis of MPA, typically the kidney, skin, sural nerve, or lung. Because of the prominence of RPGN in MPA, renal biopsy is important both diagnostically and prognostically.

Prognosis and Disease Outcomes

The prognosis of untreated MPA is poor, particularly in patients presenting with pulmonary hemorrhage. In patients with concomitant renal disease and pulmonary hemorrhage, there is a nine-fold increased risk of mortality when compared to patients with renal disease alone. Treatment with cyclophosphamide decreases the mortality five-fold when compared to treatment with corticosteroids alone (5). In individuals treated with various combinations of immunosuppressive agents, 5-year patient and kidney survival rates were 65% and 55%, respectively (6). The majority of deaths are attributed to active vasculitis complicated by renal failure or pulmonary hemorrhage and to the adverse effects of immunosuppressive and cytotoxic agents. Poor prognostic factors include age greater than 50 years and a serum creatinine greater than 4.5 mg/dL.

Management

Prompt diagnosis and treatment of MPA is crucial for optimal outcome. Rapid control of systemic inflammation and aggressive immunosuppression for induction of remission are essential management goals. The risk of relapse is significant, especially as corticosteroid and immunosuppressive therapy is withdrawn, and presents a major challenge in treatment.

Pharmacological Therapy

As with PAN, initial management of MPA with major organ involvement consists of high-dose corticosteroids (e.g., prednisone 1 mg/kg/d) in addition to intravenous or oral cyclophosphamide. Pulmonary hemorrhage is a life-threatening complication and should be immediately treated with "pulse" intravenous methylprednisolone (1 g/d for 3 days), cyclophosphamide, and possibly plasmapheresis. Hemodynamic and respiratory support and hemodialysis are often required, especially in the setting of fulminant MPA and pulmonary-renal failure.

Prompt treatment of glomerulonephritis with high-dose corticosteroids and cyclophosphamide induces remission in 80% of patients. Delay in treatment is a major contributor to poor renal and overall outcome. One third of patients relapse when treatment is discontinued or while corticosteroids are tapered; however, of these, two thirds can again promptly respond to the induction regimen.

In patients with MPA, no significant differences in patient survival, remission rate, time to remission, relapse rate, or outcome of renal function have been found between daily oral cyclophosphamide therapy and intermittent intravenous dosing (7). However, because oral administration (1.5-2 mg/kg/d) may be associated with increased risk of bladder toxicities, intermittent intravenous cyclophosphamide (0.5-0.75 g/m² monthly) has come into favor among many clinicians. Cyclophosphamide is generally continued monthly until a remission is achieved and maintained for at least one year, after which the dosing interval is slowly lengthened as dictated by continued clinical response. Alternatively, cyclophosphamide may be replaced by less toxic agents such as methotrexate or azathioprine to maintain disease control after it has been achieved. The recent CYCAZAREM trial has demonstrated that once a remission is induced by cyclophosphamide, azathioprine is as effective as cyclophosphosphamide in sustaining the remission (8).

Disease Monitoring

Unlike PAN, which is often a self-limited disease, MPA is generally chronic and persistent. Patients should be monitored for toxicity related to therapy, clinical response to therapy, or evidence suggesting disease relapse. Patients should be followed at least monthly while they are being treated with immunosuppressive agents. In particular, close clinical observation for disease relapse is critical during periods of dose reduction or discontinuation of immunosuppressive drugs. Moreover, because one third of patients with MPA relapse within the first two years after achieving remissions, close clinical follow-up during that period is exceptionally important (4). Monitoring should include thorough clinical evaluations, complete blood counts, markers of inflammation (ESR and CRP), serum electrolytes, renal and hepatic profiles, and urinalyses.

Hematuria may reflect either disease exacerbations or cyclophosphamide bladder toxicity (i.e., hemorrhagic cystitis or transitional cell carcinoma). Therefore cystoscopy should be performed in those patients previously or currently treated with cyclophosphamide who do not exhibit other signs or symptoms suggestive of active disease.

Mixed Cryoglobulinemia

Cryoglobulins are circulating immunoglobulins that precipitate at temperatures lower than 37°C. They can be monoclonal (arising from a single clone of genetically identical B cells) or polyclonal (several B cell populations interacting with different antigenic determinants of a specific antigen to produce a more generalized antibody response). Cryoglobulins are grouped into three categories: type 1 (composed of a single monoclonal immunoglobulin), type 2 (characterized by immune complexes of monoclonal IgM with anti-IgG rheumatoid factor activity and polyclonal IgG), and type 3 (immune complexes of polyclonal IgM with rheumatoid factor activity and polyclonal IgG). Accordingly, types 2 and 3 are considered *mixed cryoglobulins*. Mixed cryoglobulins lead to vasculitis through the deposition of immune complexes that in turn activate complement and trigger vascular inflammation. Cryoglobulinemic vasculitis predominantly affects small vessels.

Pathogenesis

Several factors are hypothesized to contribute to the pathogenesis of cryoglobulinemia: genetic susceptibility, superantigen properties of infectious agents, prolonged antigenic stimulation, cross-reactivity of various antigens, activation of proto-oncogenes, polyclonal activation of B lymphocytes, and decreased clearance of circulating immune complexes (9).

Several infectious agents have been associated with cryoglobulins, notably hepatotropic viruses. Over 90% of cases of mixed cryoglobulinemia (MC) are related to chronic hepatitis C virus (HCV) infection, but the exact pathogenic role of HCV is unclear. The incidence of MC is associated with the duration of HCV infection and is highest in patients that have been infected for 20 or more years. Although mixed cryoglobulinemia can be found in over 50% of individuals infected with HCV, the prevalence of active vasculitis is lower. Therefore the detection of mixed cryoglobulins in the serum does not necessarily indicate the presence of vasculitis. Additional conditions associated with cryoglobulin production are listed in Table 12-2.

Cryoglobulinemia has also been associated with several collagen vascular diseases as well as myeloproliferative and lymphoproliferative disorders. Sixteen percent of patients with primary Sjögren's syndrome have circulating cryoglobulins, particularly those patients with extraglandular disease. When present in systemic lupus erythematosus, cryoglobulinemia is related to disease severity and activity, particularly nephritis and hypocomplementemia. Cryoglobulinemia in rheumatoid arthritis correlates with disease severity and the presence of Felty's syndrome. Myeloproliferative and lymphoproliferative diseases associated with cryoglobulinemia include

---

Table 12-2   Conditions Associated with Cryoglobulins

Infections	Collagen Vascular Diseases
• Hepatitic C virus	• Systemic lupus erythematosus
• Hepatitis B virus	• Sjögren's syndrome
• Varicella zoster virus	• Rheumatoid arthritis/Felty's syndrome
• Cytomegalovirus	Myoproliferative Disorders
• Parvovirus B19	• Non-Hodgkin's lymphoma
• Influenza virus	• Multiple myeloma
• Epstein-Barr virus	• Waldenström's macroglobulinemia
• Bacterial endocarditis	• Chronic myeloid leukemia
• Rikettsial diseases	• Chronic lymphocytic leukemia
• Syphilis	
• Human immunodeficiency virus	

non-Hodgkin's lymphoma, multiple myeloma, Waldenström's macroglobulinemia, chronic myeloid leukemia, and chronic lymphocytic leukemia.

Case Presentation 3

A 55-year-old Caucasian male presents with 3 months of fevers to 39°C, fatigue, malaise, polyarthralgias, and rash on both of his legs. His medical history is notable for chronic hepatitis C virus infection contracted via blood transfusion 22 years ago. On examination, the patient had a temperature of 37.8°C, and palpable purpura was present over the lower extremities. The remainder of the physical examination was unremarkable. Laboratory evaluation was significant for a normochromic anemia, thrombocytosis, mildly elevated serum transaminases, and an erythrocyte sedimentation rate of 65 mm/h. Complement component C4 was low; ANCA was negative. Urinalysis was normal. Circulating cryoglobulins were detected, but immunoelectrophoresis revealed no monoclonal band. Skin biopsy was consistent with a leukocytoclastic vasculitis.

The diagnosis of type 3 mixed cryoglobulinemic vasculitis was made, and the patient was treated with a combination of interferon-alpha (3 million U three times weekly) and ribavirin (1200 mg daily) for 18 months. He did well, with resolution of his skin lesions, normalization of complement levels, decrease in circulating cryoglobulins, and elimination of HCV RNA. His disease relapsed 6 months after discontinuation of treatment, but he responded well to a repeat course of combination anti-viral therapy.

Clinical Features

Constitutional symptoms (fever, fatigue, and weakness), palpable purpura, and arthralgias are the most common presenting features of MC. Cryoglobulinemia is the most common cause of palpable purpura in adults. Frank arthritis occurs in only 9% of cases and is non-erosive.

Renal involvement is seen in up to 40% of cases. Cryoglobulinemic glomerulonephritis (most often a membranoproliferative glomerulonephritis) is almost exclusively found in type 2 cryoglobulinemia. In addition, vasculitis of small and medium-sized renal arteries occurs in about one third of patients with cryoglobulinemic glomerulonephritis, presenting as an acute nephritic syndrome or occasionally as rapidly progressive renal insufficiency and oliguria.

Liver involvement occurs in up to two thirds of patients. It is generally asymptomatic but can slowly progress to cirrhosis in a minority of cases. Gastrointestinal involvement may present as nonspecific abdominal pain, hematemesis, hematochezia, diarrhea, or intestinal infarction.

Peripheral neuropathy is seen in one third of patients and may be due to vasculitis of the vasa nervorum, immunologically mediated demyelination, hyperviscosity, or microcirculatory (i.e., capillary) occlusion. Central nervous system involvement can take the form of stroke, cerebral vasculitis, diffuse encephalopathy, or cranial neuropathy (e.g., hearing loss).

Diagnosis

Cryoglobulins are detected by incubating venous blood at 37°C for 2 hours to allow coagulation, after which the serum is removed and kept at 4°C for 96 hours in order to precipitate cryoproteins. Precipitates are quantified as the cryocrit (percent per volume) or as the protein concentration (mg/L). Cryoprecipitates can then be assayed by immunoelectrophoresis or immunofixation for the detection of polyclonal and monoclonal components. There is no correlation between cryocrit and disease severity.

Anti-HCV antibodies are found in over 90% of patients with MC, and HCV RNA is detected in 85%. HCV serologic testing should be obtained in all patients with cryoglobulinemic vasculitis. Circulating rheumatoid factors are found in over 70% of patients.

Hypocomplementemia is seen in 90% of cases and helps to distinguish cryoglobulinemic vasculitis from ANCA-associated vasculitides (which are usually normo- or hyper-complementemic). C4 levels are usually very low at baseline, whereas C3 levels tend to fluctuate with disease activity.

Histopathology of the purpuric skin lesions typically reveals leukocytoclastic vasculitis, an immune complex-mediated inflammation with prominent polymorphonuclear cell infiltration and "nuclear dust" in post-capillary venules.

Prognosis and Disease Outcomes

Although treatment with antiviral agents such as interferon-alpha (IFN-α) eliminates HCV RNA in 30% to 60% of patients, decreases cryoglobulinemia, and normalizes complement levels, the relapse rates are as high as 90% once therapy is discontinued. Long-term responses in patients with cryoglobulinemic vasculitis are achieved in no more than 22% of cases, and these agents are not associated with sustained elimination of HCV RNA. HCV genotype 1b has been associated with a less favorable response to IFN-α and a worse overall outcome in HCV-associated cryoglobulinemic vasculitis. Factors predictive of a good response to IFN-α include male sex and HCV genotypes 2 or 3. The main cause of morbidity is progressive glomerulonephritis.

Management

The clinical presentations of mixed cryoglobulinemia can be quite variable, ranging from mild musculoskeletal symptoms to life-threatening visceral organ involvement. Therefore the appropriate potency of therapy requires full appreciation of the extent and severity of disease. A distinct challenge in the treatment of mixed cryoglobulinemia is the enhanced risk of progressive HCV viremia during immunosuppressive therapy.

Pharmacological Therapy

Mild disease with arthralgias or purpura can usually be treated with brief courses of nonsteroidal anti-inflammatory drugs or low-dose corticosteroids (e.g., prednisone ≤20 mg daily). However, severe visceral organ involvement or rapidly progressive illness with deterioration of end-organ function in patients with HCV-related MC requires high-dose systemic corticosteroids in conjunction with aggressive immunosuppression using cyclophosphamide (10). Plasmapheresis or cryofiltration may be also added as adjunctive therapy in deteriorating clinical situations, especially in cases with progressive neurological disease or a rapidly progressive glomerulonephritis. Methotrexate and azathioprine are reasonable alternatives to cyclophosphamide in less severe cases.

However, although immunosuppressive therapies are often required to aggressively suppress inflammation and to prevent end-organ damage, they increase the risk of progressive viremia and generally do not induce long-term remissions. Therefore immunosuppressive approaches have been more recently superceded by the use of IFN-α as the treatment of choice in HCV-associated mixed cryoglobulinemic vasculitis and are seen more as temporary therapeutic bridges until the effects of IFN-α are realized. The clinical benefits of IFN-α in mixed cryoglobulinemia are thought to be due to its antiviral action rather than its immunomodulatory effects. Reduction of the viral load is believed to diminish the antigenic stimulus driving the inflammatory process and is manifested by decreased cryoglobulinemia and normalized complement levels. IFN-α is given as a subcutaneous injection of 3 million units three times per week. As a single agent, IFN-α is efficacious in treating skin manifestations in most patients but does not demonstrate a clear efficacy on nerve or kidney involvement. Initial biochemical, virological, and immunological (i.e., reduced cryoglobulinemia) improvement to IFN-α is seen in up to 73% of patients with mixed cryoglobulinemia (11). However, sustained remission of vasculitis following a year-long course of IFN-α is achieved in no more than 22% of patients after discontinuation of therapy (12). The benefit of longer regimens of IFN-α is under investigation. In some patients with HCV-related MC who have failed IFN-α, ribavirin (1000-1200 mg daily in divided oral doses) can be effective (13).

Recent data, however, suggest that improved responses can be obtained with concomitant IFN-α and ribavirin therapy in the treatment of joint, skin, and kidney disease, although neuropathy may remain relatively resistant to treatment (14,15). Combination therapy with IFN-α and ribavirin must be continued for at least 18 to 24 months, and side effects are common. Flu-like symptoms occur in over 50% of patients. Hematologic effects such as hemolytic anemia, leukopenia, and thrombocytopenia may necessitate dosage adjustments. Adverse psychiatric effects such as depression are the most common cause for discontinuation of treatment.

Cryoglobulinemic vasculitis associated with infectious endocarditis or other bacterial infections requires appropriate antibiotic therapy, and the role of concomitant immunosuppression is controversial. In cases secondary to lymphoproliferative or myeloproliferative diseases or due to connective tissue diseases, treatment of the underlying condition is required to control the vasculitis. Plasmapheresis may improve severe cryoglobulinemic vasculitis in these cases.

Disease Monitoring

Patients should be monitored for toxicity related to therapy, clinical response to therapy, or evidence suggesting disease relapse. In addition to thorough clinical evaluations, complete blood counts (CBC), levels of acute phase reactants (ESR and CRP), electrolytes, renal and hepatic profiles, and urinalyses should be examined on a monthly basis during the course of treatment and when an increased level of disease activity is suspected. Because of potential myelosuppression, a baseline CBC should be obtained before the start of IFN-α or ribavirin therapy and at weeks 2 and 4 after the onset of treatment. Thyroid function testing should be performed at baseline and repeated intermittently during treatment with IFN-α because of an increased risk of autoimmune thyroiditis. Patients with cardiovascular disease receiving IFN-α should have electrocardiograms and echocardiograms before and periodically during therapy because of potential cardiac toxicities such as hypotension, arrhythmias, and a reversible cardiomyopathy. Viremia and cryoglobulinemia typically recur once antiviral therapy is discontinued, resulting in clinical relapse. Disease exacerbations after withdrawal of antiviral therapies can be treated with additional courses of combination antiviral therapy.

REFERENCES

1. **Ewald EA, Griffin D, McCune WJ.** Correlation of angiographic abnormalities with disease manifestations and disease severity in polyarteritis nodosa. J Rheumatol. 1987;14:952-6.

2. **Fortin PR, Larson MG, Watters AK, et al.** Prognostic factors in systemic necrotizing vasculitis of the polyarteritis nodosa group: a review of 45 cases. J Rheumatol. 1995;22:78-84.

3. **Gayraud M, Guillevin L, le Toumelin P, et al.** Long-term follow-up of polyarteritis nodosa, microscopic polyangiitis, and Churg-Strauss syndrome: analysis of four prospective trials including 278 patients. Arthritis Rheum. 2001;44:666-75.

4. **Guillevin L, Lhote F.** Treatment of polyarteritis nodosa and microscopic polyangiitis. Arthritis Rheum. 1998;41:2100-5.

5. **Hogan SL, Nachman PH, Wilkman AS, et al.** Prognostic markers in patients with antineutrophil cytoplasmic autoantibody-associated microscopic polyangiitis and glomerulonephritis. J Am Soc Nephrol. 1996;7:23-32.

6. **Savage CO, Winearls CG, Evans DJ, et al.** Microscopic polyarteritis: presentation, pathology and prognosis. Q J Med. 1985;56:467-83.

7. **Haubitz M, Schellong S, Gobel U, et al.** Intravenous pulse administration of cyclophosphamide versus daily oral treatment in patients with antineutrophil cytoplasmic antibody-associated vasculitis and renal involvement: a prospective, randomized study. Arthritis Rheum. 1998;41:1835-44.

8. **Jayne D, Rasmussen N, Andrassy K, et al.** A randomized trial of maintenance therapy for vasculitis associated with antineutrophil cytoplasmic antibodies. N Engl J Med. 2003;349:36-44.

9. **Ferri C, La Civita L, Longombardo G, et al.** Mixed cryoglobulinaemia: a crossroad between autoimmune and lymphoproliferative disorders. Lupus. 1998;7:275-9.

10. **Lamprecht P, Gause A, Gross WL.** Cryoglobulinemic vasculitis. Arthritis Rheum. 1999;42:2507-16.

11. **Ramos-Casals M, Trejo O, Garcia-Carrasco M, et al.** Mixed cryoglobulinemia: new concepts. Lupus. 2000;9:83-91.

12. **Adinolfi LE, Utilit R, Zampino R, et al.** Effects of long-term course of alpha-interferon in patients with chronic hepatitis C associated mixed cryoglobulinaemia. Eur J Gastroenterol Hepatol. 1997;9:1067-72.

13. **Durand J-M, Cacub P, Lunel-Faiani F, et al.** Ribavirin in hepatitis C related cryoglobulinemia. J Rheumatol. 1998;25:115-7.

14. **Zuckerman E, Keren D, Slobodin G, et al.** Treatment of refractory, symptomatic, hepatitis C virus related mixed cryoglobulinemia with ribavirin and interferon-alpha. J Rheumatol. 2000;27:2172-8.

15. **Cacoub P, Costedoat-Chalumeau N, Lidove O, Alric L.** Cryoglobulinemia vasculitis. Curr Opin Rheumatol. 2002;14:29-35.

13

Wegener's Granulomatosis and Churg-Strauss Syndrome: ANCA-Associated Vasculitides

Eduardo Wainstein, MD

egener's granulomatosis (WG) and Churg-Strauss syndrome (CSS) are two systemic necrotizing vasculitides that share some pathological features that separate them from other vasculitic diseases. They affect medium and sometimes small arteries; feature granulomatous inflammatory changes; have strong predilections for lung involvement; and are associated with anti-neutrophil cytoplasmic antibodies (ANCA). However, there are important differences between the two. WG stereotypically involves the upper airways, the lower respiratory tract, and the kidneys. On the other hand, CSS is distinct in its strong association with asthma, allergic rhinitis, and marked circulating and tissue eosinophilia.

Wegener's Granulomatosis

WG is a systemic vasculitis characterized by necrotizing granulomatous inflammation of small and medium arteries. WG classically involves the upper and lower respiratory tract and kidneys, but significant involvement of other organ systems can also exist. The prevalence of WG is three to five cases per 100,000. It can occur at any age but usually presents during adulthood (mean age of onset around 40 years). Men and women are equally affected.

Pathogenesis

Although the etiology of WG is still largely unexplained, a better comprehension of its pathogenesis became apparent when a strong association between the presence of ANCA and WG was described in the 1980s. Screening for ANCA is normally performed by indirect immunofluorescence, which can identify two main patterns of fluorescence: perinuclear staining (pANCA) and granular cytoplasmic staining (cANCA). These two patterns differ in their clinical associations: cANCA is more consistently associated with WG, whereas pANCA has been observed in a wide variety of diseases, including microscopic polyangiitis, CSS, and idiopathic crescentic glomerulonephritis, among many others (Table 13-1). The two ANCA patterns also differ with regard to antigen specificity. The principal antigen associated with cANCA is proteinase 3 (PR3). In contrast, pANCA is associated with several antigens, of which myeloperoxidase has been the best characterized.

PR3 is a neutral serine protease, normally stored in the primary granules of neutrophils and monocytes. Upon cell activation, PR3 is translocated to the outer cell membrane layer, where it is exposed to the extracellular milieu. If circulating anti-PR3 antibodies (i.e., cANCA) are present, the antibody-antigen interaction that ensues on the cell surface brings about several changes in the cell, which result in fueling of the inflammatory response: a respiratory burst with production of free oxygen radicals, increased influx of calcium, degranulation of primary and secondary granules with the release of several enzymes potentially hazardous to the endothelium, upregulation of adhesion molecules on the cell surface, and release of pro-inflammatory cytokines (1).

It is likely that immunological mechanisms other than those involving ANCA contribute to the development of WG. One important observation is that tumor necrosis factor (TNF)-α expression is elevated in active WG. Because TNF-α is capable of inducing the translocation and expression of

Table 13-1   Anti-Neutrophil Cytoplasmic Antibody (ANCA)-Associated Diseases

Disease	Frequency (%)	
	cANCA	pANCA
Wegener's granulomatosis	>90	<5
Microscopic polyangiitis	<20	40-85
Polyarteritis nodosa	<10	<10
Churg-Strauss syndrome	<5	75
Giant cell arteritis	<2	<2
Takayasu's arteritis	<2	<2
Goodpasture's disease	12	25
Ulcerative colitis	<2	60-80
Crohn's disease	<2	10-27

cANCA = cytoplasmic ANCA; pANCA = perinuclear ANCA.

PR3 on the cell surface of neutrophils and monocytes, this finding suggests that TNF-α may play a pivotal role in the pathogenesis of WG and may be an attractive target for therapeutic intervention with anti-TNF-α agents.

Case Presentation 1

A 55-year-old previously healthy woman presented with 3 months of progressive malaise, low-grade fever, rhinorrhea, earache, and discharge from the ears. Treatment with multiple courses of antibiotics for presumed bacterial sinusitis and otitis media brought about no improvement. In fact, the patient began complaining of a dry cough and mild dyspnea with exertion. Laboratory analysis revealed a leukocytosis, thrombocytosis, and an elevated sedimentation rate (ESR). Renal function (serum creatinine 1.0 mg/dL) and routine urinalysis were normal. Multiple pulmonary nodules and diffuse interstitial infiltrates were seen on a routine chest X-ray (Figure 13-1) and were confirmed by high-resolution computed tomography. Serologic testing for ANCA was strongly positive in a cytoplasmic pattern. An open lung biopsy demonstrated necrotizing granulomatous vasculitis of the small and medium-sized arteries consistent with WG. Stains and cultures for acid-fast bacilli and fungi were negative.

Daily oral prednisone (1 mg/kg) was initiated, as well as oral methotrexate 10 mg/wk, with gradual escalation to 20 mg/wk. Significant clinical and laboratory improvement was observed within the first month, and the pulmonary nodules disappeared. Serum cANCA levels became negative.

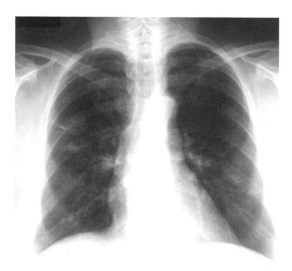

Figure 13-1   Anteroposterior chest X-ray of a patient with Wegener's granulomatosis demonstrates bilateral interstitial nodules and infiltrates. All of these changes steadily resolved after the start of corticosteroid and immunosuppressive therapy.

The prednisone was tapered off steadily over several months, and methotrexate was maintained for 2 years before being discontinued.

Three months after cessation of methotrexate therapy, the patient developed a recurrence of fever, otitis media, and lower respiratory symptoms. Chest X-ray showed reappearance of pulmonary nodules. Urinalysis revealed red cell casts, and the serum creatinine was 1.7 mg/dL. High-dose prednisone was restarted along with oral cyclophosphamide 2 mg/kg/d. Complete resolution of symptoms and laboratory abnormalities were observed after 6 weeks. Prednisone was again tapered, and cyclophosphamide was maintained for 6 months before being replaced with a maintenance therapy of oral azathioprine 2 mg/kg/d, which the patient continued for more than 1 year with no evidence of active disease.

In this case of WG, the kidneys were initially spared, and systemic corticosteroids for rapid control of inflammation and methotrexate for immunosuppression were chosen as treatments of choice. Cyclophosphamide, which carries greater toxicities, was not introduced until the appearance of renal involvement, which demands cytotoxic therapy. Once sustained control of disease was achieved, maintenance therapy with azathioprine was used to replace cyclophosphamide in order to minimize toxicities.

Clinical Features

Although WG has a predilection for involving the upper and lower respiratory tract and the kidneys, the disease can affect many organs either simultaneously or in an additive fashion over time. The ELK (where E is ear/nose/throat, L is lung, and K is kidney) classification system has been used historically to help stratify WG into a limited form in which there is no renal involvement and a generalized form in which the kidneys are affected. However, although perhaps useful for clinical studies, the ELK classification system is not as relevant in clinical practice, and it gives the impression that localized disease may not be severe and thus not warrant aggressive intervention. In fact, upper or lower respiratory tract involvement can be quite devastating, if not organ- or life-threatening. Moreover, involvement of other organs such as the nervous system will also merit aggressive treatment.

Most patients will exhibit signs and symptoms indicative of a systemic inflammatory process. These commonly include fever, fatigue, anorexia, and weight loss. An anemia of chronic disease, leukocytosis, thrombocytosis, an elevated ESR and elevations in plasma C-reactive protein (CRP) also reflect systemic inflammation. More specific manifestations reflect the variety of organ systems that may be affected.

Ear, Nose, and Throat Manifestations
92% of patients with WG will have ear, nose, and throat involvement, normally presenting with ear and/or sinus disease in the form of a non-resolving otitis media and sinusitis. Painful, crusty, and bleeding ulcers of nasal

mucosa are not uncommon. Nasal deformity secondary to necrosis of the nasal septum may lead to a saddle nose deformity. Ear involvement can often lead to permanent hearing loss.

Upper and Lower Respiratory Tract Involvement

Granulomatous inflammation of the trachea is not uncommon and may eventually lead to scarring and stenosis. Subglottic stenosis is a complication with increased morbidity and mortality and may require an endotracheal prosthesis to maintain a patent airway. Lower respiratory tract involvement may involve lungs and pleural tissue and is found in 85% of patients. This may take the form of interstitial infiltrates, pulmonary nodules (see Figure 13-1), hemoptysis or pleuritis, and its presentation can vary from an asymptomatic X-ray finding to life-threatening hemoptysis and respiratory compromise. The most characteristic radiological finding is multiple nodules that can vary in size and location and cavitate, simulating a neoplasm or infection. The cavitary lesions themselves may become super-infected with bacterial pathogens. Extensive infiltrates may reflect parenchymal bleeding due to capillaritis. This is accompanied by a decrease in the hematocrit and elevation in the serum lactate dehydrogenase.

Renal Manifestations

Forty percent of patients with WG will have renal involvement at presentation, and as many as 75% of patients will develop renal involvement at some point in the evolution of the disease. The most common form of renal disease is a focal segmental glomerulonephritis, which is not associated with the deposition of immunoglobulins and immune complexes in the glomeruli (i.e., pauci-immune glomerulonephritis). A crescentic glomerulonephritis with a clinical picture of a rapidly progressive renal insufficiency has been described in WG but is not common. Interstitial granulomatous infiltration is seldom reported and probably accounts for no more than 1% of renal findings in WG.

Ocular Manifestations

The intraocular and orbital structures are involved in approximately 50% of cases. Proptosis, occurring in as many as 15% of patients, can result from granulomatous involvement of orbital tissue (resembling an inflammatory pseudotumor) or extension of purulent sinusitis; it is more commonly unilateral but can be bilateral. The eye itself can be affected in its different layers. Scleral involvement is common and presents as an episcleritis that can eventually lead to scleromalacia and perforation. Anterior chamber uveitis and retinal vasculitis are less common manifestations.

Neurological Manifestations

Peripheral nervous system disease in the form of mononeuritis multiplex or axonal sensory-motor polyneuropathy occurs in 15% of patients. Small vessel inflammation with involvement of the vasa nervorum results in ischemia of peripheral nerves. Central nervous system involvement is less common (less than 10%), presenting as focal mass lesions, pachymeningitis, infarcts, or hemorrhages.

Cardiac Manifestations

Pericarditis and vasculitis of the coronary arteries are uncommon complications, occurring in less than 5% of patients with WG.

Cutaneous Manifestations

Cutaneous lesions are common, most frequently presenting as palpable purpura secondary to leukocytoclastic vasculitis. Skin ulcers and nodules can occur in WG with histologic specimens demonstrating lobular panniculitis with necrotizing vasculitis. Although uncommon, necrotizing granulomas can be observed in skin biopsies.

Musculoskeletal Manifestations

Diffuse symmetric polyarthralgias and polymyalgias are common and initially may resemble those of other systemic inflammatory diseases such as rheumatoid arthritis. Joint involvement, however, is non-erosive.

Diagnosis

The diagnosis of WG is made on a clinical basis with support from laboratory, radiological, and pathological data. WG should be thought of when a patient presents with refractory upper and/or lower respiratory tract inflammation with prominent constitutional systemic symptoms and especially when seen in the context of active renal disease. In addition to WG, some other notable inflammatory conditions that can present with prominent involvement of both the lungs and the kidneys include systemic lupus erythematosus, Goodpasture's syndrome, microscopic polyangiitis, and CSS.

ANCA Testing

Several studies have estimated the sensitivity of cANCA testing in WG to be 80% to 90%, whereas the specificity is 90% to 95%, with the likelihood of a positive test dependent upon the extent and activity of disease. The utility of ANCA testing in WG has been analyzed systematically for different clinical scenarios (2). As with any other diagnostic test, the positive predictive value (PPV) depends on the prevalence of the disease in the population in question. In a patient with only sinusitis and a positive cANCA, the PPV for the diagnosis of WG is only 7%, whereas the PPV is 45% in a patient with pulmonary findings. In a patient with respiratory disease and glomerulonephritis, a positive cANCA has a PPV of 98%. Overall, the PPV of a positive cANCA in WG (for active or inactive, localized or generalized disease) is 63%, suggesting that this is a good but imperfect diagnostic test and should always be placed in the context of the clinical picture. The only means to increase the PPV of a test is to increase the pre-test probability, by obtaining a thorough clinical history and physical examination.

Tissue Biopsy

The pathognomonic histopathology of WG is necrotizing granulomatous vasculitis of small and medium sized vessels. However, the yield of obtaining a definitive pathological diagnosis is highly dependent on the site and means of obtaining tissue. Biopsies from the upper respiratory tract are commonly obtained because of convenience and relative safety, but the diagnositic yield is dismally low. In an analysis of 158 WG patients, vasculitis with necrosis was found in only 23% of specimens, granulomas with vasculitis in 21%, and vasculitis in 16%.

Because of relative ease and safety, the kidneys are also often biopsied, but histological findings are usually non-specific. A pauci-immune focal segmental glomerulonephritis is the most common finding. Granulomas are reported in no more than 1% of renal biopsies. However, although less useful for diagnosis, renal biopsies may be helpful prognostically. A recent analysis of 157 patients with vasculitis found that the number of normal glomeruli at the time of biopsy was the best predictor of response to therapy. A renal biopsy is probably most useful when documentation of the absence or presence of kidney involvement aids in deciding whether to use cytotoxic or less potent therapies.

Open lung biopsy, usually done by mini-thoracotomy or video thoracoscopy, offers the best chance for specific diagnosis. The yield for histological findings indicative of WG from open lung biopsies is over 90%. In contrast, less invasive sampling by a transbronchial approach has a diagnostic yield of less than 10%.

Clearly, when there is significant question as to the diagnosis, tissue biopsy is an essential step in arriving at a more definitive answer. However, even in a situation where WG appears as the obvious diagnosis based on the clinical presentation and a positive cANCA, there are still many reasons to confirm the diagnosis histologically. Since appropriate therapy for WG normally takes the form of potent immunosuppression, exclusion of an atypical infection or a neoplastic process is important. Moreover, in a chronic disease like WG that is characterized by frequent relapses and potentially high morbidity, having a definitive diagnosis is reassuring to the physician and to the patient and would minimize confusion as the illness evolves. Lastly, as noted in the above discussion, useful prognostic information may be obtained with kidney biopsies. Nonetheless, it must be stressed that treatment should never be delayed when facing organ- or life-threatening situations even when the histologic diagnosis is unproven or unavailable. In fact, it is often the case that the diagnosis of WG is made clinically without a biopsy but supported by cANCA testing and treated accordingly, particularly in dire clinical situations when biopsies are not deemed safe or when awaiting the results of biopsies before treatment is imprudent.

Prognosis

The prognosis of WG is greatly dependent on the extent of organ involvement at the time of diagnosis. In patients presenting with renal disease or severe pulmonary disease, the prognosis *without* treatment is over 80% mortality within 1 year and nearly 100% within 2 years. The advent of systemic corticosteroid therapy only marginally improved prognosis. It was not until the introduction of cyclophosphamide immunosuppressive therapy in the 1970s that significant therapeutic strides towards achieving extended periods of disease remission were made, leading to 5-year survival rates of over 85%. Nonetheless, relapse rates remain high, ranging from 50% to 60%, and increased survival rates have unmasked adverse effects associated with therapies, particularly infections and malignancies associated with cyclophosphamide use. Data on limited disease are less clear because these cases can remain undiagnosed for many years. In one review, more than 20% of cases were diagnosed over 2 years after the onset of symptoms that were interpreted as chronic sinusitis, otitis, or asthma. This suggests significant variability in disease expression and progression.

With improved prognosis, the current challenge is to prevent disease relapses and to reduce morbidity associated with therapies.

Management

Assessing the extent and severity of WG is mandatory in order to optimally guide treatment options. In addition to a thorough clinical evaluation and routine laboratory testing, chest radiography, pulmonary function testing, and 24-hour urine studies for protein and creatinine clearance should be obtained at baseline. The goals of therapy are to rapidly control active inflammation, induce a remission of disease, and maintain the remission. In general, inflammation is initially reined with the use of systemic corticosteroids. At the same time, immunosuppressive therapy, the potency of which is determined by the breadth and severity of organ involvement, is instituted to induce remission. Once remission is achieved and sustained (typically for 6 to 12 months), an alternative, less toxic immunosuppressant is employed to maintain the remission.

Pharmacological Therapy

Initial therapy for WG typically requires corticosteroid therapy for rapid control of inflammation and a second agent for chronic immunosuppression. A "standard treatment" regimen is oral prednisone 1 mg/kg/d (or equivalent) and oral cyclophosphamide (2 mg/kg/d) (3). An initial intravenous "pulse" of methylprednisolone (1 g/d for 3 days) may be administered for more immediate and aggressive control of rapidly progressive disease. High-dose corticosteroids are maintained for at least 1 month while the disease is stabilized. The dose of cyclophosphamide is adjusted to maintain a leukocyte count of no less than 3000/mm³ and an absolute neutrophil count of no less than 1500/mm³. The corticosteroids are then slowly tapered, usually over the course of months according to the response of the individual patient, with the goal of eventually maintaining the patient on cyclophosphamide only. If a remission can be continued for more than a year without corticosteroids, then the dose of cyclophosphamide can be slowly tapered.

Variations from the "standard treatment" have been studied to reduce the frequency of relapses, to minimize adverse effects associated with oral cyclophosphamide, and to tailor therapy to the severity of disease (4). For example, one scheme is an induction/consolidation approach similar to that used in the treatment of malignant neoplasms. The recent CYCAZAREM trial showed that a protocol with high-dose corticosteroids plus oral cyclophosphamide for 3 to 6 months, followed by a corticosteroid taper and replacement of cyclophosphamide with oral azathioprine for up to 18 months, can induce and maintain disease remissions as well as traditional schedules (5). Alternatively, monthly intravenous cyclophosphamide may be as effective in inducing remissions as, and associated with fewer adverse effects than, oral cyclophosphamide. Although there appears to be a greater likelihood of relapses in patients treated intravenously, these relapses are usually not severe and are generally controlled readily with retreatment.

For cases of WG that do not involve the kidneys or severe pulmonary disease, much attention has been given to immunosuppressive agents other than cyclophosphamide. Methotrexate initially showed encouraging responses in the subgroup of patients with non-life-threatening clinical manifestations and moderately impaired renal function (serum creatinine <2 mg/dL) (6,7). Oral methotrexate given at 20 to 25 mg weekly doses was as effective as cyclophosphamide in inducing remissions. However, this initial enthusiasm has been tempered by high relapse rates ranging from 27% to 50% in different series. Nonetheless, because of its relative safety, methotrexate should still be considered in selected patients with localized non-life-threatening disease. Newer immunosuppressive agents such as leflunomide and mycophenolate mofetil have also shown promise in small studies but will require more extensive investigation in larger trials to determine their utility in WG.

Biological therapy using anti-TNF-α agents in WG has been studied in two open label studies (8,9). Significant clinical improvement was observed. Preliminary data suggest that relapses were common with etanercept therapy but less so with infliximab. Multicenter trials are currently assessing the efficacy of these agents in prospective randomized studies.

Trimethoprim/sulfamethoxazole has been reported to be of benefit in certain patients with mild WG. It has been conjectured that chronic carriage of *Staphylococcus aureus* may trigger exacerbations of WG, leading to the thought that antimicrobial agents may be useful to reduce the antigenic stimulus. One relatively large study showed that trimethoprim/sulfamethoxazole maintained disease remissions induced by immunosuppressive agents in patients with limited upper respiratory tract disease (10). However, although trimethoprim/sulfamethoxazole may be considered for the treatment of mild nasal disease, it is not recommended for treatment of active disease elsewhere.

Disease Monitoring

There are no absolutely reliable laboratory tests that correlate with disease activity. Although indicators of active systemic inflammation such as ESR elevations, thrombocytosis, or increased levels of CRP may be useful markers on a case-to-case basis, there is no substitute for close clinical observation. Monitoring for signs and symptoms of renal dysfunction is particularly important because these may be quite insidious, asymptomatic, and rapid. Although cANCA levels were initially thought to correlate closely with disease exacerbations, more recent data suggest that elevations in cANCA titers predicted disease flares in only one-fourth of patients. So, although increases in cANCA titers may prompt closer observation, they should be considered in the context of the overall clinical picture and should not reflexively lead to more aggressive intervention. Conversely, normal or stable levels of cANCA should never lull the clinician into a false sense of security when the clinical picture suggests a possible exacerbation of WG.

Churg-Strauss Syndrome

Churg-Strauss syndrome, also known as allergic granulomatous angiitis and allergic granulomatosis, is a systemic necrotizing vasculitis of unknown etiology, associated with profound peripheral and tissue eosinophilia, asthma, and/or allergic rhinitis. Although originally considered to be a subgroup of polyarteritis nodosa, the classic pathological triad of tissue eosinophilia, extravascular granulomata, and necrotizing vasculitis of small to medium size vessels was defined by Churg and Strauss in 1951 as the distinct clinical entity that now bears their names (11).

CSS is a rare disease even among the systemic vasculitides. In a recent Spanish report, it represented only 3% of all diagnoses of vasculitis. There appears to be no strong racial or age predilection, although a slight predominance in males has been shown by some. The estimated annual incidence varies from 2.4 to 18 cases per million. The annual incidence is higher in patients with asthma.

Pathogenesis

The etiology of CSS is largely unknown. A relationship with inhaled allergens has been sought, but only indirect evidence is currently available to support this hypothesis. The recent observation of CSS associated with the use of leukotriene inhibitors (zafirlukast) in asthma is intriguing. A recent National Institutes of Health workshop conjectured that the withdrawal of corticosteroids after the initiation of leukotriene inhibitor therapy might exacerbate previously unrecognized and smoldering underlying CSS (12). Although more than two-thirds of patients with CSS may have circulating pANCA, no correlations with activity or specific clinical features have been demonstrated in these individuals. At present, a significant pathogenic role for ANCA in CSS has not yet been identified.

Recently, elevated levels of soluble CD95 have been described in a group of patients with CSS (13). It is well established that that CD95 mediates efficient apoptosis of eosinophils, and so the competitive inhibition of CD95 by soluble CD95 may result in the increased survival of eosinophils and the hypereosinophilia characteristic of CSS. Overexpression of soluble CD95 is associated with oligoclonal T cell expansion, suggesting that specific antigens are involved in the stimulation of specific T cell clones. Collectively, these findings implicate exogenous agents (e.g., inhaled antigens, vaccinations, desensitization therapies) as potential triggers for the development of CSS.

Case Presentation 2

A 42-year-old man presents with fever, cough, and progressive shortness of breath. The patient had a 6-year history of allergic rhinitis and asthma, managed primarily with inhaled bronchodilators and corticosteroids, but occasionally requiring short courses of systemic corticosteroids. Two months before the current illness, he developed a low-grade fever, non-productive cough, and progressive dyspnea at rest. Multiple courses of antibiotics were not helpful. He improved slightly with low-dose prednisone, but the symptoms recurred with discontinuation of corticosteroids, and over several weeks he became increasingly dyspneic. He also complained of "tripping" frequently when he walked.

The patient had a fever of 39°C and a respiratory rate of 24 breaths/min. Diffuse dry rales were heard on auscultation of the lungs, with no evidence of consolidation. On the neurological examination, weakness of left foot extension and an absent left ankle jerk reflex were found.

The complete blood count showed a leukocytosis ($11.5 \times 10^3/mm^3$) with a marked eosinophilia (18%). The ESR was markedly elevated at 125 mm/h. Serum chemistries and urinalysis were normal. Chest X-ray showed diffuse interstitial infiltrates. Electromyography and nerve conduction studies of the left lower extremity were compatible with a mononeuritis multiplex.

Prednisone 1 mg/kg/day was started for the presumptive diagnosis of CSS. At the same time, testing for ANCA and a left sural nerve biopsy were performed. One week after the onset of corticosteroid treatment, the patient had a significant improvement in his respiratory and neurological symptoms, and he was enrolled in a rehabilitation program. ANCA testing was eventually found to be positive at a titer of 1:160 in a perinuclear pattern, and histopathology from the sural nerve biopsy revealed a necrotizing vasculitis of the vasa nervorum, with an eosinophil-rich infiltrate. By the second week of therapy, the chest X-ray abnormalities and eosinophilia completely resolved.

High-dose prednisone was maintained for 4 weeks with continued good response, but the patient began to develop weight gain, worsening hypertension, and severe hyperglycemia. Oral cyclophosphamide 2 mg/kg/d was started as a corticosteroid-sparing agent, enabling the steady reduction of the prednisone dose to 10 mg daily over 6 months without disease relapse.

Clinical Features

CSS usually but not invariably unfolds in three stages: 1) a prodromal phase characterized by asthma and/or allergic disease; 2) an eosinophilia/tissue infiltration phase in which a high peripheral eosinophil count is found, as well as eosinophilic infiltration in the lungs, the gastrointestinal tract, and eventually other tissues; and 3) a vasculitic phase in which a systemic necrotizing vasculitis occurs, affecting many organs such as the lungs, skin, peripheral nervous system, gastrointestinal tract, or kidneys.

Prodromal Phase

The prodromal phase is usually dominated by non-specific upper respiratory symptoms such as sinusitis, rhinitis, and asthma, which may mimic a viral syndrome. The duration of this prodromal phase is variable but can precede the infiltrative and vasculitic phases by many years. Eventually in the course of the disease, most patients develop asthma, which occurs in more than 95% of CSS patients. Clinically, it is identical to idiopathic asthma but tends to be more severe and progressive, usually requiring systemic steroids for its management. In most patients, asthma precedes the appearance of florid CSS. Rarely, CSS can develop simultaneously with new-onset asthma or in individuals with no previous history of asthma at all. Allergic rhinitis and sinusitis are also common early clinical findings and occur in up to 70% of patients.

Active (Infiltrative and Vasculitic) Phases

Non-specific constitutional signs or symptoms such as fever, fatigue, anorexia, and weight loss reflect the systemic inflammatory process. The specific clinical manifestations of the infiltrative and vasculitic phases in individual CSS patients depend on the presence and level of involvement of organs affected by the disease process. The following are commonly observed findings.

CUTANEOUS MANIFESTATIONS
Cutaneous lesions are very common in CSS, occurring in the majority of patients. Palpable purpura is the most common, which is described in up to

62% of patients. Other forms of cutaneous involvement are nodules, urticaria, livedo reticularis, infiltrated papules, digital ischemia, fingertip vesicles, aseptic pustules, and necrotic bullae.

GASTROINTESTINAL MANIFESTATIONS
About one third of patients with CSS will have gastrointestinal complaints. Although unexplained non-specific abdominal pain is a very common clinical feature, occurring in up to 90% of patients in one series, severe gastrointestinal consequences of vasculitis such as bleeding, perforation, and colitis are rare.

CARDIOVASCULAR MANIFESTATIONS
Several forms of cardiac involvement have been reported, including acute pericarditis (23% of patients), cardiomyopathy due to myocardial vasculitis (13%), and rarely myocardial infarction. The most common manifestation of cardiovascular involvement is hypertension thought to be due to renal infarction, which in some series have been found in 75% of patients. Cardiovascular manifestations may account for up to half of deaths in CSS.

PULMONARY AND THORACIC MANIFESTATIONS
In addition to asthma, pulmonary and thoracic involvement of CSS can include interstitial lung disease, pleural disease, and intrathoracic lymphadenopathy (14). Radiological abnormalities on routine chest X-ray or computed tomography are reported to occur in 27%-93% of patients. The most common findings are nonsegmental airspace disease in 72%, Loeffler's syndrome (eosinophilic pneumonitis) in 40%, and patchy multifocal peripheral consolidation in 67%. Nodular lesions with or without cavitation have also been reported, but cavitation is a rare phenomenon in CSS. Pleural effusions are found in 30% of patients, and the pleural fluid usually shows an exudate rich in eosinophils.

NEUROLOGICAL MANIFESTATIONS
Peripheral neuropathy is the most common manifestation of nervous system involvement and has been reported in as many as 75% of patients. Mononeuritis multiplex is the classic lesion and may be more commonly associated with CSS than other systemic vasculitides. Not infrequently, more than one peripheral nerve may become affected, resulting in a polyneuropathy. Central nervous system involvement includes cranial nerve defects and potentially fatal cerebral hemorrhages and infarcts.

RENAL MANIFESTATIONS
Some form of renal involvement is described in up to 88% of patients, generally detected as mild proteinuria and/or microscopic hematuria on routine urinalysis. Renal failure is uncommon in CSS, but it is well recognized that these patients can rarely develop a rapidly progressive glomerulonephritis.

Renal biopsy usually shows a crescentic necrotizing glomerulonephritis with eosinophilic interstitial infiltration in most of these patients.

HEAD AND NECK INVOLVEMENT

Ophthalmological findings and hearing loss are not as common in CSS as in other form of vasculitis like WG. Some of the reported clinical findings are exophthalmos and episcleritis.

MUSCULOSKELETAL MANIFESTATIONS

Migratory arthralgias and myalgias are very common in CSS, particularly during the vasculitic phase of disease. However, true inflammatory arthritis with joint effusions or erosions is fairly uncommon.

Diagnosis

CSS is a clinical diagnosis supported by laboratory, radiological, and pathological data. Hallmark characteristics of CSS include a history of asthma, peripheral and tissue eosinophilia, and pulmonary infiltrates. The peripheral eosinophilia is over 10% and commonly over 15%. Other diagnoses to be considered when faced with pulmonary disease and marked eosinophilia are listed in Table 13-2. However, extrapulmonary manifestations such as mononeuritis multiplex and palpable purpura are strong clues that point to CSS.

Laboratory Testing

Non-specific markers of inflammation are commonly abnormal such as an elevated ESR and high serum levels of CRP. A marked peripheral eosinophilia is a characteristic and diagnostic feature of CSS. Most series of CSS patients show an absolute eosinophil count over of 1500/mm^3. Some patients,

---

Table 13-2   Conditions Associated with Pulmonary Infiltrates and Eosinophila

---

- Idiopathic Loffler's syndrome

- Acute eosinophilic pneumonia

- Chronic eosinophilic pnemonia

- Allergic bronchopulmonary aspergillosis

- Infections
    Fungal (e.g., coccidioidomycosis)
    Mycobacterial (e.g., tuberculosis)
    Parasitic (e.g., *Ascaris*)

- Malignancies (e.g., non-small-cell lung cancers, lymphomas)

- Reactions to drugs, chemicals, or metals (e.g., antibiotics, nickel)

particularly those who are already taking corticosteroids for asthma, may not have such an overtly elevated count, but they almost always have counts over the normal range (i.e., >500/mm³). Many patients also have an elevated serum level of IgE. Complement levels, cryoglobulins, antinuclear antibodies, and rheumatoid factor studies are usually normal.

Patients with CSS frequently have circulating ANCA. When done by the screening indirect immunofluorescence technique, a pANCA pattern is seen in as many as 77% of patients during active phases of disease. Antigen-specific studies with enzyme-linked immunosorbent assay (ELISA) have shown that the ANCA is predominantly anti-myeloperoxidase antibodies. Isolated cases of cytoplasmic staining (c-ANCA pattern) have been reported; however, it is interesting to note that many of them fail to demonstrate the usual anti-proteinase 3 antibody by ELISA.

Biopsy

Although the diagnosis of CSS is based upon clinical findings, obtaining a tissue diagnosis can be reassuring for the physician and the patient and may be useful when response to therapy is not as expected. However, it is not strictly required for making the diagnosis. As in WG, an open lung biopsy offers the best diagnostic yield. However, a sural nerve biopsy can be diagnostic in over 50% of cases and can be more easily and safely obtained. The classical histological findings are an eosinophilic infiltrate and necrotizing vasculitis with giant cells involving medium-sized and small vessels. Perivascular or interstitial granulomatous infiltration can also be seen. However, pathological specimens can often be non-diagnostic. In a series of 162 biopsies performed in 88 patients with clinically defined CSS, vasculitis was found in only 66.7% and necrotizing vasculitis in only 40.5% of the samples. Accordingly, one should never wait for histological confirmation before treatment when facing an organ- or life-threatening condition consistent with CSS or any other systemic necrotizing vasculitis.

Prognosis

Long-term follow-up of treated patients with CSS has shown a survival rate of over 70% at 5 years. Mortality rates are closely related to disease severity as measured by the Five Factor Score (FFS): poor prognostic factors include 1) cardiomyopathy; 2) proteinuria ≥1 g/24 h; 3) serum creatinine >1.6 mg/dL; 4) severe gastrointestinal disease, defined as intestinal bleeding, perforation, pancreatitis or need for laparotomy; and 5) central nervous system involvement (15). An FFS of 0 (none of these five factors is present) is associated with an 11.9% 5-year mortality rate, whereas an FFS of 1 (one factor present) is associated with a 5-year mortality rate of 25.9%. The presence of two or more factors (FFS of 2) carries a 45.9% 5-year mortality rate. A short duration of asthma before the onset of vasculitis also seems to negatively correlate with prognosis.

Management

Pharmacological Therapy

Because of the rarity of CSS, there are no large controlled clinical trials to define the best treatment for this condition. Treatment usually starts with high doses of systemic corticosteroids (e.g., prednisone 0.5 to 1 mg/kg/day) maintained for 6 to 12 weeks to quickly suppress active inflammation, followed by a slow taper guided by clinical changes. More severe disease activity may require higher initial doses or "pulse corticosteroid therapy," such as intravenous methylprednisolone 1 g daily for 3 days before starting daily maintenance prednisone therapy. Although many clinical manifestations respond quickly to corticosteroids, premature reduction of dose frequently results in disease relapse. The addition of immunosupressive agents is often necessary in organ- and life-threatening situations or in corticosteroid-dependent or corticosteroid-refractory disease. Cyclophosphamide enjoys the largest experience and is generally the agent of choice when potent immunosuppression is required (16). Oral doses of 2-3 mg/kg/d or monthly intravenous doses of 0.5-0.75 g/m² body surface area have been used with comparable efficacy in small short-term studies. Oral dosing appears to carry more urological complications such as hemorrhagic cystitis and bladder cancer.

Other agents that have shown benefit in some patients include azathioprine and intravenous gammaglobulin. There are also recent anecdotal reports of the benefits of plasmapheresis and interferon-α (17).

Disease Monitoring

There is no single laboratory test that reliably reflects disease activity, and monitoring of disease and therapeutic response is made predominantly on clinical grounds. A markedly high eosinophil count and laboratory evidence of systemic inflammation (e.g., ESR or CRP) should alert the physician to a possible disease exacerbation, but it is important to always adjust treatment to the clinical picture and not to chase after abnormal laboratory tests. Conversely, the peripheral eosinophil count usually decreases very quickly upon the initiation of corticosteroid therapy, and so a normal eosinophil count does not necessarily mean that the disease is under control.

REFERENCES

1. **Russell KA, Specks U.** Are antineutrophil cytoplasmic antibodies pathogenic? Experimental approaches to understand the antineutrophil cytoplasmic antibody phenomenon. Rheum Dis Clin North Am. 2001;27:815-32.
2. **Wiik AS.** Clinical use of serological tests for antineutrophil cytoplasmic antibodies. What do the studies say? Rheum Dis Clin North Am. 2001;27:799-813.
3. **Hoffman GS, Kerr GS, Leavitt RY, et al.** Wegener granulomatosis: an analysis of 158 patients. Ann Intern Med. 1992;116:488-98.

4. **Reinhold-Keller E, Beuge N, Latza U, et al.** An interdisciplinary approach to the care of patients with Wegener's granulomatosis: long term outcome in 155 patients. Arthritis Rheum. 2000;43:1021-32.

5. **Jayne D, Rasmussen N, Andrassy K, et al.** A randomized trial of maintenance therapy for vasculitis associated with antineutrophil cytoplasmic antibodies. N Engl J Med. 2003;349:36-44.

6. **Sneller MC, Hoffman GS, Talar-Williams C, et al.** An analysis of forty-two Wegener's granulomatosis patients treated with methotrexate and prednisone. Arthritis Rheum. 1995;38:608-13.

7. **Stone JH, Tun W, Hellmann DB.** Treatment of non-life threatening Wegener's granulomatosis with methotrexate and daily prednisone as the initial therapy of choice. J Rheumatol. 1999;26:1134-9.

8. **Stone JH, Uhlfelder ML, Hellmann DB, et al.** Etanercept combined with conventional treatment in Wegener's granulomatosis: a six-month open-label trial to evaluate safety. Arthritis Rheum. 2001;44:1149-54.

9. **Lamprecht P, Voswindel J, Lilienthal T, et al.** Effectiveness of TNF-alpha blockade with infliximab in refractory Wegener's granulomatosis. Rheumatology. 2002; 41:1303-7.

10. **Stegeman CA, Tervaert JW, de Jong PE, Kullenberg CG.** Trimethoprim-sulfamethoxazole (co-trimoxazole) for the prevention of relapses of Wegener's granulomatosis. Dutch Co-Trimoxazole Wegener Study Group. N Engl J Med. 1996;335: 16-20.

11. **Churg J, Strauss L.** Allergic granulomatosis, allergic angiitis and periarteritis nodosa. Am J Pathol. 1951;27:277-301.

12. **Weller PF, Plaut M, Taggart V, Trontell A.** The relationship of asthma therapy and Churg-Strauss syndrome: NIH workshop summary report. J Allergy Clin Immunol. 2001;108:175-83.

13. **Müschen M, Warskulat U, Perniok A, et al.** Involvement of soluble CD95 in Churg-Strauss syndrome. Am J Pathol. 1999;155:915-25.

14. **Choi YH, Im JG, Han BK, et al.** Thoracic manifestation of Churg-Strauss syndrome: radiologic and clinical findings. Chest. 2000;117:117-24.

15. **Gayraud M, Guillevin L, le Toumelin P, et al.** Long-term follow-up of polyarteritis nodosa, microscopic polyangiitis, and Churg-Strauss syndrome. Arthritis Rheum. 2001;44:666-75.

16. **Guillevin L, Cohen P, Gayraud M, et al.** Churg-Strauss syndrome. Clincal study and long-term follow-up of 96 patients. Medicine (Baltimore). 1999;78:26-37.

17. **Tatsis E, Schnabel A, Gross WL.** Interferon-alpha treatment of four patients with the Churg-Strauss syndrome. Ann Intern Med. 1998;129:370-4.

14

■ ■ ■

Polymyalgia Rheumatica, Giant Cell Arteritis, and Takayasu's Arteritis

Robert F. Spiera, MD

Giant cell arteritis (GCA; also known as temporal arteritis) and Takayasu's arteritis (TA) are necrotizing vasculitides that are distinctly characterized by granulomatous inflammation that affect large arteries. They differ notably in the age of the patients that are affected. GCA almost always occurs in individuals over the age of 50 (usually over 60), whereas TA typically occurs in young women under the age of 40. Also, while the two conditions may share many nonspecific clinical features of systemic inflammation (e.g., fever, weight loss, fatigue), TA patients most commonly present with upper extremity claudication and diminished peripheral pulses. In contrast, patients with GCA characteristically complain of manifestations reflecting ischemia of the external carotid artery and its branches, such as headache, scalp tenderness, jaw claudication, and tongue pain. Many patients with GCA also develop symptoms of polymyalgia rheumatica (PMR), a clinical syndrome marked by prominent morning stiffness and aching in the large muscles around the neck/shoulder and hip/thigh regions. However, while up to half of patients with GCA have PMR, most cases of PMR are idiopathic and are not associated with a pathologically defined vasculitis.

Polymyalgia Rheumatica

Polymyalgia rheumatica (PMR) is a systemic inflammatory condition characterized by prominent shoulder and hip girdle pain, aching and stiffness with prolonged inactivity, and laboratory evidence of systemic inflammation. It is relatively common, with an estimated prevalence of up to 1% in persons over the age of 50. PMR usually occurs in isolation, but in approximately 10% to 15% of patients it is found in association with giant cell arteritis (GCA). PMR is a clinically defined syndrome, without a single definitive laboratory or biopsy finding that establishes the diagnosis.

Pathogenesis

The etiology of PMR is unknown. Pathophysiologically, evidence of a low-grade synovitis and tendon inflammation has been demonstrated in the shoulder and hip girdles, and elevated plasma levels of pro-inflammatory cytokines such as interleukin-2 and interleukin-6 have been recognized in this disease. There is also a genetic association with HLA-DR4.

Case Presentation 1

A 64-year-old woman is seen for a four-month history of diffuse musculoskeletal pain. Initially, she noted a relatively abrupt onset of pain in her neck and stiffness in her shoulder girdle without any antecedent history of trauma. An orthopedic surgeon diagnosed degenerative disc disease and treated the patient with anti-inflammatory medications and physical therapy. At first, the patient felt some mild improvement but, over the ensuing months, her symptoms progressed. She now complains of up to two hours of severe generalized morning stiffness not only in her neck/shoulder girdle but in the hip/thigh girdle as well. In general, her symptoms improve over the course of the day but are exacerbated by prolonged sitting such as at a movie or on a long car ride. In the two weeks prior to her visit, she had developed pain and some mild swelling in her hands, which were also more uncomfortable in the morning hours.

The patient denied any significant past medical history. She had a recent bone densitometry test that showed normal bone density. Other than her anti-inflammatory medication, she takes only supplemental calcium and a daily multivitamin. The review of systems revealed no fevers, weight loss, headaches, scalp tenderness, jaw claudication, facial pain, visual disturbances, or tongue symptoms.

She appeared physically well but uncomfortable. Her vital signs were normal. There was no appreciable scalp tenderness or temporal artery prominence or discomfort. Heart, lung, and abdominal examinations were normal. There was minimal fullness in the metacarpophalangeal joints bilaterally but no overt proximal interphalangeal joint or wrist swelling. Her grip strength was minimally diminished bilaterally. Active abduction of the shoulders was limited to 90 degrees, but the shoulders had full range of motion passively. The hips had painless and full range of motion. There was tenderness in the deltoids and thighs to palpation but no diffuse trigger point tenderness suggestive of fibromyalgia. The neurological examination was nonfocal other than mildly reduced strength in the shoulder abductors and forward flexors due to pain.

The complete blood count revealed a mild anemia (hemoglobin 11.0 mg/dL) but was otherwise normal. The erythrocyte sedimentation rate (ESR) was elevated at 54 mm/h. Serum chemistries including muscle enzymes (e.g., creatine phosphokinase) were all within normal limits. The rheumatoid factor was negative. The diagnosis of polymyalgia rheumatica was made.

Prednisone therapy was started at a dose of 10 mg in the morning and 5 mg in the evening. Within one day of starting therapy, the patient noted a dramatic improvement in her myalgias and arthralgias, which were nearly completely resolved. Corticosteroid therapy was subsequently consolidated to a single morning 15 mg dose for one week, then tapered off slowly over the ensuing year without relapse of her symptoms. The ESR and anemia both normalized.

Clinical Features

Patients with PMR complain of severe pain and stiffness predominantly in the shoulder and pelvic girdles. The symptoms are generally symmetrical and more prominent in the early morning hours and with inactivity, lessening with activity. Classically, peripheral small joint synovitis was not felt to be a feature of PMR and, when present, was considered to be more consistent with a diagnosis of rheumatoid arthritis (RA). This distinction may be semantic, however, because it is now well recognized that there are RA patients with PMR-like symptoms and peripheral synovitis in whom rheumatoid factor (RF) is not detectable. These patients do not ultimately demonstrate erosive joint disease over time and respond dramatically to low doses of corticosteroids. Unlike classical RA, these patients generally do not require the use of disease-modifying anti-rheumatic drugs (DMARDs).

PMR patients frequently complain of feeling systemically unwell with fatigue and malaise. Findings such as significant weight loss or high fevers are uncommon and should sensitize the clinician to the possibility of a more sinister underlying diagnosis such as GCA or an occult infection or malignancy. On physical examination, patients generally have discomfort with movement or palpation of the shoulder and thigh girdle musculature. Frank muscle weakness is not typically seen in PMR, although the tenderness and pain can make it difficult to assess formal muscle strength with the patient's arms and legs giving way due to discomfort.

Diagnosis

PMR is a clinically defined syndrome, diagnosed by eliciting a characteristic history in a patient over the age of 50 and supported by the finding of an elevated ESR. Laboratory studies usually reflect nonspecific findings of systemic inflammation such as an elevated sedimentation rate (ESR) or C-reactive protein (CRP). Similarly, a low-grade anemia of chronic disease and/or mild thrombocytosis may be present. Serum levels of muscle enzymes such as creatine phosphokinase and lactate dehydrogenase are not elevated. Serologic testing for RF and antinuclear antibodies (ANA) is negative.

Although an elevated ESR is typical, it is now recognized that PMR can occur in the context of a normal ESR in as many as 10% of patients (1). In some of these patients, an elevated CRP can still be demonstrated and taken as laboratory evidence of systemic inflammation. Even so, the presence of a normal ESR or CRP in an otherwise typical clinical setting should not exclude the diagnosis of PMR. In these cases, a trial of low-dose corticosteroids can be a helpful additional diagnostic tool. A rapid and dramatic response (often within hours of the initial dose) to low-dose corticosteroids is characteristic and supports the diagnosis of PMR.

Differential Diagnosis

The clinician must consider potential PMR mimics, particularly in this older population in whom co-morbidities are common. Differential diagnostic considerations include subacute bacterial endocarditis, hypothyroidism, myositis, seronegative rheumatoid arthritis, drug effects (notably "statins"), and even fibromyalgia. Multiple myeloma can also cause musculoskeletal discomfort and is associated with anemia and an elevated ESR. Accordingly, serum protein- and immunoelectrophoreses are recommended in the initial laboratory assessment. Although no specific associations have been recognized between PMR and malignancy, it is important to verify that the patient is up to date in terms of an age-appropriate cancer screening.

Prognosis and Disease Outcomes

A dramatic and prompt response to low-dose corticosteroids is typical and, in fact, is considered by some to be diagnostic for PMR. PMR is generally a self-limited disease, although later relapses can occur. The duration of corticosteroid treatment generally lasts for several months to two years, although in a minority of patients miniscule doses of corticosteroids may be necessary for longer periods. In the absence of associated GCA, PMR is not a life- or organ-threatening disease. Long-term complications arising from chronic corticosteroid use may outweigh those associated with the illness itself.

Many patients with PMR are not identified and are left untreated for years, their myalgic symptoms attributed to the aging process. These individuals may develop complications related to overall inactivity and disuse of muscle, but there is no evidence that untreated patients are at increased risk of developing GCA.

Although up to 15% of patients with PMR may have GCA, in the absence of clinical signs suggesting the latter a temporal artery biopsy is *not* routinely recommended. However, in a patient who does not seem to be responding appropriately to low-dose corticosteroids (less than 20 mg of daily prednisone or equivalent), underlying GCA is a possibility and a biopsy should be considered.

Management

PMR is a functionally limiting and miserably uncomfortable disease prior to initiating therapy, but it is exquisitely treatment-responsive and thus a gratifying disorder to diagnose and treat. It is commonly treated by primary care physicians. A major challenge of management is to balance the risks of therapy with achieving an acceptable therapeutic response. The mainstay of treatment is low-dose corticosteroids. Generally, therapy is initiated with 10 to 20 mg of daily prednisone or its equivalent, initially in divided doses and then consolidated later when a therapeutic response is observed. A dramatic response is typically achieved within hours to the first few days of therapy.

Different corticosteroid tapering schedules can be used. For example, the daily dose of prednisone can be tapered from 20 mg by 2.5 mg weekly to 10 mg by the fourth week. The daily dose can then be reduced by 1 mg weekly to 5 mg and thereafter by 1 mg monthly unless symptoms recur or until prednisone is tapered off completely. However, there is tremendous variability in patient response, and it is the clinical response that should guide the rapidity of the taper.

Although laboratory tests such as ESR and CRP can be followed serially during treatment, the clinical response, *not* laboratory values, should be used as the primary guide in determining the rate of corticosteroid taper. In some patients, adequate symptom control is maintained despite persistent mild elevations of ESR, and further reductions of corticosteroid dosage can be continued. Conversely, in patients with recurrent symptoms despite normal or stable laboratory tests, the corticosteroid dosage should be maintained or even increased. As discussed above, at any time when a patient does not appear to be responding appropriately to treatment adjustments, caution should be taken to exclude co-morbid conditions such as infections. Occasionally, some patients who do not respond to prednisone may respond to other corticosteroids such as methylprednisolone, and it is reasonable to try these alternatives in such cases.

There are no proven steroid-sparing interventions in PMR. Methotrexate has not reliably shown a steroid-sparing/disease-modifying benefit in clinical studies, although it has been used occasionally in patients in whom corticosteroid therapy is excessively morbid and continued disease activity is present. Non-steroidal anti-inflammatory drugs (NSAIDs) in full anti-inflammatory doses can be helpful in controlling symptoms in PMR but only rarely can be employed as the sole therapy.

As with other corticosteroid-treated diseases, a baseline determination of bone mineral density is recommended and measures to prevent osteoporosis should be taken. For patients who will be taking >5 mg/d for >3 months of prednisone or its equivalent, evaluation and treatment of potential bone loss is necessary. (See Chapter 23, the section on "Corticosteroid-Induced Osteoporosis," for more information.) All patients should be treated with adequate calcium and vitamin D supplementation while on corticosteroid therapy, and, when appropriate, medications such as oral bisphosphonates should be administered to prevent bone resorption. Moreover, regular blood pressure monitoring and screening for diabetes mellitus should be maintained. Immunizations should be kept current.

Giant Cell Arteritis

Giant cell arteritis (GCA), also known as temporal arteritis, is a systemic vasculitis affecting large and medium sized arteries that occurs almost exclusively in individuals over age 50 and usually over age 60. It has a predilection for affecting branches of the ascending aorta but tends to spare intracranial vessels. Among the vasculitides, GCA is one of the more common entities, with a prevalence of approximately 20 per 100,000 individuals over the age of 50 in some populations.

Pathogenesis

The etiology of GCA is unknown. Host factors seem to play a role, as GCA can cluster in families, and as with PMR there is an association with the presence of HLA-DR4. Environmental factors, particularly viral infections, have been hypothesized but not proven as possible triggers. GCA is pathologically characterized by an occlusive pan-arteritis, with giant cells and granuloma formation and disruption of the internal elastic lamina. A distinctive feature of GCA is that affected arteries tend to have "skipped" lesions with areas of vasculitis directly adjacent to normal tissue.

Case Presentation 2

A 74-year-old woman is seen for fever, headache, and pain with chewing. Five years ago, she was diagnosed with polymyalgia rheumatica (PMR) after presenting with neck/shoulder and hip/thigh girdle pain and stiffness and an erythrocyte sedimentation rate (ESR) of 44 mm/h. She responded to low-dose prednisone that was tapered off over 18 months without complications. The patient did well until three months before the current evaluation, at which time she developed recurrent myalgias in the neck/shoulder and hip/thigh areas reminiscent of her past PMR. She also reported low-grade fevers. Ibuprofen did not relieve her symptoms. She subsequently developed increasing neck pain, prompting treatment with prednisone 15 mg daily. Although there was modest improvement in her myalgias, the response was not as complete nor as dramatic as her prior treatment for PMR. Over the past three weeks, she has developed severe headaches, mostly in the occipital and left temporal areas. She also describes scalp sensitivity, manifesting as severe pain while brushing her hair. In addition, chewing bagels had become difficult because of left-sided jaw pain. She denied any visual symptoms but admitted to increasing fatigue and a 14-pound weight loss over the previous few months.

She was febrile to 38.7°C, but her vital signs were otherwise within normal limits. Light palpation of her scalp was very uncomfortable, particularly in the left temporal area. The temporal arteries were not tender and had normal pulsations. There was no scleral injection, and the funduscopic and visual field examinations were normal. There were no carotid bruits. Heart, lung, and abdominal examinations were normal. There was neither peripheral synovitis nor edema, but there was moderate proximal shoulder and hip girdle tenderness to palpation. The neurological examination was nonfocal. Her vascular exam was without appreciable abdominal aneurysms or peripheral bruits.

A mild anemia (hemoglobin 10.2 g/dL) and thrombocytosis (platelet count 502,000/mm^3) were found on the complete blood count, and the ESR was 114 mm/h. The basic biochemical profile was otherwise normal. Serum immunofixation did not reveal a monoclonal spike.

Giant cell arteritis was suspected, and the patient was treated empirically with prednisone 40 mg qAM and 20 mg qPM and was referred for a temporal artery biopsy. Within two days of beginning corticosteroid therapy, the patient had a dramatic improvement in her symptoms. One week later, the ESR was 50 mm/h. A left temporal artery biopsy obtained two weeks after the start of corticosteroid therapy revealed a necrotizing arteritis with disruption of the internal elastica, giant cell infiltration, and granuloma formation.

The prednisone was subsequently consolidated to a single morning dose and tapered off slowly over the ensuing 18 months without recurrence of symptoms.

Clinical Features

The clinical manifestations of GCA result from the systemic inflammatory nature of the disorder and from local ischemic complications of discrete arterial involvement. Constitutional symptoms such as fatigue, weight loss, and fever are frequent. Anemia, usually normochromic and normocytic, is common and may be substantial. In some instances, these systemic symptoms may be the only presenting complaint, and GCA should always be considered in the differential diagnosis of unexplained fever and/or anemia in the elderly individual, particularly once infection and malignancy have been reasonably excluded. Proximal musculoskeletal symptoms reminiscent of PMR are common, occurring in up to half of patients with GCA at presentation.

Localizing symptoms related to arterial inflammation are more specific for GCA. Of these, the most common presenting complaint is headache. The headache is often severe and inescapable and typically localized to the temporal areas but can be occipital as well. Even in patients with a tendency to headache, the pain is usually qualitatively and quantitatively distinguishable from prior complaints. Jaw claudication is a common ischemic complaint, and tongue pain or even throat pain can also occur. Scalp tenderness is a suggestive complaint, with patients often mentioning discomfort while brushing or combing their hair. Although scalp and lingular necrosis can occur, they are rare complications due to the presence of collateral circulation.

Ophthalmic involvement, however, remains the most dreaded clinical feature of GCA. Vision loss, either partial or complete, can occur in up to 20% of patients and, once vision loss occurs, it is generally irreversible because it represents an end-organ ischemic complication of the disease. Vision loss is often abrupt but may be partial or fluctuating initially and can clinically resemble amaurosis fugax. When not treated promptly, progression to complete loss of vision in the affected eye and even loss of vision in the contralateral eye is common, often within 24 hours. Any visual symptoms, therefore, require emergency intervention that should be instituted even *without* pathologic diagnosis. Rare ophthalmologic complications include diplopia and ptosis, both resulting from ischemia of the extraocular muscles.

Involvement of other branches of the aortic arch such as axillary or subclavian vessels can lead to claudication, ischemia, or asymmetric peripheral pulses of the upper extremities. Aortic aneurysms can occur but are usually late complications (2). In studies of repaired aortic aneurysms, pathologic findings consistent with GCA have been found in approximately 2% of individuals who did not have previously recognized arteritis.

It is unusual for GCA to affect intracranial vessels. Thus cerebral vascular accidents are not common complications and should signal the clinician to consider alternative diagnostic possibilities. Peripheral neuropathy can uncommonly occur. A minority of patients complain of upper respiratory symptoms such as cough or sore throat.

Diagnosis

The diagnosis of GCA is best made by maintaining a high index of suspicion, particularly in elderly patients presenting with complaints such as fever, headache, visual loss, prominent shoulder and hip girdle symptoms, and anemia. It is crucial that the diagnosis be established promptly, because permanent ischemic ocular complications can easily be prevented if therapy is initiated in a timely fashion. Conversely, failure to recognize and appropriately treat GCA can rapidly result in blindness.

A thorough physical examination should be performed, with palpation of the temporal areas, looking for nodularity, tenderness, or diminished pulsations of the temporal arteries. Scalp tenderness can be a telling finding. The carotid and subclavian arteries should be auscultated for the presence of bruits. In patients with PMR symptoms, tenderness of the proximal musculature or pain on range of motion testing may be present.

Laboratory Testing

Laboratory investigations are helpful in GCA but are not specific. The ESR is substantially elevated, usually greater than 50 mm/h and often greater than 100 mm/h. Although isolated PMR can occur in the context of a normal ESR, this would be extraordinarily rare in GCA, except in patients already being treated with corticosteroids for PMR or other indications. It should be kept in mind that some conditions such as polycythemia vera can artifactually lower the ESR. Other acute-phase reactants such as CRP are also elevated in plasma and may be more reliable in that setting. Anemia is common and may be substantial, and platelet counts are often elevated. Mild serum alkaline phosphatase elevations can occur in up to 30% of patients but are not usually clinically important. Serologic evaluations such as ANA, RF, and anti-neutrophil cytoplasmic antibodies are negative.

Temporal Artery Biopsy

GCA is unusual among the vasculitides in that the diagnosis can most often be readily confirmed pathologically. Obtaining temporal artery biopsy is advocated in all patients suspected of having GCA, because the mainstay of treatment, namely substantial doses of corticosteroids, is associated with significant morbidity, especially in this age group. In patients with localizing signs or symptoms, the biopsy should be taken from the involved side. In the absence of palpable temporal artery abnormalities, it is important to obtain a segment of substantial length (at least 3.5 cm) to maximize the yield of the procedure. The sensitivity of temporal artery biopsies is approximately 70%; 30% of adequate biopsies are negative. In some cases, due to the patchy nature of arterial involvement, re-examination of multiple sections of a specimen initially read as negative can reveal evidence of GCA. Biopsy of the contralateral side can also increase the diagnostic yield (3). However, in the setting of a characteristic clinical presentation of GCA, systemic corticosteroids should be initiated even if the temporal artery biopsy is unrevealing or unavailable.

Radiologic Studies

Angiography is generally not utilized in the diagnosis of GCA. False-positive results are common in this age group in whom atherosclerosis can cause vascular irregularities. It can be helpful documenting disease, however, in patients with symptoms of large-artery involvement such as subclavian disease. Other vascular imaging modalities, such as magnetic resonance angiography, may be helpful for documenting large vessel disease and are less invasive.

Color duplex high-frequency ultrasonography of the temporal arteries can reveal stenoses, occlusions, or "halos" surrounding the vessel lumen in most patients with GCA. The presence of the halo suggests inflammatory changes in the vessel wall and has been championed by some as being specific for GCA. It is not clear, however, whether results of the published studies can be generalized, due to variable experience in the use of this technology in the diagnosis of GCA. In our experience, ultrasonography has not been generally helpful and, given the relative accessibility and safety of temporal artery biopsies, histologic confirmation of a diagnosis is always preferred if possible.

Differential Diagnosis

When presenting stereotypically (e.g., an elderly patient with fever, headache, visual disturbance, and jaw claudication), it is difficult to confuse GCA for any other condition. On occasion, other forms of necrotizing vasculitis such as polyarteritis nodosa may atypically involve branches of the external carotid artery and mimic GCA. Takayasu's arteritis, like GCA, affects large vessels but is seen in a distinctly younger patient population. The differential diagnosis for GCA is wider when symptoms are few or unusual. A fever of unknown origin in an older patient in the absence of other specific signs or symptoms should raise the possibility of GCA, but an occult infection or an occult malignancy (especially lymphoma) should also be suspected. Atypical presentations of GCA, such as diplopia or ptosis, are particularly challenging to diagnose.

Prognosis and Disease Outcomes

GCA is often a gratifying diagnosis to make because it is very responsive to corticosteroid therapy and potentially serious problems can be prevented. For example, when the ophthalmologic complications are identified early, prompt intervention will spare the patient from permanent loss of visual acuity. Most studies suggest that the majority of patients with GCA are able to discontinue corticosteroid therapy after two years. It must be cautioned, however, that an overly rapid corticosteroid taper or an inadequate corticosteroid dose contributes to increased risk of disease relapse. Therefore rote adherence to strict tapering schedule without adequate assessment of clinical status should be avoided, and close clinical monitoring is necessary to determine the appropriate rate of dose reduction.

Management

Systemic corticosteroids are dramatically effective in controlling the inflammatory processes and preventing the complications of GCA. When clinical suspicion is high and particularly when ocular complaints are present, therapy should be instituted immediately, even before histologic confirmation of the diagnosis. Optimally, the biopsy should be done as soon as possible, generally within two weeks of initiating corticosteroid therapy, to ensure a high diagnostic yield (4). Nonetheless, positive biopsies can occasionally be seen even after prolonged corticosteroid therapy.

There is no consensus regarding the optimal corticosteroid regimen in treating GCA. Treatment is generally tailored to the particular clinical circumstance. Often an initial dosage of 40 to 60 mg of daily prednisone or an equivalent is used, although in patients with visual loss, "pulse" intravenous methylprednisolone (1000 mg IV daily for 3 consecutive days) is often used initially before the onset of daily oral therapy. In some centers, an initial dosage of as little as 20 mg of daily prednisone has been used to treat GCA without ocular signs or symptoms, recognizing that if adequate control of the inflammatory signs and symptoms is not rapidly achieved, higher doses of corticosteroids should be quickly utilized.

In general, we initially employ divided doses of corticosteroids but consolidate to a single daily dose when a good therapeutic response is seen. Alternate-day corticosteroid regimens are not recommended in the treatment of this disorder, because vision loss has occurred with these regimens in some series (5). Control of inflammatory disease is typically rapid, and a taper of corticosteroids and consolidation to a single daily dose can usually be started within two weeks. There are no firm guidelines, but the corticosteroid dosage can generally be tapered to 30 mg of daily prednisone or an equivalent by the second month of treatment. Further tapering of corticosteroids is guided by clinical and laboratory evidence of disease activity. Often, in the lower dose ranges (i.e., less than 15 mg of daily prednisone), more gradual corticosteroid tapers are required. Relapses can occur but usually respond to small increases in the corticosteroid dose. Most patients can be tapered off corticosteroid medications entirely within the first or second year of therapy, although in some patients, particularly those with associated PMR, small corticosteroid doses (prednisone 5 mg or less daily) are required for symptomatic control for longer periods. Some studies have suggested that the addition of low-dose aspirin may further reduce the risk of cranial ischemic events.

Although ESR and CRP are valuable tools in assessing disease activity, decisions regarding corticosteroid dose or taper should be based on the overall clinical picture and never solely on laboratory data. Inappropriate reliance on the ESR or CRP can lead to inadequate or excessive corticosteroid therapy and their attendant morbidities.

The morbidity of high-dose and/or long-term corticosteroid therapy is substantial, particularly in this elderly group of patients. Corticosteroid-related side effects such as hypertension, hyperglycemia, mood changes, and alterations in lipid profile require close monitoring and should be managed aggressively. All patients should be treated with adequate calcium (1500 mg daily) and vitamin D (400-800 U daily) supplements. A baseline bone mineral density determination should be obtained. In patients with significant osteopenia or osteoporosis, anti-resorptive agents such as bisphosphonates can be effective in preventing corticosteroid-induced osteoporosis.

A number of agents have been considered as possible "steroid sparing"/disease-controlling interventions in GCA including cyclophosphamide, dapsone, and azathioprine, even though there are no convincing trials demonstrating their efficacy. In recent years, it has been suggested that methotrexate may have a role in the management of this disorder. One controlled trial suggested that the addition of weekly oral methotrexate (10 mg) to standard corticosteroid therapy resulted in fewer relapses (6), but two other controlled studies using up to 20 mg weekly did not suggest a steroid-sparing or disease-controlling benefit (7).

Clinical trials assessing the role of biologic agents such as tumor necrosis factor inhibitors and interleukin-1 receptor antagonists in the management of GCA are in progress.

Takayasu's Arteritis

Pathogenesis

Like GCA, Takayasu's arteritis (TA) is a granulomatous large vessel vasculitis primarily affecting the aorta and its primary branches. It predominantly affects young women less than 40 years of age as opposed to GCA, which is a disease of older individuals. It has a higher incidence in Asians but occurs worldwide. It is relatively uncommon in the United States. Little is known of the pathogenesis of TA. Cell-mediated mechanisms driven by as yet undefined antigens are felt to promote the ongoing systemic inflammatory process.

Case Presentation 3

A 34-year-old woman is evaluated for progressive left arm pain. At age 23, the patient was diagnosed with Takayasu's arteritis after presenting with a three-month history of fatigue, low-grade fevers, a 17-pound weight loss, and arthralgias of the knees and wrists. At that time, she had been found to have a blood pressure differential in her upper extremities, as well as an erythrocyte sedimentation rate (ESR) of 90 mm/h and a normocytic anemia (hemoglobin 10.2 g/dL). Serologic testing for antinuclear antibodies, rheumatoid factor, and syphilis was negative. Angiography demonstrated narrowing of the left subclavian artery, consistent with Takayasu's arteritis. The patient responded to treatment with prednisone 60 mg daily, which was tapered over the ensuing year to 5 mg daily. She subsequently was maintained on prednisone 5 mg on alternate days for three months, after which time corticosteroid therapy was discontinued.

The patient remained well until her current presentation. Four months ago, she developed progressive discomfort in her left arm. Her symptoms were related to exertion, generally becoming prominent as she used the arm in the course of doing housework. She denied more generalized musculoskeletal symptoms. She also denied fevers, fatigue, recent weight loss, and other constitutional symptoms.

On physical examination, she was well appearing. Her blood pressure was 140/100 mm Hg in the right arm and 90/60 in the left arm. Pulse was 84 and regular. The general physical examination of her skin, head, heart, lungs, and abdomen was unremarkable except for a right renal bruit. Her extremities were without synovitis, edema, or cyanosis at rest. She had markedly diminished brachial and radial pulses on the left side compared with the right side. There was a bruit over the left subclavian area. The pedal pulses were 1+ on the left and trace on the right. The neurological examination was nonfocal.

Laboratory studies showed a mild normocytic anemia (hemoglobin 11.4 g/dL), but the white blood cell and platelet counts were well within normal limits. The ESR was 24 mm/h. Her biochemical profile and urinalysis were normal.

Angiography of the upper and lower extremities revealed changes consistent with Takayasu's arteritis. There were prominent areas of stenosis in the left subclavian artery. Narrowing in the right femoral artery was also demonstrated, but significant collateral circulation contributing to distal flow was visualized.

The patient was empirically treated with 60 mg of daily prednisone for the possibility of active arteritis. After three weeks of therapy, however, there was no improvement in her symptoms, the left subclavian bruit, or blood pressure differential. Moreover, she developed steroid-induced hyperglycemia and complained of increased appetite, weight gain, and poor sleep.

The corticosteroids were tapered completely off over the ensuing two weeks. The patient was referred for a vascular surgery evaluation and eventually underwent a left subclavian bypass procedure.

Clinical Features

Two phases of the disease are generally appreciated: an early inflammatory phase and a late "pulseless" phase. In the early phase, clinical features reflect ongoing systemic inflammatory disease and can include fatigue, weight loss, low-grade fevers, arthralgias, and myalgias. Manifestations of the "pulseless" phase relate to ischemic complications due to irreversibly compromised vasculature. Claudication, particularly of the upper extremities, is common, and ischemic ulcerations or gangrene can occur. Diminished cerebral perfusion secondary to carotid and vertebral involvement can result in vertigo, syncope, headaches, or visual impairment. Pulmonary artery involvement can result in dyspnea. Angina can result from aortitis or coronary arteritis.

Diagnosis

Diagnosing TA can be difficult, particularly in the early systemic phase; many of the clinical features are nonspecific, and often there is no evidence of distal vascular compromise. Arterial bruits, particularly in the carotid, subclavian, and abdominal regions, should be sought on physical examination. Patients in the early phase may also present with tenderness over an involved artery, particularly of the carotid arteries. Such vascular findings in a young female patient should raise a high index of suspicion for TA. Hypertension due to renal artery stenosis or aortic disease is common but may not be fully appreciated late in the disease when blood pressure readings may be deceptively reduced due to the presence of fixed proximal occlusive lesions in the arms. Detecting differential blood pressure findings in the two upper extremities and measuring blood pressure in the lower extremities can be helpful. Funduscopic findings may include hypertensive changes.

Laboratory Testing

There are no laboratory abnormalities specific for TA. In the inflammatory phase, markers of active inflammatory disease are usually present, including an elevated ESR or plasma CRP level, and often there is a mild leukocytosis or a mild anemia of chronic disease. Autoantibodies are not typical of TA. In the later phase of the disease, the absence of inflammatory marker abnormalities can be helpful in distinguishing whether new symptoms are related to an acute flare of active inflammatory disease or to vascular occlusion related to prior damage. The converse, however, is not necessarily true; ESR can be elevated in as many as half of patients with quiescent TA.

Radiologic Studies

Arteriography is usually the most helpful imaging modality in confirming the diagnosis of TA and determining the extent of involvement. Typical findings include smooth-walled, tapered, and narrowed areas often beginning at the origin of the vessel. Noninvasive modalities have been utilized as well, including magnetic resonance angiography (MRA) (8), Doppler ultrasonography, and helical computed tomographic scanning angiography (9). In addition to being safer than conventional angiography, MRA offers the advantage of assessing arterial wall thickening (Figure 14-1). Transthoracic echocardiography to assess changes in the aorta and its ascending branches and transesophageal echocardiography to assess the descending aorta have also been used. In general, arteriography remains the gold standard, particularly in establishing the diagnosis. Noninvasive imaging modalities may prove useful, however, in following patients over time and in assessing response to therapy safely.

Differential Diagnosis

GCA can similarly affect large vessels and is pathologically also a granulomatous vasculitis. The clinical context, however, generally makes these entities readily distinguishable because TA generally affects young females whereas GCA is exceedingly uncommon in patients under the age of 50. Other considerations in the differential diagnosis may include arterial spasm secondary

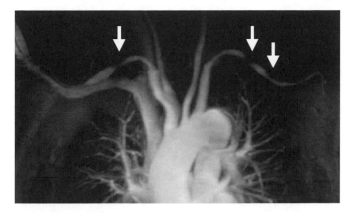

Figure 14-1   Magnetic resonance angiography in Takayasu's arteritis demonstrates multiple areas of marked stenosis, notably in both subclavian arteries (*arrows*). (Courtesy of Dr. Michael Lockshin.)

to excessive intake of sympathomimetic agents, Buerger's disease, and even Ehlers-Danlos syndrome, which can be associated with vascular abnormalities and aneurysms. A comprehensive history and physical examination are usually adequate to distinguish many of these entities. Syphilitic aortitis should also be considered and can be assessed with appropriate serologic testing.

Prognosis and Disease Outcomes

With early recognition and appropriate therapy, the short-term prognosis of TA is excellent, with a 5-year survival of over 90% reported. TA, however, is a chronic and unpredictable disease characterized by alternating periods of exacerbations and remissions. Thus careful vigilance is needed both for disease flares and for potential toxicities and adverse effects associated with therapies in order to reduce long-term complications. Minimizing co-morbidities is a major component of optimizing outcome in patients with TA. Appropriate treatment of hypertension, cessation of smoking, and close attention to achieving an optimal lipid profile are helpful in maximizing arterial health.

Management

A rheumatology consultation should generally be obtained upon diagnosis. Corticosteroids can be dramatically effective in controlling the systemic and ischemic symptoms early in the disease course or during exacerbations when active inflammatory disease is the primary problem. Initially, high-dose oral corticosteroids are utilized, generally on the order of prednisone 1 mg/kg/d or its equivalent. Corticosteroids are tapered gradually when control of active inflammatory symptoms is achieved. Some have advocated long-term low-dose corticosteroid maintenance to prevent flares of disease or progression of vascular compromise. In general, however, corticosteroids can be tapered completely if a remission is achieved, recognizing that reinstitution of therapy may be necessary for relapses. Many patients do not seem to achieve full remission.

The substantial morbidity of high-dose and long-term corticosteroid therapy has prompted the use of various steroid-sparing/disease-modifying interventions. Azathioprine and cyclophosphamide have been used in patients unresponsive to prednisone alone or in those with high corticosteroid requirements. Methotrexate (mean dose 17 mg/week) and mycophenolate mofetil (1 g bid) have more recently been shown to have disease-controlling benefits (10,11).

During the late stenotic phase of the disease, revascularization procedures may be necessary. Angioplasty has been less commonly helpful because diseased vascular segments can be very lengthy, but arterial bypass procedures can be very effective. Aneurysm repairs or even aortic valve surgery may be needed in some patients.

REFERENCES

1. **Helfgott SM, Kieval RI.** Polymyalgia rheumatica in patients with a normal erythrocyte sedimentation rate. Arthritis Rheum. 1996;39:304-7.

2. **Evans JM, O'Fallon WM, Hunder GG.** Increased incidence of aortic aneurysm and dissection in giant cell (temporal) arteritis: a population-based study. Ann Intern Med. 1995;122:502-7.

3. **Boyev LR, Miller NR, Green WR.** Efficacy of unilateral versus bilateral temporal artery biopsies for the diagnosis of giant cell arteritis. Am J Ophthalmol. 1999;128: 211-5.

4. **Achkar AA, Lie JT, Hunder GG, et al.** How does previous corticosteroid treatment affect the biopsy findings in giant cell (temporal) arteritis? Ann Intern Med. 1994;120:987-92.

5. **Hunder GG, Sheps SG, Allen GL, Joyce JW.** Daily and alternate-day corticosteroid regimens in treatment of giant cell arteritis: comparison in a prospective study. Ann Intern Med. 1975;82:613-8.

6. **Jover JA, Hernandez-Garcia C, Morado IC, et al.** Combined treatment of giant-cell arteritis with methotrexate and prednisone: a randomized, double-blind, placebo-controlled trial. Ann Intern Med. 2001;134:106-14.

7. **Spiera R, Mitnick HJ, Kupersmith M, et al.** A prospective, double-blind randomized, placebo controlled trial of methotrexate in the treatment of giant cell arteritis (GCA). Clin Exp Rheumatol. 2001;19:495-501.

8. **Hata A, Numano F.** Magnetic resonance imaging of vascular changes in Takayasu's arteritis. Int J Cardiol. 1995;52:45-52.

9. **Yamada I, Nakagawa T, Himeno Y, et al.** Takayasu's arteritis: evaluation of the thoracic aorta with CT angiography. Radiology. 1998;209:103-9.

10. **Hoffman GS, Leavitt RY, Kerr GS, et al.** Treatment of glucocorticoid-resistant or relapsing Takayasu's arteritis with methotrexate. Arthritis Rheum. 1994;37:578-82.

11. **Daina E, Schieppati A, Remuzzi G.** Mycophenolate mofetil for the treatment of Takayasu's arteritis: report of three cases. Ann Intern Med. 1999;130:422-6.

SECTION V

INFECTIONS

15

■ ■ ■

Infections of the Musculoskeletal System

Barry D. Brause, MD

Infections of the musculoskeletal system are urgent, if not emergent, conditions that demand prompt recognition and intervention. Taken together, acute infectious arthritis, septic bursitis, and osteomyelitis occur with an annual incidence of up to 30 cases per 100,000 in the general population (1). However, select patient groups (e.g., those who are immunocompromised, have underlying joint or bone damage, with joint prostheses or internal fixation devices, or with co-morbid medical conditions) are at greatly increased risks.

The clinical presentation of infections of the musculoskeletal system is quite variable and is determined by the intrinsic characteristics of the specific pathogens, as well as the interaction between the microbes and the host defense responses within the synovial tissue, cartilage and bone. Thus, while an acute *Staphylococcus aureus* infection of a joint will demonstrate the stereotypical tetrad of inflammation (acute pain, edema, erythema, and warmth), a mycobacterial or fungal infection can be relatively indolent and slowly progressive.

Coordinated care between the internist, infectious disease specialist, and orthopedic surgeon is essential for optimal management. Early diagnosis and treatment can effectively neutralize the destructive process and optimize functional outcomes. Conversely, delayed intervention can result in the sequestration or dissemination of the infectious agent, leading to diminished response to antibiotic therapy and potentially resulting in irreparable local damage to joint or bone, progression to chronic infection, or even death.

Infectious Arthritis

Pathogenesis

Invasion of the synovial membrane by microorganisms defines septic arthritis and is the initial event in all pyogenic arthritides involving native (i.e., nonprosthetic) articulations. Subsequently, infection extends into the joint space where a paucity of phagocytes, antibodies, and complement permits a closed-space infection to be established. As the pathological process continues, bacterial and leukocyte enzymes degrade the avascular cartilage. The infection progresses at a rate determined by the virulence of the pathogen, the nature and extent of the inflammatory reaction, and the vulnerability of the underlying host tissue. Polymorphonuclear leukocytes, recruited by microbial chemotactic factors, appear to be essential for evolution of tissue destruction. Phagocytosis and neutrophil autolysis release lysozomal enzymes that subsequently damage synovium and cartilage.

The articular cartilage is also degraded by bacteria that bind to and fragment the collagen fibrils of cartilage, enabling microbial invasion of the tissue. This leads to a cascade of other mechanisms by which microbial products promote cartilage damage, including inhibition of proteoglycan synthesis, induction of intravascular thrombosis of subsynovial vessels, and activation of host proteolytic processes. The synovial inflammatory response includes synovial membrane proliferation that becomes an aggressive form of granulation tissue (pannus), which expands throughout the entire articulation. Irreversible loss of joint function is related to the extent of cartilaginous dissolution and joint deformity due to ensuing secondary osteoarthritis.

Microbial arthritis can arise via three routes of infection: hematogenous seeding, extension from sepsis in adjacent tissue, and direct inoculation. Infections of the skin and soft tissues, genitourinary tract, respiratory tract, and gastrointestinal tract can spread to the synovial membrane through the bloodstream. Local septic processes in tissue contiguous to the joint such as cellulitis, infected skin ulcerations, paronychia, infected synovial cysts, and osteomyelitis can invade synovial membranes by direct extension. Lastly, microorganisms can be introduced into articular tissue through penetrating trauma, arthrocentesis/intra-articular injections, and orthopedic procedures.

Patients are generally prone to joint infections on the basis of either local factors at their articulations or systemic factors that increase the risk of bacteremia. Thus, while the annual incidence of septic arthritis is 2 to 5 cases per 100,000 in the general population, the annual incidence is 28 to 38 per 100,000 among patients with rheumatoid arthritis (2). Factors predisposing to the development of septic arthritis include one or more of the following (with approximate frequencies appearing in parentheses):

- Immunosuppressive or corticosteroid therapy (50%)
- Extra-articular infection (50%)
- Previous damage to joint architecture – for example, as the result of rheumatoid arthritis, degenerative joint disease, crystal-induced arthritis, systemic lupus erythematosus, neuropathic arthropathy, trauma, or surgery (27%)
- Serious underlying chronic illness associated with impaired immunological defenses and/or recurrent bacteremias, including malignancy, diabetes mellitus, renal insufficiency, hepatic cirrhosis, and parenteral drug abuse (19%)

Case Presentation 1

A 62-year-old woman with a history of well-controlled non-insulin dependent diabetes mellitus and degenerative knee arthritis was seen for fever, cough, and a swollen left knee. The patient was in her usual state of health until four days before evaluation when she developed a cough and a low-grade fever. Over the next two days, her fever rose to 38.9°C and she developed chills, rigors, and pleuritic chest pain. Her cough became productive of thick yellow sputum. The next day, her left knee became warm, swollen, erythematous, and painful, and she found it increasingly difficult to bear weight. She was brought in by wheelchair to the emergency room.

On physical examination, the patient appeared ill, dyspneic, and diaphoretic. Her blood pressure was 110/65 mm Hg; her pulse was 100/min; her respiratory rate was 24/min; her temperature was 39.2°C. Bronchial breath sounds and coarse rhonchi were heard in the area of the right middle lobe. The left knee was very warm and erythematous. There was a large intra-articular effusion that extended into the suprapatellar pouch. The joint line was markedly tender, and the knee was painful with minimal passive or active movement. The rest of the physical examination was noncontributory but notable for the absence of stigmata of septic emboli. No other joint was inflamed.

Laboratory testing demonstrated a peripheral leukocytosis and thrombocytosis. Plain chest radiography revealed a right middle lobar pneumonia. Arthrocentesis of the left knee removed 80 cc of purulent synovial fluid (95×10^3 white blood cells/mm^3; 99% polymorphonuclear neutrophils). The synovial fluid showed many neutrophils with intracellular gram-positive cocci and diplococci.

After a day of intravenous vancomycin therapy the patient remained febrile but was breathing more comfortably. There was reaccumulation of the left knee effusion; 40 cc of synovial fluid was removed and revealed 50 $\times 10^3$ white blood cells/mm^3. *Streptococcus pneumoniae* was isolated from cultures of the original arthrocentesis and was subsequently found to be sensitive to penicillin. Peripheral blood cultures were negative. Vancomycin was discontinued, and intravenous penicillin G was initiated.

The patient defervesced after three days of intravenous antibiotic therapy, and her respiratory status and knee symptoms and signs improved steadily. Repeat aspiration of the knee yielded significantly less fluid, the leukocyte count of which was also improved. After one week of intravenous antibiotics, the patient was started on oral antibiotics without further complications.

Clinical Features

Bacterial infection should be considered in any patient with an acute monoarticular arthritis. The sudden onset of joint pain is the most characteristic symptom, with increasing severity upon movement or weight bearing. Articular pain is induced by even minimal degrees of passive or active joint motion. Swelling, tenderness, erythema, and warmth along the joint line accompany restriction in range of motion. Pain that is produced only by extreme flexion or extreme extension is more suggestive of periarticular inflammation, as seen in septic bursitis.

Fever is an almost constant feature of pyarthrosis (90% of cases), and systemic sepsis with septic shock can occur with particularly virulent pathogens in vulnerable patients. Synovial effusions are present in over 90% of cases. Bacterial arthritis typically affects only one joint; however, infection in more than one joint is seen in 10% of patients and usually reflects concomitant bacteremia. The knees and hips are the most commonly infected joints, but atypical sites such as the glenohumeral, tibiotalar, sternoclavicular, and sacroiliac joints can also be involved, especially in predisposed individuals such as parenteral drug abusers. Sepsis within the hip joint can be particularly difficult to diagnose, because focal symptoms may be minimal and joint effusions may be difficult to appreciate. Subacute or chronic, slowly progressive monoarthritis should raise suspicion for possible mycobacterial or fungal infections.

Viral arthritides (e.g., rubella, parvovirus B19, and hepatitis B) commonly produce oligo- or poly-articular arthritis, typically involving the hands and wrists and often resembling rheumatoid arthritis and other immune-mediated inflammatory conditions. The vast majority of viral arthritides is self-limited, but some patients may develop a chronic inflammatory arthropathy.

Certain pyarthroses are characteristically accompanied by dermatologic manifestations. Infectious arthritis due to *Neisseria gonorrhoeae* often is associated with prodromal or concomitant migratory tenosynovitis (68% of cases) and erythematous papules, vesiculopustules, or petechial skin rashes (44% of cases) during the disseminated stage of gonococcemia. *Haemophilus influenzae* pyarthrosis can be associated with tenosynovitis and erysipeloid, pustular, or petechial rashes. Similar presentations have been described for bacterial arthritis due to *Neisseria meningitidis, Streptobacillus moniliformis* (rat-bite fever), and *Moraxella catarrhalis*. Inflammation of the tendon sheaths adjacent to the infected articulation is also seen with rubella, atypical mycobacteria, and sporotrichosis. As discussed in Chapter 16, erythema chronicum migrans is pathognomonic of early *Borrelia burgdorferi* infection (Lyme disease), which can later develop into an inflammatory arthritis.

Diagnosis

Arthrocentesis and Synovial Fluid Studies

Synovial fluid analysis is the essential element in the evaluation of any suspected joint infection. Initial joint aspiration should be performed with a needle lumen of sufficient size (typically no smaller than 20 gauge) to permit recovery of potentially large volumes of thick, purulent material. In most cases, aspiration can take place at the bedside. However, arthrocentesis under radiographic guidance may be preferred in certain circumstances such as for deeply located joints like the hip or when there is suspicion of intra-articular loculations due to ongoing inflammation and fibrosis. In these situations, early orthopedic surgical evaluations are also appropriate, because arthroscopic or open surgical joint drainage may be necessary.

The results of the synovial fluid analysis form the basis for initial therapy and confirmation of the specific microbiologic diagnosis (Table 15-1). In septic arthritis, the synovial fluid cell count and differential commonly reveal a leukocytosis with predominance of neutrophils, but the leukocyte count can range widely. Nonbacterial joint infections may demonstrate a predominance of mononuclear cells. The probability of infection increases with higher leukocyte counts. Forty percent of patients with bacterial arthritis have a synovial fluid white blood cell greater than 100,000 cells/mm^3;

Table 15-1   Synovial Fluid Analysis from Normal, Rheumatoid, and Septic Joints

	Normal Joints	Rheumatoid Joints	Septic Joints
Color	Colorless to straw	Yellow	Yellow
Turbidity	Clear	Turbid	Turbid to purulent
Typical leukocyte count/mm^3	<1000	1000-50,000	10,000->100,000
Cell type	Mononuclear	Neutrophilic	Neutrophilic
Synovial fluid/blood glucose ratio	0.8-1.0	0.5-0.8	<0.5
Gram stain	No organisms	No organisms	Positive in 65% of cases
Culture	Negative	Negative	Positive

rheumatoid arthritis and crystal-induced arthritis rarely produce these counts. It should be noted that septic arthritis can result in the "strip-mining" of urate and calcium pyrophosphate crystals within the joint, resulting in concomitant acute gout or pseudogout. Therefore the identification of such crystals should not deter continued evaluations for joint infection.

Synovial fluid Gram stain results are available shortly after arthrocentesis and therefore become the cornerstone of initial antibiotic selection while awaiting the results of cultures (Table 15-2). Countercurrent immuno-electrophoresis (CIE) can rapidly detect antigens from pneumococci, meningococci, and *H. influenzae* in joint fluid (and urine) and can also be helpful in establishing the microbiologic diagnosis, especially when prior antibiotic therapy interferes with routine cultures.

Synovial fluid cultures represent the definitive approach to establishing the diagnosis of septic arthritis. Optimally, the fluid should be inoculated onto media directly after aspiration or promptly delivered to the micro-biology laboratory for immediate plating and incubation. Media should be selected for gram-positive and gram-negative aerobes (including *N. gonor-rhoeae* and *H. influenzae*), anaerobes, and, if indicated, fungi and myco-bacteria. Cultures of synovial fluid are highly likely (85% to 90% sensitivity) to confirm the specific etiologic microorganism in all bacterial arthritides except in gonococcal infection where only 25% to 50% sensitivity is found. Gonococcal infection is often established on the basis of urethral, cervical, pharyngeal, and rectal cultures or diagnosed clinically by the presence of tenosynovitis and the characteristic skin lesions of disseminated gonococ-cemia. Synovial fluid cultures for mycobacteria and fungi should be con-sidered in immunocompromised patients and in patients with persistent joint effusions or chronic monoarticular arthritis with negative bacterial cultures. Synovial biopsies for bacterial, mycobacterial, and fungal culture

Table 15-2   Initial Antibiotic Therapy for Pyogenic Arthritis Based on Gram Stain Results of Synovial Fluid

Gram Stain Results	Initial Antibiotic Therapy	Alternative Antibiotic Therapy
Gram-positive cocci*	Nafcillin or oxacillin	Vancomycin
Gram-negative cocci**	Ceftriaxone, cefotaxime, or ceftizoxime	Spectinomycin or ciprofloxacin
Gram-negative bacilli***	Gentamicin	Ceftazidime
Unrevealing Gram stain with a clinical picture consistent with infection	Ampicillin/sulbactam plus gentamicin	Vancomycin plus ceftizoxime

* Vancomycin should be used if methicillin-resistant *Staphylococcus aureus* is prevalent.
** Ceftizoxime and spectinomycin should not be used if *Neisseria meningitidis* is a possible pathogen.
*** Gentamicin should be used if the patient is a compromised host (e.g., hepatic cirrhosis, diabetes melli-tus, intravenous drug abuse, neoplastic disease, immunosuppression).

(in addition to histopathology) can be diagnostic in cases of unexplained chronic synovitis.

The age-related incidence of bacterial pathogens in septic arthritis is presented in Table 15-3. *Staphylococcus aureus* is a frequent cause of septic arthritis in all age groups (Fig. 15-1). Streptococci are important etiologic agents in children under 15 years of age due to bacteremic upper respiratory infections with *S. pneumoniae* and *S. pyogenes*. *Haemophilus influenzae* biotype II, previously a significant cause of hematogenous joint sepsis for the same reason in children under 6 years of age, is now rarely seen since the advent of routine *Haemophilus* conjugate vaccination in infancy. Although gonococcus is still the most frequent cause of bacterial arthritis in the most sexually active age groups, the incidence of *N. gonorrhoeae* infection has markedly declined with increased use of safer sex techniques (3). The population at risk for gram-negative bacillary arthritis reflects those

Table 15-3   Age-Related Frequency of Specific Pathogens in Infectious Arthritis

Microorganism	Under age 2	Age 2-15 years	Age 16-50 years	Over age 50 years
Staphylococcus aureus	45%	50%	15%	70%
Streptococci	25%	30%	5%	15%
Haemophilus influenzae*	30%	9%	—	—
Neisseria gonorrhoeae	—	5%	75%	—
Gram-negative bacilli	3%	5%	5%	8%

* *Haemophilus* infections are seen less frequently in children vaccinated with *Haemophilus influenzae* biotype II.

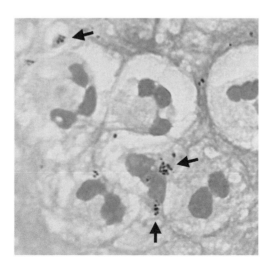

Figure 15-1 Gram stain of synovial fluid from a patient with *Staphylococcus aureus* septic arthritis demonstrates polymorphonuclear neutrophils with intracellular clusters of gram-positive cocci (*arrows*).

predisposed to gram-negative bacteremia including immunosuppressed patients and intravenous drug abusers. Two thirds of these patients have debilitating diseases, and most joint infections are caused by hematogenous spread from urinary tract foci.

Other Laboratory Studies

In 49% of cases, the same organism is cultured from an extra-articular site as well as from the infected joint. Therefore it is helpful to obtain cultures from all possible foci of infection as appropriate for the individual patient's history and physical examination (including proper consideration of sputum, urine, skin lesions, oropharynx, urethra, uterine cervix, and rectum). In addition, at least two blood cultures should be drawn. Specific culture media for gonococci (Thayer-Martin or chocolate agars) should be employed in addition to routine media for specimens from mucosal surfaces and skin lesions.

The peripheral leukocyte count is typically elevated but is nonspecific and may actually be normal in 30% of patients with septic arthritis.

Radiographic Imaging

Plain radiographs of the joint are useful to document extent of previous damage, observe for evidence of osteomyelitis, and provide a baseline for follow-up studies. The earliest radiographic sign of joint infection is periarticular soft tissue swelling with displacement of the adjacent fat pads by synovial edema or an articular effusion during the first week of pyarthrosis. After this period, periarticular osteopenia develops due to local hyperemia as well as bone atrophy secondary to relative immobility. With more fulminant infection, uniform joint space narrowing becomes visible by X-ray as a consequence of articular cartilage dissolution. Subsequently osseous erosions and loss of cortical bone *on both sides of the joint,* induced by pannus, can be seen subchondrally or in peripheral areas between the joint capsule insertion and the joint cartilage where the synovium is in direct contact with bone (Fig. 15-2). Eventually, fibrous or bony ankylosis may develop in chronic infections. Radiologic evaluation of the infected joint is generally helpful but not diagnostic, because these anatomic changes are not specific for septic processes.

Radioisotope bone scans can be of value in diagnostic problems involving deep-seated joints such as the hip, shoulder, or spine and in detecting multiple sites of infection. However, the findings are often not specific, and these scans usually have little role in the initial evaluation of acute infectious arthritis. Although magnetic resonance imaging (MRI) is useful in delineating peri-articular abscesses and avascular necrosis in adjacent bone, this technique is not sufficiently specific to diagnose a septic joint.

Prognosis and Disease Outcomes

Acute bacterial arthritis is a rheumatologic emergency, and immediate intervention is crucial to prevent joint damage, local spread to contiguous structures,

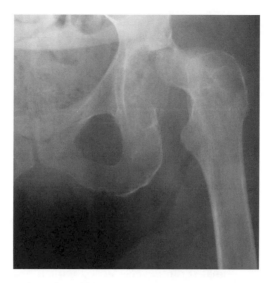

Figure 15-2   X-ray of an infected left hip in a patient with underlying rheumatoid arthritis. The patient complained of several weeks of progressive disproportionate left groin pain that ultimately caused her to be unable to bear weight on her left hip. The X-ray shows extensive destruction of the cortical bone on both the acetabular and femoral sides of the joint. Cultures of synovial fluid obtained via fluoroscopic aspiration grew out *Peptostreptococci.*

or even systemic sepsis. Several factors have been identified to correlate with the overall prognosis for full recovery of articular function after pyarthrosis:

1. *Prompt Intervention*—Appropriate therapy instituted within seven days is associated with the best outcome.

2. *Serial Synovial Fluid Leukocyte Counts*—Appropriate response to therapy should be accompanied at least a 50% to 75% reduction in synovial fluid white blood cell count within 5 to 7 days.

3. *Synovial Fluid Sterility*—Optimally, the synovial fluid should be sterile within 5 days of therapy.

4. *Virulence of the Pathogen* (Table 15-4)—*S. aureus* and gram-negative bacilli infections carry poor prognoses.

5. *Host Factors*—Patients with hip or shoulder involvement, with more than three joints infected, who are over 60 years old, with rheumatoid arthritis, or with diabetes mellitus appear to recover less completely.

Management

Initial Treatment
Antibiotic therapy, empirically determined on the basis of clinical presentation and Gram stain results, should be initiated promptly (see Table 15-2).

Table 15-4   Prognosis for Recovery of Baseline Articular Function Related to Specific Pathogens Causing Joint Infection

Microorganism	Patients (%) Recovering Baseline Articular Function after Appropriate Therapy
Neisseria gonorrhoeae	>95%
Streptococcus pneumoniae	94%
Streptococcus pyogenes (Group A)	85%
Staphylococcus aureus	73%
Gram-negative bacilli	21%

Several oral antimicrobial agents achieve sufficient serum and tissue levels to be effective in treating septic articulations. Because reliable gastrointestinal absorption must be assured, however, initial therapy is usually parenteral to ensure optimal serum levels. Most antimicrobial agents achieve effective synovial fluid levels with parenteral dosing. Intra-articular instillation of, or irrigation with, antimicrobial agents is not indicated and may even be hazardous; direct injection of antibiotics into the joint space can cause a chemical synovitis or lead to systemic absorption resulting in potentially toxic serum levels.

Relative joint immobilization (maintained in the functional position) should be employed initially until joint pain begins to resolve (usually within 1 to 3 days). Weight bearing should be avoided initially to reduce the risk of further damage to articular cartilage in lower extremity joints. Subsequently, range of motion exercises should be started (without weight bearing) to prevent the development of joint contractures. This technique may also enhance nutritional diffusion to cartilage and assist in restoring natural cartilage repair mechanisms inhibited by prolonged immobilization.

Analgesics that do not affect fever, such as opiates without acetaminophen, should be used as necessary. For the same reason, non-steroidal anti-inflammatory drugs should be avoided initially if possible.

Disease Monitoring
Daily assessment of patient status includes monitoring the fever curve and constitutional symptoms, changes in range of motion of the joint, peripheral leukocyte counts, and the resolution of any extra-articular foci of infection. Selection of definitive antibiotic therapy is made as final microbial culture results become available (Table 15-5). The duration of antibiotic therapy varies with different types of bacterial arthritis. Gonococcal arthritis can generally be treated with 7 days of therapy (4), whereas other bacterial pathogens may require 2 to 4 weeks of antibiotic therapy depending upon the microorganism, the response to therapy, and the health of the underlying articular tissues. Treatment of infections in prosthetic joints (which are

Table 15-5   Antibiotic Therapy Based on Culture Identification of Organism

Organism	Antibiotic	Alternative
Staphylococcus aureus	Nafcillin	Vancomycin
Methicillin-resistant S. aureus	Vancomycin	Linezolid or quinupristin/ dalfopristin
Non-enterococcal streptococci	Penicillin	Cefazolin, ceftriaxone, or vancomycin
Enterococci	Penicillin plus gentamicin	Vancomycin plus gentamicin, linezolid, or quinupristin/ dalfopristin
Neisseria gonorrhoeae (penicillin-sensitive)	Ampicillin	Third-generation cephalosporin or spectinomycin
Neisseria gonorrhoeae (penicillin-resistant or unknown sensitivity)	Third-generation cephalosporin	Spectinomycin or ciprofloxacin
Enterobacteriaceae	Third-generation cephalosporin	Aminoglycoside, ciprofloxacin, or aztreonam
Haemophilus influenzae	Third-generation cephalosporin	Trimethoprim/sulfamethoxazole or chloramphenicol
Pseudomonas	Aminoglycoside	Third-generation cephalosporin or anti-Pseudomonas penicillin

usually considered as special forms of osteomyelitis) is discussed later in this chapter.

Serial Joint Aspiration

Because septic arthritis is a closed-space infection, drainage procedures are essential to decrease intra-articular pressure and to reduce leukocyte enzyme activity. Serial arthrocenteses and synovial fluid aspirations are performed as frequently as prompted by the rate of reaccumulation of effusions and are commonly adequate to accomplish this aspect of therapy. Serial synovial fluid leukocyte counts can also be used to monitor the response to therapy. After 5 to 7 days of effective treatment, the joint fluid WBC should decline by 50% to 75%. Failure to achieve such a reduction should be viewed as an indication of inadequate therapy, and surgical drainage should be considered.

Surgery

Surgical drainage, often with synovectomy, is indicated in the treatment of many hip and shoulder infections (particularly with S. aureus or gram-negative bacilli) due to the mechanical difficulty encountered in percutaneous needle aspiration of these deep articulations. Operative debridement of any joint is essential when pyarthrosis is inadequately responsive to serial arthrocentesis or in the event of loculation of infection caused by intra-articular adhesions or underlying joint disease. The development of loculations is often suspected when the synovial fluid leukocyte counts demonstrate great variability according to the site of aspiration. Arthroscopic techniques have generally replaced open arthrotomy for debridement in these situations. Arthroscopy may provide more complete visualization of the tissue (by magnification and access to posterior compartments), decreases morbidity (lower complication rate), increases joint mobility (earlier post-operative motion due to decreased incision size and associated pain), and is more economical (allows a shorter hospitalization period).

In general, indications for surgical drainage include

1. Hip or shoulder infection (with the exception of gonococcal arthritis)

2. Failure of serial needle aspirations to adequately drain the joint

3. Development of intra-articular loculations

4. Lack of local or systemic response to therapy (e.g., failure to sterilize the joint fluid, continued fever or persistent peripheral leukocytosis after 72 to 96 hours of appropriate antibiotic therapy)

5. Gram-negative bacillary arthritis in a compromised host

Septic Bursitis

Pathogenesis and Etiology

Bursae are closed sacs with a synovial lining that facilitate the smooth gliding of adjacent connective tissue structures against each other during musculoskeletal motion. Many different forms of trauma can induce a bland (aseptic) bursitis, an accumulation of sterile synovial fluid within the bursal sac. Occupations and activities that cause impact, pressure, abrasions, contusions, or lacerations at the elbows or knees increase the risk for developing bursitis around these joints. Underlying inflammatory conditions such as gout, pseudogout, and rheumatoid arthritis also increase the risk of developing bursal effusions. Bacteria, once given access, grow easily within these effusions. Infection of the bursal sac (septic bursitis) typically develops as a consequence of *direct* bacterial seeding of the bursa at the time of trauma or by *contiguous spread* from adjacent cellulitis. The annual incidence of septic bursitis in the general population is roughly 10 to 20 cases per 100,000. Due to their superficial locations and susceptibility to trauma, the olecranon, prepatellar, and superficial infrapatellar bursae are the most frequently infected. A clear history of prior bursal area trauma is reported in as many as 77% of cases. Hematogenous infection can also occur but is much less common and generally involves the deep bursae (5,6).

Clinical Features

The diagnosis of septic bursitis is supported by histories of prior trauma to the area (49%-77%) and/or prior bursal disease (30%-40%) (7). Patients uniformly complain of focal bursal swelling. Tenderness is found in 82% to 100% of patients, surrounding erythema and cellulitis are seen in 60% to 100%, and a skin lesion (such as a laceration or abrasion) is observed in 50% to 60%. Pain is evident on palpation of the bursa and on extreme flexion and extreme extension of the adjacent joint but not on limited or passive motion; this distinguishes "extra-articular" septic bursitis from "intra-articular" septic arthritis.

Infection of the superficial bursae (e.g., olecranon, peripatellar) does not imply involvement of the underlying joints, because there is normally no communication between the two compartments. Infrequently, however, infection can involve both the joint and the bursa when a communication has been created by underlying disease (e.g., rheumatoid arthritis) or trauma (e.g., penetrating wound, fracture). In contrast, infections that affect specific deep bursae more frequently involve the adjacent joint, such as the popliteal (Baker's) cyst and the knee, the subacromial bursa and the glenohumeral joint, or the iliopsoas bursa and the hip.

Diagnosis

As for septic arthritis, aspiration and examination of bursal fluid are essential for the diagnosis and treatment of septic bursitis. Fluid analysis reveals abnormalities similar to infected joint fluid. The etiologic pathogen is *S. aureus* in over 90% of cases.

Radiologic studies are rarely indicated for bursal infections unless clinical response to therapy is not progressing as expected or a concomitant joint or bone infection is suspected.

Prognosis and Disease Outcomes

Generally, septic bursitis responds readily to antibiotic therapy and needle drainage without complications or residua. Aspiration of the bursa should be repeated as often as necessary to remove reaccumulated fluid, but care must be taken to avoid introducing infection into the neighboring joint. Full recovery of function can be anticipated. Systemic complications include bacteremia (in approximately 6% of patients) and rare cases of toxic shock syndrome. Local complications include necrotizing fasciitis, fistula formation, septic arthritis, and osteomyelitis. Bursal sepsis can be recurrent, especially if predisposing conditions persist.

Management

Treatment involves drainage of the purulent fluid and antibiotic therapy. Clinically mild infections without evidence of systemic illness can be treated with oral antibiotics for 10 to 28 days, if the patient is compliant and can be trusted to report lack of improvement or progression of the infection. If within two days such patients fail to improve, parenteral therapy should be instituted with intravenous treatment for 2 weeks, followed by 2 weeks of oral therapy. Immunocompromised patients and those with evidence of systemic sepsis should be treated with parenteral therapy from the outset for at least 2 weeks.

Because *S. aureus* is the overwhelmingly predominant pathogen in septic bursitis, empiric treatment should always include an anti-staphylococcal agent unless the results of the Gram stain or culture reveal a different organism. Options for oral therapy include dicloxacillin 500 mg every 6 hours or, in penicillin-allergic individuals, cephalexin 500 mg every 6 hours or levofloxacin 750 mg daily plus rifampin 300 mg twice daily. When intravenous therapy is necessary, nafcillin 2 g every 4 hours or oxacillin 2 g every 4 hours or, in penicillin-allergic patients, cefazolin 1 g every 8 hours or vancomycin 1 g every 12 hours are appropriate regimens.

Since septic bursitis is a closed-space infection, drainage procedures are essential. Percutaneous needle aspirations are usually effective and should be repeated as needed with reaccumulations of bursal fluid. Bursal effusions are generally sterilized with appropriate antibiotic therapy and percutaneous drainage within 5 days in immunocompetent patients and within a mean of 12 days for immunocompromised patients.

If the usually thin bursal lining is thickened by prior disease or edematous by persistent infection, percutaneous aspirations become increasingly difficult and potentially inadequate. Surgical drainage with bursectomy is indicated for deep bursal sacs that are percutaneously inaccessible or for persistent infections.

Osteomyelitis

Pathogenesis

Osteomyelitis represents invasion of microorganisms into osseous tissue. Three potential routes of infection define the major forms of osteomyelitis, with pathogens reaching osseous tissue by 1) hematogenous seeding, 2) contamination accompanying surgical and non-surgical trauma (termed *introduced infection*), or 3) spread from infected contiguous tissue (8).

Bacteria are the usual pathogens, among which staphylococci are the most prominent etiologic agents. *Staphylococcus aureus* causes approximately 60% of hematogenous and introduced infections and is also a principal agent when osseous sepsis spreads contiguously. *Staphylococcus epidermidis* has become a major pathogen in bone infections associated with indwelling prosthetic materials such as joint implants and fracture fixation devices and is responsible for 30% of these cases. In other specific clinical settings, streptococci, gram-negative bacilli, anaerobes, mycobacteria, and fungi are also potential pathogenic agents (Table 15-6).

Hematogenous Osteomyelitis

With hematogenous osteomyelitis, sites of increased perfusion are more likely to become infected. Accordingly, in childhood hematogenous osteomyelitis (from birth to puberty), the initial infective site is usually the long bone metaphysis. In contrast, in adult hematogenous osteomyelitis, the vertebral bodies are more commonly infected, particularly at the vascular anterior end plates (9). Infection commonly involves two adjacent vertebral bodies and the intervening intervertebral disk space. This results in compromised nutrient supply to the disk, resulting in necrosis and disk space narrowing,

Table 15-6   Forms of Osteomyelitis

Form	Predisposing Conditions	Common Sites	Prominent Pathogens
Childhood hematogenous	None	Long bones	*Staphylococcus aureus,* streptococci, *Haemophilus influenzae*
	Sickle cell disease and hemoglobinopathies	Multiple	*Salmonella* sp., *S. aureus*
Adult hematogenous	Urinary tract infection or instrumentation	Vertebral	GNB, streptococci
	Skin infection	Vertebral	*S. aureus,* streptococci
	Respiratory tract infection	Vertebral, hip, knee	Streptococci, *Mycobacterium tuberculosis*
	Intravenous catheterization or drug abuse	Vertebral, clavicle, pelvis	GNB, staphylococci, *Candida albicans*
	AIDS	Multiple	Fungi, mycobacteria
	Endocarditis	Vertebral	Streptococci, staphylococci
Introduced	Fractures	Fracture site	*S. aureus, Staphylococcus epidermidis,* GNB
	Prosthetic joint	Prosthesis	*S. aureus, S. epidermidis*
Contiguous	Skin ulcers (e.g., diabetic, decubitus, stasis, vasculitic)	Foot, leg	Polymicrobial, staphylococci, streptococci, GNB, anaerobes
	Sinusitis	Skull	Streptococci, anaerobes
	Dental abscess	Mandible, maxilla	Streptococci, anaerobes
	Human or animal bites	Site of bite	Streptococci, anaerobes, *Pasteurella multocida*
	Felon	Finger	*S. aureus*
	Gardening	Hand	*Sporothrix schenkii*

GNB = gram-negative bacilli; AIDS = acquired immunodeficiency syndrome.

which is often the earliest radiologic sign of vertebral osteomyelitis. Table 15-6 lists examples of clinical conditions that predispose to the development of blood-borne bone infection.

Bacteremias seed the medullary bone and produce intraosseous edema by inducing local acidosis and inflammation. As the septic process spreads, local thrombophlebitis develops, further increasing intraosseus edema and pressure that eventually result in ischemic necrosis of large areas of bone termed *sequestra*. If the osseous cortex is breached, subperiosteal abscesses can develop with periosteal inflammation that induces new bone formation in adjacent soft tissue. If the infection extends beyond the periosteum, abscesses can form in surrounding soft tissues. Finally, with chronicity the infection can spread to produce a drainage tract or sinus that eventually reaches the skin surface and creates a draining cutaneous sinus orifice.

Introduced Infections

Osseous tissue is at risk for infection whenever the skin and soft tissues overlying and protecting the bone are breached by trauma or surgery. Approximately 70% of compound fractures are contaminated by skin and soil microflora but, with effective debridement and perioperative antibiotic therapy, osteomyelitis develops in only 2% to 9%. Prophylactic antibiotics and extensive antiseptic operative techniques allow complex reparative and reconstructive orthopedic surgery, often accompanied by insertion of foreign materials, with infection rates below 2%. In the introduced form of osteomyelitis, direct septic trauma breaches all protective tissue around the bone, allowing microorganisms into the osseous matrix. Implanted metallic fixation devices or prosthetic joints decrease the size of the innoculum of bacteria necessary to establish infection in bone. These artificial avascular surfaces permit pathogens to persist, frequently within host or pathogen-derived "biofilms" that are sequestered from circulating immune factors and systemic antibiotics.

Contiguous Extension

Osteomyelitis can occur by contiguous extension from infected adjacent soft tissue when the soft tissue process is inadequately controlled. For example, chronic diabetic foot infections reflect the persistence of neuropathic and vasculopathic processes that initiate skin ulceration and interfere with wound healing. Chronic infections of these soft-tissue ulcers can eventually spread to the periosteum and then to the underlying bone. Osteomyelitis develops by contiguous spread in 30% to 68% of diabetic patients with foot ulcers, and it is notable that more in-hospital days are spent treating foot infections than treating any other complication of diabetes.

Clinical Features

In *children,* hematogenous osteomyelitis signs and symptoms of systemic inflammation, such as fever, chills, and malaise, are typically present. The annual incidence is about 10 per 100,000 (10). Localized bony pain is a characteristic feature of osteomyelitis, with overlying erythema, warmth, and swelling variably observed. Limb motion may be limited if infection is near an articulation. When the epiphyseal cartilage is intact, the joint is usually spared from infection, although sterile sympathetic joint effusions can occur.

In *adults,* hematogenous vertebral osteomyelitis often presents subacutely with back pain, spine tenderness, and low-grade fever. The annual incidence is approximately 2 to 3 per 100,000 (11). Frequently, a source of infection can be identified: after urinary tract instrumentation or infection in 30% of cases, skin infection in 13%, or respiratory infection in 11% (9). Fever is present in fewer than 50% of patients and is commonly low-grade. Extension of the septic process beyond the vertebral column can result in retropharyngeal abscesses, mediastinitis, empyema, subdiaphragmatic and iliopsoas abscesses, and meningitis. If paresis, sensory deficits, or bowel or bladder dysfunction develops, a spinal epidural abscess – the most feared complication – should be suspected and evaluated immediately. *Mycobacterium tuberculosis* should be considered in relatively indolent infections of vertebrae.

Osteomyelitis after trauma or bone surgery is usually associated with persistent or recurrent fevers, increasing pain at the operative site, and poor incisional wound healing, which is often accompanied by protracted wound drainage, dehiscence, cellulitis, suture abscesses, and wound hematomas or seromas. Bone infection should also be considered in cases of persistent fracture nonunion and failed arthrodesis.

Bone involvement by contiguous spread from an overlying chronic ischemic or neuropathic foot ulcer typically occurs in patients with long-standing insulin-dependent diabetes (12) or other neuropathic or vascular diseases and frequently involves the metatarsals (44%) or the proximal phalanges (32%). It is characterized by local cellulitis with inflammation and necrosis, but pain is only variably found due to the presence of sensory neuropathy. Osseous extension is common when the skin ulcer is more than 2 cm^2 in area with a depth more than 3 mm or when bone is visibly exposed. Osteomyelitis by contiguous spread also develops from infected decubitus ulcers, venous stasis ulcers, and vasculitic ulcers. Additional examples of osteomyelitis from contiguous spread of infection are listed in Table 15-6.

Diagnosis

The diagnosis of osteomyelitis is dependent upon the compilation of 1) clinical observations (history and physical examination), 2) findings from well-chosen imaging studies (13), and 3) sound clinical judgment to give appropriate weight to the data collected. It is essential to be mindful of the pathogenesis attributed to the specific clinical situation being evaluated.

Establishing the presence of osteomyelitis includes both confirmation of the site of bone involvement and identifying the causative microorganism(s). Osseous infection should be differentiated from septic arthritis and bursitis, cellulitis, soft tissue abscesses, bone fractures, and neoplasms, as well as from bone infarcts as seen with sickle cell disease, hemoglobinopathies, or Gaucher's disease.

Microbiological Studies

Every effort should be made to identify the specific pathogen, because the diversity of potential organisms does not readily allow routine presumptive therapy. Moreover, antibiotic sensitivity of the isolated causative bacterium is essential to design optimal therapy. Blood cultures are positive in 25% to 50% of children with acute hematogenous osteomyelitis but in less than 10% of other forms of bone infection. If septic arthritis or soft tissue abscess accompanies the osseous infection, arthrocentesis or abscess aspiration cultures can be diagnostic. However, superficial cultures of open wounds, wound drainage, or skin ulcerations and cultures of cutaneous sinus tracts often reflect colonizing flora and do not reliably identify the true bone pathogen(s). In patients with deep chronic skin ulcers by which infection has spread to bone, curettage cultures from the base of the ulcer have a 75% correlation with osseous tissue cultures. Bone aspirate cultures are positive in 50% to 60% of patients, whereas bone biopsy cultures are positive in 70% to 93% of cases and should always be sought when there is no overlying skin ulcer and when the pathogen has not been otherwise determined. Specific culture techniques for mycobacteria, fungi, and anaerobes should be considered when routine bacterial cultures are negative.

Plain Radiography and Computed Tomography

Radiologic imaging techniques are essential in delineating the anatomy of bone infection (Table 15-7). In hematogenous infections, the earliest osseous X-ray changes are medullary lucencies, which require 30% to 50% decalcification to be seen and take 2 to 4 weeks to develop. As sepsis progresses, periosteal elevation, thickening, and new bone formation may be seen with sequestra and sclerosis occurring in chronic cases. Vertebral osteomyelitis appears initially as disc space narrowing with subsequent cortical degradation at the adjacent vertebral end-plates. With the introduced form of osteomyelitis, bone resorption is evident at the site of the fracture, the fixation device, or the bone-cement interface of a joint prosthesis. Periosteal reaction is commonly seen in patients with chronic, deep ulcerations overlying bone and does not definitively make the diagnosis of osteomyelitis. Only late in contiguous infections do specific findings for osteomyelitis such as cortical erosions, subperiosteal bone lucencies, and lytic medullary lesions appear.

There is commonly a delay in radiographic improvement during the healing phase of bone infection, and 30% of patients have worsening X-rays while improving clinically on therapy. X-ray is the most specific and least

Table 15-7   Sensitivity and Specificity of Different Imaging Techniques for the Diagnosis of Complicated Osteomyelitis*

Technique	Sensitivity	Specificity
X-ray	69%	82%
Technetium bone scan	77%	36%
Gallium scan	95%	38%
Indium-labeled leukocyte scan	74%	69%
Sequential indium/technetium scans	86%	72%
Magnetic resonance imaging	83%	75%

* Complicated cases include diabetes, neuropathic (Charcot's) arthropathy, cellulitis, and recent trauma (e.g., orthopedic surgery, fractures).

expensive imaging technique for diagnosing osteomyelitis. However, in patients with acute and fulminant infections, X-rays may not be sufficiently sensitive to reveal diagnostic abnormalities at the time of presentation and additional studies are needed. Nonetheless, because most cases of bone infection present subacutely with adequate time for demineralization to occur, plain radiographic techniques are useful. Computed tomography can be a useful adjunct in demonstrating small osseous changes, sequestra, and extraosseous extension of infection.

Radionuclide Scans
Technetium diphosphonate bone scans, gallium citrate scans, and indium-labeled leukocyte scintigraphy are much more sensitive than X-rays and usually demonstrate increased radionuclide uptake at the onset of symptoms. However, these imaging methods are plagued by inadequate specificity and spatial resolution and thus cannot be relied upon to be definitively diagnostic. Inflammatory and degenerative processes in surrounding soft tissues, recent orthopedic surgery or trauma, bone fractures, and neoplasms produce abnormal nuclide scans in the absence of osteomyelitis. Table 15-7 lists the approximate sensitivity and specificity of these imaging techniques when used in clinical situations where the diagnosis is ambiguous due to the presence of a pathological process in adjacent tissues (e.g.. cellulitis, edema) or a co-morbid state in the osseous tissue (e.g.. diabetic osteoarthropathy, bone infarction, recent trauma).

Magnetic Resonance Imaging
MRI can detect osteomyelitis earlier than X-rays and with equal or greater sensitivity and much better spatial resolution than scintigraphy. Negative MRI findings can be taken as strong evidence against the presence of osteomyelitis. However, MRI lacks sufficient specificity to be the optimal imaging techinque for the detection of bone infection.

Increased MRI signals represent small increases in tissue water content and edema. Gadolinium is deposited in the extracellular fluid compartment in areas of increased vascular permeability and thereby increases the sensitivity of MRI for inflammation of any etiology. MRI easily detects the bone edema of osteomyelitis, but differentiation from other causes of edema (e.g., sterile inflammation, edema in tissues adjacent to bone, bone infarction, recent trauma, diabetic osteoarthropathy, heterotopic bone formation, neoplasm, local radiation therapy) is often not possible. This lack of specificity for osteomyelitis significantly undermines the utility of MRI. Recently developed MRI techniques using fat suppression have increased specificity but not yet to the level needed to be sufficiently diagnostic.

Prognosis and Disease Outcomes

Acute osteomyelitis is curable with adequate antimicrobial therapy accompanied by surgical debridement when necessary. Intravenously administered antibiotics are commonly used, but oral agents are also effective when the pathogen is sufficiently susceptible and when gastrointestinal absorption and compliance are ensured. Failure of therapy for acute osteomyelitis results in relapsing infection and progression to chronic osteomyelitis. Therefore definitive treatment of the acute infection is obligatory.

Due to the presence of gross and microscopic foci of avascular bone, chronic osteomyelitis is not curable with systemic antibiotics and surgical debridement. Definitive cure can be obtained only by radical resection and occasionally amputation. Acute exacerbations of these persistent infections can be suppressed successfully by debridement of identifiable sequestra followed by protracted courses of parenteral and/or oral antimicrobial agents. Rare complications of chronic bone infection include pathologic fractures, squamous cell carcinoma at the sinus tract cutaneous orifice, and secondary amyloidosis.

Management

The exact potency and duration of antimicrobial therapy necessary to eradicate bone infections are not known. Antibiotics that produce trough serum bactericidal activity at a 1:2 titer are associated with highly successful outcomes; therapy should generally be administered for at least 4 to 6 weeks. Designing a therapeutic regimen for osteomyelitis is decidedly dependent on the sensitivity of the isolated pathogen to specific antimicrobial agents, underscoring the utmost importance of identifying the pathogen.

Surgery is indicated to drain abscesses, debride necrotic tissues, remove foreign materials, and provide skin closure of chronic unhealed wounds. Surgery is also important when neurologic structures are threatened (e.g., cord compression in vertebral osteomyelitis). In osteomyelitis associated with peripheral vascular disease, amputation of the affected area is frequently required if the infection does not respond to parenteral antibiotics.

Prosthetic Joint Infections

One to five percent of prosthetic joint arthroplasties eventually becomes infected (14). These infections are calamitous events, associated with significant morbidity and occasionally leading to death. They usually involve osseous tissue adjacent to the foreign body and therefore are a special form of osteomyelitis. Prior surgery at the site of the prosthesis, rheumatoid arthritis, immunocompromised states, diabetes mellitus, poor nutritional status, obesity, psoriasis, and extremely advanced age are associated with increased risks of prosthetic joint infections.

Pathogenesis

Infection of the joint can be locally introduced or seeded hematogenously. The locally introduced route is typically the result of wound sepsis contiguous to the prosthesis or of operative contamination. Factors that delay wound healing increase the risk of infection. Ischemic necrosis, infected wound hematomas, wound infection (with or without identifiable cellulitis), and suture abscesses are common preceding events for joint replacement sepsis. During the early post-implantation period, when these superficial infections develop, the fascial layers have not yet healed, and the deep periprosthesis tissue is not protected by the usual physical barriers. Generally, these infections are caused by a single pathogen, but polymicrobial sepsis can also occur. Coagulase-negative staphylococci are the most common etiologic agents in this clinical setting. Infrequently, latent foci of chronic quiescent osteomyelitis are reactivated by the disruption of tissue associated with implantation surgery. For example, latent *Staphylococcus aureus* and *Mycobacterium tuberculosis* infections can recrudesce post-operatively, even when the intraoperative bone cultures are often sterile.

Any bacteremia can cause infection of a joint replacement by the hematogenous route, which accounts for 20% to 40% of cases. Dento-gingival infections and manipulations are known causes of viridans streptococcal and anaerobic (e.g., *Peptococcus, Peptostreptococcus*) infections in prostheses. Pyogenic skin processes can cause staphylococcal (*S. aureus* or *S. epidermidis*) and streptococcal (groups A, B, C, and G streptococci) infections of joint replacements. Genitourinary and gastrointestinal tract procedures or infections are associated with gram-negative bacillary, enterococcal, and anaerobic infections of prostheses. Staphylococci (coagulase-negative staphylococci and *S. aureus*) are the principal causative agents and are isolated in 40% to 50% of cases; aerobic streptococci, enterococci, and gram-negative bacilli are each responsible for 15% to 20%; and anaerobes represent up to 10% of these infections. The spectrum of microbial agents capable of infecting prosthetic joints is unlimited and includes organisms ordinarily considered "contaminants" of cultures such as corynebacteria, propionibacteria, and *Bacillus* spp. Infections with fungi (particularly *Candida*) and mycobacteria have been described rarely.

Case Presentation 2

A 58-year-old woman with long-standing rheumatoid arthritis was seen for fever and acute left knee pain. The patient has had rheumatoid arthritis for fifteen years and underwent total joint arthroplasties of both hips and both knees several years ago. Over the past five years, the patient had been treated with subcutaneous etanercept 25 mg twice weekly with excellent control of her disease. She had been taking no corticosteroids or anti-inflammatory drugs.

Two days ago, the patient did some moderately exertional housework during which she bumped her left knee against some furniture. The next morning, she noted some discomfort in the knee but did not notice any grossly apparent changes. Over the course of the day, the patient developed a fever to 39.0°C and some chills, and the left knee became increasingly swollen. By the evening, she could no longer bear weight on her left leg, and the knee was very warm, swollen, and tender. The patient was brought to the emergency room.

Her temperature was 39.4°C, but other vital signs were normal. Her left knee was markedly inflamed with a large effusion, and its range of active and passive movement was severely limited by extreme pain (Fig. 15-3, *A*). There was overlying cellulitis that tracked up to the distal thigh and down to the proximal tibial region (Fig. 15-3, *B*). The rest of the musculoskeletal examination revealed only some chronic rheumatoid changes in the small joints of the hands but no evidence of synovitis in any other joint. There were no stigmata of embolic disease, and no heart murmur was appreciated. Laboratory testing was remarkable for a peripheral leukocyte count of 28×10^3 white blood cells/mm^3.

Seventy-five (75) cc of grossly purulent fluid were aspirated from the left knee prosthesis. The synovial fluid white cell count was 85×10^3 white blood cells/mm^3; Gram stain revealed many neutrophils with intracellular gram-positive cocci in clusters. Intravenous vancomycin was administered after blood and synovial fluid cultures were sent for microbial cultures.

The following day, the patient underwent surgical removal of the left knee prosthesis and placement of an antibiotic-impregnated spacer. Methicillin-sensitive *Staphylococcus aureus* (MSSA) eventually grew out from synovial fluid and blood cultures, and vancomycin was replaced with intravenous cefazolin.

The patient showed initial clinical improvement but, after several days of antibiotic therapy, she continued to have a fever to 38.8°C and peripheral leukocyte count remained elevated at 18×10^3 white blood cells/mm^3. The patient's right hip (also prosthetic) now had anterior capsular tenderness on palpation. Cultures were obtained from the right hip as well as other prosthetic joints, and MSSA subsequently grew out from the right hip fluid.

After explantation of the right hip prosthesis, the patient steadily defervesced, and her peripheral leukocyte count normalized. After removal of the second prosthesis, the patient received six weeks of intravenous cefazolin, during which time the patient had an unremarkable course. She remained afebrile for two weeks after discontinuation of cefazolin with no relapse of knee swelling and subsequently underwent successful reimplantation of the knee and hip prostheses.

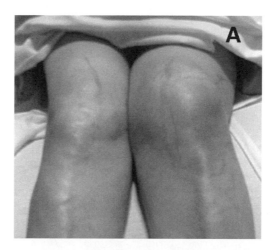

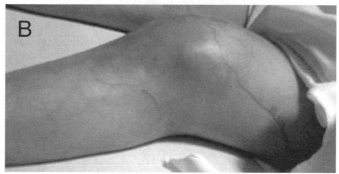

Figure 15-3   Acute infection of a left knee prosthesis. This patient with underlying rheumatoid arthritis and two total knee arthroplasties presented with acute inflammation of the left knee (Panel A). The right knee prosthesis was not affected. *Staphylococcus aureus* was cultured out of the joint fluid. Local cellulitis (the margins of which are outlined in Panel B) was thought to be the source of the infection.

Clinical Features

Prosthetic joint sepsis produces the cardinal symptoms of inflammation but with a wide spectrum of severity. Many patients present with a long indolent course characterized by persistent joint pain or effusions (95% of cases). Occasionally, draining cutaneous sinuses may form (32%). Often, there is no fever or evidence of systemic toxicity. However, in contrast, other patients may present with an acute and fulminant illness with severe joint pain, local swelling and erythema, and high fever, or rarely with frank systemic sepsis. This fulminant pattern of onset is usually seen only with highly virulent pathogens such as *S. aureus,* beta-hemolytic streptococci, or gram-negative bacilli.

Infection should always be presumed when faced with a painful prosthesis accompanied by fever and local signs of inflammation, warranting confirmatory testing. Fortunately, although infection is the most serious potential diagnosis in this setting and should be sought promptly and thoroughly, aseptic and mechanical processes (e.g., hemarthrosis, gout, bland loosening, dislocation, debris-induced synovitis, osteolysis) are more common causes of prosthetic joint pain and inflammation.

Diagnosis

Peripheral leukocytosis, markers of inflammation (e.g., elevated sedimentation rates), radiography, bone scans, and leukocyte scans are usually too nonspecific to differentiate between septic and aseptic etiologies for painful prosthetic joints. The specific diagnosis depends prominently on isolation of the pathogen by arthrocentesis or surgical debridement (15). Joint aspiration demonstrates the pathogen in 85% to 98% of patients. If initial cultures reveal a relatively avirulent organism (e.g., coagulase-negative staphylococci, corynebacteria, propionibacteria, or *Bacillus* spp.), a second arthrocentesis should be considered to confirm the bacteriologic diagnosis and to reduce the possibility that the isolate is a culture contaminant. However, sequestered foci of infection are not uncommon, and surgical debridement is often necessary for diagnosis when sampling by arthrocentesis is unrevealing.

Management

Eradication of the pathogen in prosthetic joint infection most commonly requires removal of the prosthesis. Excision of the prosthesis followed by 6 weeks of bactericidal antimicrobial therapy and subsequent reimplantation is successful in 90% to 97% of cases. Explantation of the infected joint and reimplantation of a new prosthesis in a one-stage procedure with antibiotic-impregnated cement can be successful in 70% to 80% of patients. When removal of the prosthesis cannot be performed but the prosthesis is not loose, chronic suppressive oral antibiotic therapy is an option (16,17).

However, suppressive therapy is successful in only 62% of hip and in 26% of knee prostheses.

Prevention of Infection

Because prosthetic joint infection is a catastrophic event for the patient, prevention is of considerable importance. In anticipation of elective total joint arthroplasty, patients should be evaluated and, if appropriate, treated for pyogenic dentogingival pathology, obstructive uropathy, and dermatologic conditions that might predispose to surgical site infection or bacteremia. Intravenous anti-staphylococcal antibiotics such as cefazolin or vancomycin are frequently administered at the time of arthroplasty to reduce the risk of infections originating from the surgical incision site.

After arthroplasty, the use of prophylactic antibiotics in patients with prosthetic joints for events or procedures associated with anticipated bacteremia is controversial, and no data are available with which to determine the adequacy or the cost-effectiveness of such intervention. The American Dental Association and the American Academy of Orthopaedic Surgeons (18) have jointly advised that prophylactic antibiotics be given to selected patients with joint prostheses undergoing dental procedures associated with significant bleeding. The American Urologic Association has also issued an advisory statement jointly with the American Academy of Orthopaedic Surgeons recommending consideration of antibiotic prophylaxis for selected urinary tract procedures in patients with indwelling joint prostheses.

Special Problems and Conditions

Polyarticular Septic Arthritis

Simultaneous infection of multiple joints is usually the result of bacteremic spread and is generally seen in older patients (mean age 62 years). Underlying rheumatoid arthritis is the most important risk factor, accounting for over half of cases. *Staphylococcus aureus* is the etiologic pathogen in two thirds of cases. Streptococci including *S. pneumoniae* and groups B, C, and G species are other common culprits. Prognosis is generally poor. Full recovery of joint function occurs in only 58% of cases, and mortality approaches 30%.

Rheumatoid Arthritis

Joint infections occur with a yearly incidence of 0.3% to 3% in patients with rheumatoid arthritis (RA) and constitute approximately half of all cases of non-gonococcal bacterial septic arthritis. A disproportionately inflamed joint in an RA patient should always trigger suspicion for possible infection and be addressed accordingly. Recurrent joint infections occur in 16% to 22% of cases. Only one third of cases regain full recovery of prior joint function. There is a 15% to 22% mortality rate in monoarticular infections, while polyarticular infections are associated with 47% to 56% mortality rates.

Intravenous Drug Use

Intravenous drug use is accompanied by increased risks of recurrent transient bacteremia and hematogenous septic arthritis. While the knee is the most frequently affected joint, atypical sites of infection, notably the wrists and sternoclavicular joints, are also common in these patients. Common pathogens are *S. aureus* and gram-negative bacilli.

Neisseria gonorrhoeae (Gonococcal) Arthritis

Gonococcal monoarthritis and migratory polyarthritis occur in approximately equal proportions at presentation. Migratory tenosynovitis is also characteristic, observed in over two thirds of cases. Pustulovesicular skin lesions, often with central necrosis, occur in 44% of cases. The diagnostic yield is greatly enhanced by culturing multiple body sites; positive cultures can be obtained from the urethra (81%), synovial fluid (25%-50%), blood (24%), pharynx (17%), and rectum (13%). Polymerase chain reaction and ligase chain reaction techniques are much more sensitive than microbial cultures but do not provide necessary data regarding antibiotic resistance.

Because host defenses against *N. gonorrhoeae* involve complement-mediated mechanisms, complement deficiencies (mainly C5-C8) are associated with increased risk for infection.

Tuberculous and Other Mycobacterial Infections

Mycobacterium tuberculosis infection of the musculoskeletal system is typically a chronic monarthritis or spondylitis (Pott's disease) and is commonly a concomitant osteomyelitis and arthritis involving adjacent structures (19). The chest X-ray is often normal, and constitutional symptoms may not be present. The tuberculin skin test is almost always positive. Synovial fluid analysis reveals a leukocytosis (usually 10,000-20,000/mm^3) with neutrophil predominance in 80% of cases. Acid-fast stains of joint effusions are positive in only 27% and, although joint fluid culture is positive in 83%, cultivation requires 4 to 8 weeks incubation. Synovial biopsy is the procedure of choice for immediate diagnosis, because histopathology demonstrates granuloma formation in 95%, caseation in 55%, and the tubercle bacillus in 10% of cases.

Mycobacterium marinum is the most common cause of atypical mycobacterial arthritis. Presentation is usually a subacute or chronic interphalangeal or metacarpophalangeal monoarthritis. Symptoms commonly develop several weeks after local traumatic contact with marine life (e.g., fish, fishing equipment, fish tanks). Diagnosis is assisted by synovial biopsy revealing granulomas or acid-fast bacilli. Mycobacterial cultures of synovial tissue are diagnostic. However, the microbiology laboratory should be alerted to incubate specimens at 30°C for optimal results.

Fungal Arthritis

Fungal arthritis usually presents as a chronic monarticular infection, but acute polyarticular disease can be seen. Hematogenous seeding in an immunocompromised host is the most common setting, although direct extension from a contiguous source can also occur. Diagnosis is dependent on synovial tissue histopathology and mycotic stains and cultures. Erythema nodosum is a not uncommon associated finding.

REFERENCES

1. **Lidgren L, Lindberg L.** Orthopaedic infections during a 5-year period: analysis of a patient material from an orthopaedic clinic, 1963-1967. Acta Orthop Scand. 1972;43:325-34.

2. **Kaandorp CJ, van Schaardenburg D, Krijnen P, et al.** Risk factors for septic arthritis in patients with joint disease: a prospective study. Arthritis Rheum. 1995; 38:1819-25.

3. **Cucurull E, Espinoza LR.** Gonococcal arthritis. Rheum Dis Clin North Am. 1998; 24:305-22.

4. Sexually transmitted diseases treatment guidelines, 2002. Centers for Disease Control and Prevention. MMWR Recomm Rep. 2002;51:1-78.

5. **Garcia-Porrua C, Gonzalez-Gay MA, Ibanez D, Garcia-Pais MJ.** The clinical spectrum of severe septic bursitis in northwestern Spain: a 10-year study. J Rheumatol. 1999;26:663-7.

6. **Laupland KB, Davies HD, Calgary Parenteral Therapy Program Study Group.** Olecranon septic bursitis managed in an ambulatory setting. Clin Invest Med. 2001;24:171-8.

7. **Zimmermann B 3rd, Mikolich DJ, Ho G Jr.** Septic bursitis. Semin Arthritis Rheum. 1995;24:391-410.

8. **Lew DP, Waldvogel FA.** Osteomyelitis. N Engl J Med. 1997;336:999-1007.

9. **Carragee EJ.** Pyogenic vertebral osteomyelitis. J Bone Joint Surg Am. 1997;79: 874-80.

10. **Dahl LB, Hoyland AL, Dramsdahl H, Kaaresen PI.** Acute osteomyelitis in children: a population-based retrospective study, 1965 to 1994. Scand J Infect Dis. 1998;30:573-7.

11. **Beronius M, Bergman B, Andersson R.** Vertebral osteomyelitis in Goteborg, Sweden: a retrospective study of patients during 1990-95. Scand J Infect Dis. 2001;33:527-32.

12. **Lipsky BA.** Osteomyelitis of the foot in diabetic patients. Clin Infect Dis. 1997;25:1318-26.

13. **Crim JR, Seeger LL.** Imaging evaluation of osteomyelitis. Crit Rev Diagn Imaging. 1994;35:201-56.

14. **Hanssen AD, Rand JA.** Evaluation and treatment of infection at the site of a total hip or knee arthroplasty. J Bone Joint Surg Am. 1998;80:910-22.

15. **Atkins BL, Athanasou N, Deeks JJ, et al.** Prospective evaluation of criteria for microbiological diagnosis of prosthetic-joint infection at revision arthroplasty. The OSIRIS Collaborative Study Group. J Clin Microbiol. 1998;36:2932-9.

16. **Goulet JA, Pellicci PM, Brause BD, Salvati EM.** Prolonged suppression of infection in total hip arthroplasty. J Arthroplasty. 1988;3:109-16.

17. **Segreti J, Nelson JA, Trenholme GM.** Prolonged suppressive antibiotic therapy for infected orthopedic prostheses. Clin Infect Dis. 1998;27:711-3.

18. Antibiotic prophylaxis for dental patients with total joint replacements. Advisory Statement of the American Dental Association and the American Academy of Orthopaedic Surgeons. J Am Dental Assoc. 1997;128:1004-8.

19. **Watts HG, Lifeso RM.** Tuberculosis of bones and joints. J Bone Joint Surg Am. 1996;78:288-98.

16

■ ■ ■

Lyme Disease

Steven K. Magid, MD

Lyme disease is a multisystem inflammatory disorder caused by *Borrelia burgdorferi,* a treponeme-like spirochete, transmitted through the bite of the deer tick. It is the most commonly reported vector-borne disease in the United States, with 17,730 cases reported to Centers for Disease Control (CDC) during 2000, more than in any previous year. This represents an incidence of 6.3 cases/100,000, an 8% increase from 1999. Twelve states reported a higher incidence than the national average and accounted for 95% of cases reported nationwide: Connecticut, Rhode Island, New Jersey, New York, Delaware, Pennsylvania, Massachusetts, Maryland, Wisconsin, Minnesota, New Hampshire, and Vermont. As of 2000, Lyme disease has been reported in all states except Montana and in the District of Columbia, although in certain instances there is question whether acquisition of the disease occurred in places different from where it was reported. There is a bimodal age distribution, with the highest incidence occurring in children 5-9 years old and in adults 50-59 years old. Peak incidence occurs from late spring to early fall. In 2000, more than 57% of cases were diagnosed in June and July, and fewer than 6% of cases were identified in December, January, and February.

Pathogenesis

Lyme disease was first described in 1972 after investigation of an unusual cluster of patients with intermittent inflammatory oligoarthritis, mostly children, in a small area around Lyme, Connecticut (1). Of particular interest, 25% of those affected had a history of an expanding annular erythematous rash. It was soon recognized that the rash was very similar to a rash that had previously been described in Europe as erythema chronicum migrans

(ECM), which was thought to be transmitted by the bite of the sheep tick, *Ixodes ricinus,* and which had been successfully treated with antibiotics. In the northeastern United States, the vector was eventually shown to be the deer tick, *I. dammini* (also known as *I. scapularis*). Subsequently, Willy Burgdorfer isolated a treponeme-like spirochete (now known as *Borrelia burgdorferi*), which, when allowed to infect rabbits, caused the characteristic skin lesion (2). Furthermore, sera from patients with Lyme disease were shown to contain antibodies against antigens from these spirochetes. Lyme disease was soon reported in three distinct areas of the United States — the Northeast, the Midwest, and the Northwest — that correlated closely with the distribution of *I. dammini* and a related species, *I. pacificus.* Subsequently, other characteristic manifestations, including cardiac and neurological involvement, became recognized as part of the clinical syndrome.

Lyme disease has also been reported in Europe and Asia, where two other species of ticks serve as vectors: *I. ricinus* and *I. persulatus.* There are three varieties of *Borrelia* included within the *Borrelia burgdorferi sensu lato* group: *B. burgdoferi sensu stricto, B. afzelii,* and *B. garinii.* Of these, only the *sensu stricto* variety has been reported in the United States, and it has been postulated that this may account for some clinical differences observed between cases seen in North America versus those seen in other continents (3).

Tick Life Cycle

The *Ixodes* tick life cycle spans 2 years and involves three life stages. The ticks take one blood meal during each of these stages. In the first stage, larvae hatch from eggs, during the spring season. The larvae then feed on many different small animals, usually in late summer. During the subsequent fall and winter, they stay dormant. Then in the second spring of the life cycle, they molt into the nymphal stage. The nymphs feed during the spring and early summer, after which they molt to become the adult ticks. Some data suggest that immature larvae and nymphs can parasitize as many as 31 different species of mammals and 49 species of birds. *Ixodes dammini* shows a strong preference for feeding on the white-footed mouse (*Peromyscus leucopus*). This is crucial because the white-footed mouse is the most important animal reservoir for *Borrelia.* In certain areas during the summer months, as many as 100% of these mice can be infected with spirochetes. In summer and fall of the second year, the adult ticks feed on the white-tailed deer (*Odocoileus virginianus*). Accordingly, *I. dammini* is often referred to as the "deer tick." All three stages feed on humans, but the nymph is the major vector for the transmission of *Borrelia* because nymphs are voracious, very small, and difficult to detect. Human infection in the late spring and early summer are usually due to the nymph. Transmission by adult tick usually occurs in the fall.

Case Presentation

A 25-year-old male telephone line repairman from upstate New York presented with a swollen right knee. He had been well until approximately 6 months earlier, in May, when he had transient "flu-like" symptoms of severe intermittent headache and diffuse myalgias and arthralgias. Shortly thereafter, he developed a Bell's palsy and transient palpitations, both of which largely resolved after 6 weeks without specific intervention. On questioning, he recalls that in early May he noticed an expanding red rash in his right axilla at the site of a tick bite but had ignored it.

At the time of presentation, he appeared well. He had a very swollen, warm, and erythematous right knee and a slight right facial droop, but his general physical and neurological examinations were otherwise normal. The complete blood count and serum biochemistry screen were normal, and serological testing for rheumatoid factor and antinuclear antibodies was negative. The erythrocyte sedimentation rate was mildly elevated at 46 mm/h.

Arthrocentesis of the right knee was performed; the synovial fluid was cloudy and revealed a white blood cell count of 20,000/mm^3. Stains, polarized light microscopy, and cultures of the fluid revealed no evidence of bacterial, fungal, or mycobacterial infection or crystalline arthritis. The screening enzyme-linked immunosorbent assay (ELISA) for Lyme disease was positive. Western blot analysis revealed multiple positive IgG bands for *Borrelia burgdorferi,* but the IgM Western blot was negative.

The diagnosis of Lyme disease was made, and the patient was prescribed oral doxycycline 100 mg twice daily for 6 weeks. Although the patient continued to have moderate synovitis of the right knee at the completion of therapy, the patient's knee steadily returned to normal within 6 months.

Clinical Features

A number of clinical classification systems for Lyme disease have been proposed, but the clinical course has been generally divided into three stages: *early localized, disseminated* (comprising early and late disseminated), and *late persistent* (Table 16-1). Although these classifications are not absolute, they provide a useful framework with which to view the natural history of the disease. Many clinically affected patients will only display the first stage, while others will present with the later stages, not having exhibited manifestations of the earlier ones.

Early Localized Disease

Erythema migrans (EM) (formerly called erythema chronicum migrans) is virtually pathognomonic for Lyme disease (Figure 16-1). In the localized

Table 16-1   Common Manifestations of Lyme Disease

Early localized disease (typically within 1 week after tick bite, but up to 1 month)
- Erythema migrans

Early disseminated disease (days to weeks after tick bite)
- Flu-like constitutional symptoms
- Secondary erythema migrans
- Migratory polymyalgias and polyarthralgias

Late disseminated disease (weeks to months after tick bite)
- Carditis and heart blocks
- Neurological disease (Bell's palsy and other cranial neuropathies, meningitis, peripheral neuropathies)
- Intermittent migratory monoarticular or oligoarticular inflammatory arthritis

Late persistent disease (months to years after tick bite)
- Chronic monoarticular or oligoarticular inflammatory arthritis
- Neurological disease (encephalopathy, sensorimotor polyneuropathies, demyelinating disease)
- Cutaneous disease (acrodermatitis chronicum atrophicans, lymphocytoma)

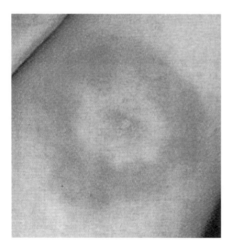

Figure 16-1 Erythema migrans (EM) is virtually pathognomonic for Lyme disease and characteristically expands steadily over several days, often becoming very large (median diameter about 15 cm), around a central punctum at the site of the bite. Secondary EM lesions lack the central punctum. This example shows a classic bull's-eye pattern, but the rash is more commonly uniformly red or displays a central area of redness.

form, the rash occurs at the site of the tick bite. However, most patients will not even be aware of the bite. In a third of patients, EM will not occur or will be overlooked. When present, primary EM occurs within days to a month after the bite, usually within the first week. The hallmark of EM is that it expands over several days and can attain a very large size (median diameter about 15 cm) around a central punctum at the site of the bite. Although classically described as exhibiting a central clearing, or even a bull's-eye pattern, more recent studies suggest that the rash is most often uniformly red or actually displays a central redness. Other patterns of rash that have been described include those with a bluish central discoloration, vesiculation, and central necrosis. Although frequently asymptomatic, there may be dysesthesias, burning, itching, or even pain at the site of EM. Primary EM typically occurs in the groin areas, axillae, popliteal fossae, belt, or brassiere lines. These areas are warm and moist and may serve as preferred sites for ticks to feed.

Early Disseminated Disease

Days to weeks after a tick bite, many patients will develop a flu-like illness characterized by fever, chills, malaise, headaches, arthralgias, and myalgias. It is during this time that there is spirochetemia, and secondary EM lesions may occur due to hematogenous spread. Secondary EM lesions may occur on any part of the body. Because they are not at the site of a tick bite, they lack the central punctum. They also tend to be smaller and can be multicentric.

Migratory polyarthralgias and polymyalgias and other musculoskeletal symptoms are common in early disseminated Lyme disease. Discomfort may develop in joints, bursae, tendons, muscle, and bones. The symptoms generally involve only one or a few areas at a time and may last only a few hours or days in a given area before occurring at another site.

Late Disseminated Disease

Even without treatment, the cutaneous and musculoskeletal manifestations of early disseminated disease resolve completely. However, many (but not all) untreated patients will develop findings of disseminated disease that can include cardiac, neurological, or articular involvement.

Cardiac Manifestations

Cardiac disease occurs in approximately 10% of all untreated patients, usually within a few weeks to months. Patients may complain of chest pain, palpitations, or dyspnea. Conduction system disease is the most common abnormality, usually presenting as fluctuating heart block. The block occurs at the level of the AV node and is unresponsive to atropine. Rapid changes in rhythm have been described, with first-degree heart block evolving to complete heart block within minutes or hours and then back again. Up to 30% of these patients will require temporary pacemakers, but permanent pacers are rarely needed after appropriate antibiotic treatment. Myocardial and pericardial manifestations are unusual and mild. Congestive heart failure has been described. Most patients recover completely, but chronic cardiomyopathy and even death have been rarely reported.

Neurological Manifestations

The neurological manifestations of Lyme disease are protean, occurring weeks to months after infection. Early features may include headache, lethargy, photophobia, and irritability. Lyme meningitis presents with intense headache, stiff neck, photophobia, and meningeal signs. The cerebrospinal fluid (CSF) analysis usually shows a lymphocytic pleocytosis. Bell's palsy is the most frequent cranial nerve manifestation of Lyme disease. It must be emphasized that even in areas endemic for *B. burgdorferi,* the majority of cases of unilateral adult Bell's Palsy in an adult is not the result of Lyme disease. However, sequential or bilateral Bell's palsy is most often caused by Lyme disease. Involvement of other cranial nerves occurs but is less common. Both painful sensory and motor peripheral neuropathies may occur. Electrophysiological testing demonstrates a sensorimotor, axonal polyradiculoneuropathy. A mononeuritis multiplex may be seen. Conjunctivitis is the most common ophthalmological manifestation of Lyme disease, but anterior and/or posterior uveitis can also occur.

Arthritis

As described above, early in the course of the disease arthralgias and myalgias are brief, intermittent, and migratory, a pattern that may persist for months. Afterwards, if untreated, up to 60% of patients will develop an overt monoarticular or oligoarticular (four or fewer joints) inflammatory arthritis. The knee is frequently affected, although involvement of most other large joints has been reported. Synovial effusions are typically very large, particularly in the knee, and evidence of direct spirochetal infection of the joint can be shown through polymerase chain reaction (PCR) testing. The synovial fluid is inflammatory with white blood cell counts reaching 25,000/mm³ and a predominance of polymorphonuclear neutrophils. The arthritic attacks wax and wane and may last days to weeks during flares but typically diminish in intensity and duration with time.

Late Persistent Disease

Manifestations of late persistent Lyme disease occur after months to years in the inadequately treated or untreated patient. There can be prominent joint, nervous system, or skin involvement.

Arthritis

The inflammatory monoarthritis or oligoarthritis seen in late disseminated disease can continue into the late persistent period (3). Erosive, destructive disease is unusual but can occur in a small minority of patients. Chronic arthritis appears to be associated with the HLA-DR4 and -DR2 haplotypes. Although the arthritis is still responsive to antibiotic therapy in the vast majority of cases, rare patients may continue to have persistent synovitis, despite the apparent eradication of the *Borrelia* organism as demonstrated by sensitive tests such as PCR. These cases may actually reflect a reactive process as opposed to a direct infection. It has been postulated that an autoimmune process may be triggered by molecular mimicry between the *Borrelia* OspA protein, a major surface antigen of the spirochete, and human lymphocyte function-associated antigen 1. Cases of chronic inflammatory arthritis have been reported after vaccination of human subjects with recombinant OspA.

Neurological Manifestations

Chronic neurological syndromes may also occur months to years after infection. The most common presentation is an insidious encephalopathy that can manifest in many apparently non-specific ways such as memory impairment, mood disorders, sleep disturbances, and cognitive changes. Neuropsychiatric and cognitive testing can be useful to document abnormalities but are not specific. Examination of CSF reveals evidence of chronic inflammation. Sensorimotor polyneuropathies presenting as focal motor defects, distal paresthesias, or radicular pain can be documented by nerve conduction velocity and electromyographic studies. Somatosensory evoked potentials can also be useful in making a diagnosis. Rarely, a demyelinating multiple sclerosis-like illness can occur.

Cutaneous Manifestations

Chronic Lyme disease can be associated with two distinct skin lesions. Acrodermatitis chronicum atrophicans occurs primarily in Europe and is characterized by an insidious purplish discoloration and swelling in acral areas that results in atrophy over years. In addition, a benign lymphoma-like skin lesion has been described called *Borrelia* lymphocytoma. It often occurs on the ear lobe and has been reported at other sites such as the breast, scrotum, and shoulder.

Diagnosis

The diagnosis of Lyme disease is a clinical one that is supported but not made by laboratory data. A variety of laboratory tests, including serological studies, bacterial cultures, and PCR for *Borrelia* DNA, have been developed for the detection and diagnosis of Lyme disease.

Serological Testing

Detection of anti-*Borrelia* antibodies is the most useful and readily accessible approach to the laboratory diagnosis of Lyme disease. ELISA is considered to be the best screening test (sensitivity about 90% and specificity about 70%), although indirect immunofluorescence assay (IFA) is also commonly employed. IgM antibodies to *B. burgdorferi* can be detected within 2 weeks of infection, and peak serum levels occur at 3 to 6 weeks before returning to baseline by 6 months. IgG antibodies may be detected within 4 to 6 weeks. Levels peak after several months, and circulating IgG can be detected years after infection. When late manifestations such as inflammatory arthritis or neurological complications are present, the ELISA is expected to be positive.

In the past, inter-laboratory variability had been an important problem. At present there is better standardization, but false-positive and false-negative results continue to be a source of diagnostic uncertainty. Common causes of false-positive ELISA results include cross-reactivity with epitopes on other spirochetes and non-specific general activation of immunity in systemic infections (e.g., subacute bacterial endocarditis) or rheumatological disorders (e.g. systemic lupus erythematosus). False-negative tests can occur early in the course of the illness when there may be clinical findings (such as EM), but the IgM immune response may not have had a chance to develop. Early antibiotic intervention that rapidly decreases the *Borrelia* antigen load can lead to a diminished immune response and is another cause of false-negative results.

Because of these inherent deficiencies in screening, the CDC developed a two-stage procedure for the diagnosis of Lyme disease in 1994. If the screening test is positive, then Western blot testing should be obtained to confirm the finding (4-6). This assay can detect specific antibodies directed against *B. burgdorferi* antigens. The IgM Western blot is considered positive if at least two of the following bands are demonstrated: 23 kDa, 39 kDa, and 41 kDa. The IgG immunoblot is considered positive if at least five of the following 10 bands are present: 18 kDa, 23 kDa, 28 kDa, 30 kDa, 39 kDa, 41 kDa, 45 kDa, 58 kDa, 66 kDa, and 93 kDa.

Bacterial Cultures

Cultures from biopsy specimens of EM rashes have a diagnostic sensitivity of 60% to 80% for isolating *B. burgdorferi,* but because the lesion is clinically quite characteristic, this is rarely necessary for making the diagnosis of Lyme disease. Yield from other tissue and body fluids, however, is notoriously low. This has led to the hypothesis that many of the manifestations of Lyme disease are due to the immune response to *B. burgdorferi* rather than direct infection of tissue.

Polymerase Chain Reaction

PCR detects genetic material specific to the organism and has been used to evaluate blood, skin, synovial fluid, cerebrospinal fluid, and urine. It is extremely sensitive, and strict laboratory controls must be in place to minimize false-positive results. It is important to note that the mere presence of genetic material does not necessarily prove that the spirochete is viable and capable of causing ongoing infection or further dissemination. However, it does raise the possibility that in some genetically predisposed patients antigenic stimulation from dead organisms may lead to an inflammatory "reactive" process resulting in end-organ manifestations such as carditis or arthritis. At present, the FDA has yet to approve PCR for the diagnosis of Lyme disease, but its use may be considered in cases where the clinical picture and standard diagnostic methods still do not reveal a clear diagnosis.

Cerebrospinal Fluid Analysis

A lumbar puncture and CSF analysis should be performed whenever meningeal irritation is present to exclude potentially life-threatening causes of acute meningitis. In the setting of Lyme disease, CSF analysis is not typically recommended for isolated Bell's palsy, but it should be considered when other neurological manifestations are present, particularly when the diagnosis remains in doubt. Central nervous system (CNS) involvement of Lyme disease typically shows a mild lymphocytic pleocytosis and elevation in protein in the CSF suggestive of chronic inflammation. Local anti-*Borrelia* antibody production within the CSF reflects CNS infection and is inferred by an elevated CSF-to-serum anti-*Borrelia* antibody ratio (7). Increased CSF anti-*Borrelia* antibody production is considered a nearly universal finding in Lyme meningitis.

Screening for Lyme Disease

Screening for Lyme disease is one of the most important and challenging issues facing clinicians and remains the subject of ongoing debate. As for all screening tests, the usefulness of serological studies for Lyme disease is dependent on the pre-test likelihood of having the disease. For example, if a patient from a non-endemic area presents with very non-specific complaints such as headache, myalgias, and fatigue, then a positive *B. burgdorferi* serology should be viewed skeptically. It has been suggested that if the pre-test likelihood of Lyme disease is less than 20%, then screening should not be performed because the probability of a false-positive test result is greater than the probability of having the disease.

Differential Diagnosis

The differential diagnosis of Lyme disease is broad because of the protean manifestations of the disease and because of the varying patterns of organ involvement from patient to patient.

Skin Disease

Erythema migrans must be distinguished from several skin diseases and lesions, such as cellulitis, tinea, granuloma annulare, erythema annulare centrifugum, erythema multiforme, and drug reactions.

- Cellulitis is associated with fever, toxicity, leukocytosis, and lymphangitic streaking with lymphadenopathy and is acute in onset.

- Tinea is pruritic and characterized by thin raised borders with scaling. It is stable in size over weeks to months, as opposed to EM, which expands rapidly.

- Granuloma annulare is sometimes associated with rheumatic diseases. It expands slowly over weeks to months and is frequently present for years.

- Erythema annulare centrifugum consists of scaling pruritic expanding lesions with gyrate borders. This lesion is associated with drug reactions and malignancies.

- Erythema multiforme involve palms and soles, often have target lesions, and can have mucous membrane involvement.

- Drug reactions frequently occur on the face and genital areas.

Neurological Disease

A variety of illnesses may mimic neuroborreliosis, but a key clue leading to the correct diagnosis is that Lyme disease frequently involves multiple levels of the neural axis (8). For example, Lyme disease should be strongly considered in a patient living in an area endemic for *B. burgdorferi* presenting with Bell's palsy (i.e., cranial nerve), a thoracic radiculopathy (nerve root), and a sensory peripheral neuropathy. Sarcoidosis is a notable condition that can also involve multiple levels of the neural axis. It is often difficult to distinguish viral meningitis from Lyme meningitis, although characteristically Lyme disease tends to wax and wane and is associated with milder meningeal signs. Demyelinating forms of neuroborreliosis should be distinguished from multiple sclerosis and related disorders.

Joint Disease

The typical acute or subacute large joint monoarthritis or oligoarthritis of Lyme disease should be distinguished from spondyloarthropathies, septic arthritis, gout and pseudogout, and rheumatoid arthritis.

- Seronegative inflammatory arthritides such as psoriatic arthritis, reactive arthritis, and arthritis associated with inflammatory bowel disease often present with large joint oligoarthritis. Extra-articular manifestations such as characteristic rashes, urethritis, uveitis, abdominal symptoms, or antecedent infections aid in making the diagnosis.

- Septic arthritis is generally more inflammatory, and patients appear more toxic. However, infections with more indolent organisms such as mycobacteria or fungi may be quite difficult to distinguish clinically from Lyme arthritis. Synovial fluid or tissue culture should be diagnostic but may require long-term cultures to assess.

- Crystalline diseases such as gout or pseudogout tend to be more acute, but chronic forms exist. Diagnosis can be made by direct examination of synovial fluid under polarized light microscopy.

- Rheumatoid arthritis (RA), while characteristically symmetric and polyarticular, may present initially with monoarthritis or oligo-arthritis. Small joint involvement and a positive serologic test for rheumatoid factor favor it.

"Pseudo-Lyme Disease"

Many patients with fibromyalgia, chronic fatigue, or depression often believe that they are suffering from Lyme disease (9). Non-specific symptoms such as diffuse myalgias, headaches, burning pain, and trouble concentrating are common complaints. However, even in the absence of supportive epidemiological data or convincing clinical or serological evidence of Lyme disease, many patients have been treated with prolonged and recurrent courses of antibiotics, often with *significant* side effects and complications. One study estimated that empiric intravenous treatment of patients with chronic fatigue and myalgias with positive anti-*Borrelia* serologies caused 29 cases of drug toxicity for one case of true Lyme disease (10).

Published studies have demonstrated that most patients referred to Lyme disease clinics with the putative diagnosis of Lyme disease failed to meet diagnostic criteria (11). Retrospectively, these patients probably suffered from fibromyalgia or other non-inflammatory diseases. In fact, the most common reason for lack of response to antibiotics is an incorrect diagnosis. This underscores the imperative for a carefully established diagnosis before the onset of treatment.

Prognosis

Most patients will have a complete recovery with appropriate therapy, but early diagnosis offers the best chance for a prompt response. The best outcomes can be expected from an accurate diagnosis and exclusion of other conditions from the outset. It has been demonstrated that if antibiotics are given early in the course of the illness, EM resolves more quickly and the later manifestations of the disease are less likely to occur. As described above, however, persistent chronic arthritis may occur in spite of antibiotic therapy, possibly reflecting a reactive immunological process that may require anti-inflammatory or immunomodulatory therapy.

Management

Many internists are comfortable diagnosing and treating Lyme disease. Referrals to subspecialists (such as rheumatologists, cardiologists, neurologists, or infectious disease specialists) can be considered on a case-by-case basis. It must be emphasized that Lyme disease is a bacterial infection that is, in fact, very responsive to antibiotic therapy. Treatment regimens have been developed on the basis of both empirical experience and the results of well-designed clinical trials (Table 16-2). Early manifestations like EM can be treated with short courses of oral antibiotics, while later manifestations may require several weeks of parenteral antibiotics. Symptoms may sometimes be slow to resolve completely even with successful treatment, particularly if the initial presentation was severe or if there was a delay in initiating treatment. In cases that are atypical or do not respond to treatment as expected,

---

Table 16-2   Recommended Treatment Regimens for Adult Lyme Disease

Primary erythema migrans (EM)
- Doxycycline* 100 mg PO bid, amoxicillin 500 mg PO tid, cefuroxime 500 mg PO bid, or erythromycin 250 mg PO qid for 2 to 3 weeks. (A recent study has suggested that as little as 10 days of therapy may be sufficient [12].)

Disseminated erythema migrans or acrodermatitis
- Oral antibiotic options as per primary EM for 3 to 4 weeks.

Inflammatory arthritis
- Oral antibiotic options as per primary EM for 4 to 6 weeks.
- If refractory to oral antibiotics, ceftriaxone 2 g IV qd, cefotaxime 2 g IV tid, or penicillin G 5 million U IV qid for 6 weeks.
- If refractory to intravenous antibiotics, consider intraarticular corticosteroid injections, nonsteroidal anti-inflammatory drugs, and/or disease-modifying antirheumatic drugs (e.g., hydroxychloroquine or methotrexate). Arthroscopic synovectomy may rarely be necessary.

Carditis
- If hemodynamically unstable, temporary pacemaker.
- For first- or second-degree atrioventricular block, oral antibiotic options as per primary EM for 4 to 6 weeks.
- For third-degree atrioventricular block or if refractory to oral antibiotics, intravenous antibiotic options as per inflammatory arthritis for 6 weeks.

Neurological disease
- For Bell's palsy, oral antibiotics as per primary EM for 4 to 6 weeks.
- For meningitis, neuropathies, and other neurological manifestations, ceftriaxone 2 g IV qd or penicillin G 5 million U IV qid for 6 weeks.

Asymptomatic *Ixodes* bite in endemic areas (antibiotic prophylaxis)
- Consider single dose of doxycycline* 200 mg within 72 hours of tick bite.

* Doxycycline should not be administered to pregnant women or to children.

the presence of a concomitant tick-borne disease such as ehrlichiosis or Rocky Mountain spotted fever should be considered.

Skin Disease

Primary EM can be treated with oral doxycycline 100 mg twice daily or amoxicillin 500 mg three times daily for 2 to 3 weeks (13,14). A recent study showed that 10 days of therapy may be equally effective (12). Doxycycline is contraindicated for children under the age of 12 and for pregnant women, but the advantage of this medication is that it is also effective treatment for ehrlichiosis. Alternatives include cefuroxime 500 mg twice daily or erythromycin 250 mg four times daily. Disseminated EM and acrodermatitis may require up to a month of oral antibiotic therapy.

Arthritis

Initial treatment of the arthritis of Lyme disease is 4 to 6 weeks of oral antibiotics as with disseminated EM. Resolution may be gradual, particularly if the arthritis has been well established. Failure of response to oral antibiotics may warrant a course of intravenous therapy with, for example, ceftriaxone 2 g daily for up to 6 weeks. Other choices for intravenous therapy include cefotaxime 2 g every 8 hours or penicillin G 5 million U every 6 hours. Antibiotic-resistant arthritis should be regarded as inflammatory but not infectious and can be treated with corticosteroid injections, non-steroidal anti-inflammatory drugs, or immunomodulatory agents like hydroxychloroquine or methotrexate. Arthroscopic synovectomy may be required in refractory cases.

Carditis

Carditis may spontaneously remit. If heart block is present, it will sometimes require a temporary pacer especially if the patient is symptomatic. Permanent pacing is only rarely required. First- and second-degree heart block can be treated with oral antibiotic regimens similar to those for Lyme arthritis. Third-degree heart block requires intravenous therapy, which can be changed to oral antibiotics when the patient is no longer in the higher-degree heart block.

Neurological Disease

Isolated Bell's palsy can be treated with oral regimens as described for arthritis. However, although most patients with Bell's palsy do not have more extensive neurological disease, care must be taken to ensure that other neurological manifestations that would warrant intravenous therapy are excluded. It is generally accepted that central nervous system involvement should be aggressively sought, no matter how subtle, and treated when present with intravenous antibiotics, in order to avoid undertreatment and to prevent late neurological sequelae.

Encephalopathy, meningitis, radiculoneuropathies, and peripheral neuropathies require intravenous therapy. Resolution of CSF abnormalities such as pleocytosis lag behind clinical resolution. Radiculoneuropathies notably do not respond as well to antibiotic treatment as other manifestations of neurological Lyme disease; slow resolution may occur over time but may be incomplete.

Special Considerations

- Herxheimer reactions upon initiation of antibiotic therapy have been reported in Lyme disease and are similar to the reactions reported during treatment of other bacterial illnesses. Symptoms include fever, rash, hypertension, or hypotension.

- Tetracyclines should be avoided in children and pregnant women due to the risk of dental staining.

- Tetracyclines are also associated with an increased risk of photosensitivity. Care should be used during the summer months. Common sunscreens do not effectively protect against this problem.

- Patients with penicillin allergies may be treated with macrolides like erythromycin or azithromycin, but these agents appear be less effective. If the allergy is mild, cefuroxime may be a better choice.

- There is ongoing controversy in the lay literature regarding prolonged antibiotic treatment in patients who have persistent symptoms. Patients have been known to receive years of continuous intravenous antibiotic therapy. A recent placebo-controlled study of previously treated patients with persistent complaints clearly demonstrates that there is no benefit to a 90-day course of additional antibiotic therapy (15).

Pregnancy

Most women who develop Lyme disease during pregnancy have normal obstetrical outcomes. In one study of 58 patients who developed EM during pregnancy, 51 had normal, full-term deliveries. Stillbirths, missed abortions, neonatal deaths, and congenital heart abnormalities have been reported in the setting of Lyme disease, but there is no good evidence for a causal relationship. Previous episodes of Lyme disease or asymptomatic seropositivity are probably not associated with adverse fetal outcomes. Nonetheless, it seems prudent to recognize and treat Lyme disease early during pregnancy (16). Again, it is worth restating that tetracyclines are contraindicated during pregnancy.

Prevention

The best way to avoid Lyme disease is to avoid exposure as much as possible. Exposure to tick habitats such as the woods, forest, or brush in endemic areas should be limited, especially during the spring and summer. Light-colored clothing allows for easier visualization of ticks, which can be very small. Long sleeves and pants (with pant legs tucked into socks) minimize adherence of the tick. For adults, insect repellent containing N,N-diethyl-meta-toluamide (DEET) on exposed skin and clothing is effective. It is very important to inspect the skin thoroughly after potential exposure, particularly in axillae, groin areas, popliteal fossae, between toes, and in areas of constriction (such as belt or brassiere lines). If an embedded tick is discovered, pointed tweezers should be used to gently apply steady upward pressure without twisting at the embedded head part. Care should be taken to avoid exerting pressure on the engorged body because this may inoculate infected fluid.

Asymptomatic Tick Bites and Antibiotic Prophylaxis

Deciding how to manage a patient who has sustained an asymptomatic tick bite depends on a number of considerations. If the tick can been identified to be not of the Ixodes family, then it is obvious that no treatment is needed. Furthermore, because it is believed that ticks must be attached for 24 to 48 hours in order to transmit infection, non-engorged ticks that have been attached for shorter periods are of much less concern. It is generally accepted that the risks of adverse drug reactions and the attendant cumulative economic costs outweigh the benefit of treating all patients who have had tick bites with full courses of antibiotics. However, certain circumstances may influence this decision, such as extreme patient (or physician) anxiety or a patient who is unlikely to follow up or report subsequent symptoms.

The prevalence of infected ticks in a particular area may eventually prove to be a very important factor in the management of the asymptomatic tick bite. A recent study from a highly endemic area reported on a strategy to treat patients with tick bites with a single prophylactic dose of doxycycline (17). Patients who were treated with a single dose of doxycycline 200 mg within 72 hours of a tick bite were much less likely to develop EM. Some experts have adopted this strategy. A reassuring observation is that no asymptomatic seroconversions occurred.

Recombinant OspA Vaccine

In 1998, the Food and Drug Administration approved the use of a recombinant OspA protein as a vaccine against Lyme disease. The controlled trials demonstrated both general safety and effectiveness. However, post-marketing concerns that the vaccine itself might be associated with a reactive arthritis were raised. The vaccine has since been withdrawn from the market because of poor sales.

REFERENCES

1. **Steere AC, Malawista SE, Snydman DR, et al.** Lyme arthritis: an epidemic of oligoarticular arthritis in children and adults in three Connecticut communities. Arthritis Rheum. 1977;20:7-17.

2. **Burgdorfer W, Barbour AG, Hayes SF, et al.** Lyme disease: a tick-borne spirochetosis? Science. 1982;216:1317-9.

3. **van Dam AP, Kuiper H, Vos K, et al.** Different genospecies of *Borrelia burgdorferi* are associated with distinct clinical manifestations of Lyme borreliosis. Clin Infect Dis. 1993;17:708-17.

4. **Engstrom SM, Shoop E, Johnson RC.** Immunoblot interpretation criteria for serodiagnosis of early Lyme disease. J Clin Microbiol. 1995;33:419-27.

5. **Tugwell P, Dennis DT, Weinstein A, et al.** Laboratory evaluation in the diagnosis of Lyme disease. Ann Intern Med. 1997;127:1109-23.

6. **Nowakowski J, Schwartz I, Liveris D, et al.** Laboratory diagnostic techniques for patients with early Lyme disease associated with erythema migrans: a comparison of different techniques. Clin Infect Dis. 2001;33:2023-7.

7. **Kaiser R, Lucking CH.** Intrathecal synthesis of specific antibodies in neuroborreliosis. Comparison of different ELISA techniques and calculation methods. J Neurol Sci. 1993;118:64-72.

8. **Halperin JJ, Luft BJ, Anand AK, et al.** Lyme neuroborreliosis: central nervous system manifestations. Neurology. 1989;39:753-9.

9. **Sigal LH.** Pseudo-Lyme disease. Bull Rheum Dis. 1995;44:1-3.

10. **Lightfoot RW Jr, Luft BJ, Rahn DW, et al.** Empiric parenteral antibiotic treatment of patients with fibromyalgia and fatigue and a positive serologic result for Lyme disease. A cost-effectiveness analysis. Ann Intern Med. 1993;119:503-9.

11. **Steere AC, Taylor E, McHugh, Logigian EL.** The overdiagnosis of Lyme disease. JAMA. 1993;269:1812-6.

12. **Wormser GP, Ramanathan R, Nowakowski J, et al.** Duration of antibiotic therapy for early Lyme disease. Ann Intern Med. 2003;138:697-704.

13. **Luft BJ, Dattwyler RJ, Johnson RC, et al.** Azithromycin compared with amoxicillin in the treatment of erythema migrans. A double-blind, randomized, controlled trial. Ann Intern Med. 1996;124:785-91.

14. **Dattwyler RJ, Luft BJ, Kunkel MJ, et al.** Ceftriaxone compared with doxycycline for the treatment of acute disseminated Lyme disease. N Engl J Med. 1997;337:289-94.

15. **Klempner MS, Hu LT, Evans J, et al.** Two controlled trials of antibiotic treatment in patients with persistent symptoms and a history of Lyme disease. N Engl J Med. 2001;345:85-92.

16. **Maraspin V, Cimperman J, Lotric-Furlan S, et al.** Treatment of erythema migrans in pregnancy. Clin Infect Dis. 1996;22:788-93.

17. **Nadelman RB, Nowakowski J, Fish D, et al.** Prophylaxis with single-dose doxycycline for the prevention of Lyme disease after an *Ixodes scapularis* tick bite. N Engl J Med. 2001;345:79-84.

17

■ ■ ■

Whipple's Disease

Stephen A. Paget, MD

Whipple's disease (WD) is a rare systemic disorder caused by *Tropheryma whippelii,* a gram-positive actinomycete. Although abdominal pain, diarrhea, and malabsorption are prominent features because of infection of the gastrointestinal tract, many organs (such as those of the musculoskeletal, cardiovascular, respiratory, and central nervous systems) may become involved.

In 75% of cases, weight loss, diarrhea, and arthropathy are present at the time of diagnosis (1). However, in almost two-thirds of cases, the arthropathy (typically a seronegative, migratory, non-erosive, inflammatory arthritis) precedes gastrointestinal and other manifestations by many years (2), and it is generally not until gastrointestinal symptoms appear that the diagnosis of WD is even entertained. Therefore, WD exemplifies the diagnostic challenge common to many systemic inflammatory diseases that frequently present in incomplete, undifferentiated, highly variable, or slowly evolving forms. Only constant vigilance and reassessment can help the clinician arrive at the correct diagnosis in a timely fashion. With an appropriate level of clinical suspicion, supported by newly available confirmatory laboratory modalities, cases may become more readily identified.

Pathogenesis

In 1907, Whipple described a young physician who died after an insidious illness presenting as weight loss, weakness, cough, joint pains, diarrhea, and an abdominal mass. Autopsy revealed pleuropericarditis, aortic valve endocarditis, and enlarged mesenteric and retroperitoneal lymph nodes with "polyblasts in the jejunal mucosa and lymph nodes."

More than 40 years later, particles in intestinal mucosal macrophages were shown to be periodic acid-Schiff (PAS) stain-positive, and in 1961 electron micrographs of intestinal tissue demonstrated bacilliform bodies (3), leading to the conjecture that the cause of this illness was infectious and to the first use of antibiotic treatment in 1964. Until recently, the pathological diagnosis of Whipple's disease (WD) was made based on these histological features.

In 1992, a novel 1321-base nucleotide sequence amplified by polymerase chain reaction (PCR) from the duodenal tissue of five patients with WD eventually led to the identification of *Tropheryma whippelii*, a grampositive actinomycete, as the causative agent of this disease (4). The nucleotide sequence of the 16S ribosomal RNA of *T. whippelii* has proven to be highly sensitive and specific in PCR analysis and has been useful in confirming the diagnosis of WD, identifying inconclusive and suspicious cases, and monitoring response to therapy. Specimens from various tissues such as the small intestine, eye, and central nervous system, and from fluids such as blood, synovial fluid, vitreous, pleural fluid, and cerebrospinal fluid can be used for analysis. The pathogen itself has been successfully isolated and propagated by using interleukin-4-deactivated macrophages but subculturing has been unsuccessful (5). Recently, specific antibodies have been generated in mice, setting the stage for a serological test for WD. The availability of serological and PCR testing will probably eventually help to define a different clinical spectrum of WD because of the possibility of early disease detection.

The pathogenesis of WD, however, remains poorly understood. Immune defects in T cells and macrophages and reduced levels of interleukin-12 and interferon (IFN)-γ production have been described in patients with WD. These abnormalities suggest that impaired ability to contain and clear intracellular bacteria is important in the evolution of the disease and could explain the long-standing presence of the *T. whippelii* in macrophages in WD patients that can last for years. This hypothesis is supported by the successful use of IFN-γ in treatment of a patient with a 10-year history of antibiotic-refractory disease (6). Nevertheless, many questions remain about host and pathogen factors, their interactions, and their role in WD and continue to generate active interest and research.

Case Presentation 1

A 48-year-old man presents with memory lapses, right-sided weakness, and uncontrollable movements of his arms and legs of 6 months duration.

At age 40, he had developed migratory polyarthritis, where joint inflammation would jump from one joint to another every few days. He also noted increasing fatigue, pleuritic pain, and cervical lymphadenopathy. Three years later, he developed recurrent episodes of fever and chills and pericarditis and was diagnosed as having disseminated tuberculosis. Treatment with anti-tuberculous medications and a short course of prednisone led to clear clinical improvement.

At age 45, the patient developed severe abdominal pain and distension, chronic diarrhea, and a 35-pound weight loss without loss of appetite. Physical examination revealed prominent adenopathy, leg edema, and temporal wasting. A lymph node biopsy demonstrated PAS-positive macrophages, and a diagnosis of Whipple's disease was made. The patient was treated with sulfamethoxazole-trimethoprim (co-trimoxazole) with a clinical improvement in 1 month. Co-trimoxazole therapy was maintained for a year. However, several months after antibiotics were discontinued, the patient developed a recurrence of his symptoms. A jejunal biopsy revealed many PAS-positive macrophages consistent with active Whipple's disease, and the patient again responded to another year of co-trimoxazole treatment.

He was well until 6 months ago, when he developed numbness of the buttocks, clonic movements, focal seizures, right-sided weakness, hesitant speech, memory lapses, and a positive Babinski's test on the right side. He was treated with multiple antibiotics, including co-trimoxazole, this time without significant improvement. A jejunal biopsy did not show histological evidence of active Whipple's disease. However, the presence of the *T. whippelii* 16S ribosomal RNA (rRNA) gene was detected by PCR. Cerebrospinal fluid revealed PAS-positive macrophages and was also PCR-positive. The patient was treated for 2 months with a combination of intravenous co-trimoxazole, gentamicin, and ceftriaxone, with a significant improvement in his neurological problems. He has remained on chronic suppressive co-trimoxazole therapy without recurrent disease exacerbations.

Case Presentation 2

A 38-year-old woman presented to an emergency room with fever and hypotension and was intubated, stabilized, and admitted to intensive care. Her husband and physicians described a prolonged illness beginning at age 31, when she developed migratory polyarthritis and was diagnosed with seronegative rheumatoid arthritis. She was treated with nonsteroidal anti-inflammatory drugs but continued to have arthritis that became more fixed in the joints of the lower extremities.

At age 36, she developed iritis, peptic ulcer disease, and episodic cramping abdominal pain. At this time, she was found to be positive for HLA-B27, and a seronegative spondyloarthropathy became the putative diagnosis. A year later, the patient developed hepatomegaly, hypercalcemia, and parotid enlargement. A liver biopsy demonstrated non-caseating granulomata. The diagnosis was revised to sarcoidosis, and systemic corticosteroid treatment was instituted with moderate clinical improvement.

Several months before her acute presentation, the patient developed severe diarrhea, weight loss, and anemia. One day, as an out-patient evaluation for possible inflammatory bowel disease was ongoing, the patient was found minimally responsive by her husband and was brought by ambulance to the emergency room, where she was found to be febrile to 39°C and hypotensive with a systolic blood pressure of 60 mm Hg. She was intubated, hydrated, and started on broad-spectrum antibiotics.

The patient showed a rapid clinical improvement over the first 24 hours. She became afebrile, her vital signs normalized, and she was extubated and became fully alert. All cultures were negative. The possibility of Whipple's disease was considered because of the systemic nature of her illness, the recent development of diarrhea, and the rapid improvement on antibiotic treatment. A jejunal biopsy was performed on day four and revealed foamy PAS-positive macrophages infiltrating the lamina propria typical of Whipple's disease. Upon eventual discharge from the hospital, the patient was treated with a 1-year oral course of co-trimoxazole and had no further disease manifestations.

Clinical Features

Although the terms "protean" and "great masquerader" have been used to describe diseases such as systemic lupus erythematosus, human immuno-deficiency virus infection, syphilis, and tuberculosis, WD fills these attributions as well as all the rest. Patients can be infected with *T. whippelii* for decades with a waxing and waning course and without rapidly succumbing to it. Nearly every organ system can be involved, and WD can march through many different clinical phases, with multiple misdiagnoses and their attendant inappropriate therapies, demonstrated in the patients described above. Prominent features of WD are presented in Table 17-1.

In the past, WD has been a predominantly white male disorder (10:1 male to female) with some reports of family clusters. This gender ratio may change with better detection through the use of sensitive screening tests such as PCR and serological testing. Eventually, WD may lose its label as a rare disorder, especially because some patients who present with seronega-tive rheumatoid arthritis, fever of unknown origin, ill-defined systemic in-flammatory disorders, and inflammatory bowel diseases may ultimately be diagnosed with WD.

The clinical course of WD often begins with a prodromal or collagen vascular/immune phase in which all the cardinal features are intermittent and can occur over many years: arthritis, abdominal discomfort and bloat-ing, diarrhea, cough, weight loss, and asthenia. The arthritis can occur 10 to 20 years before the telltale malabsorption diarrhea occurs. The next phase is called the period of decline or the gastrointestinal phase in which the bulk of the evolving and cumulative disease leads to organ dysfunction and possible death, if left undiagnosed and untreated. These patients pre-sent with an Addisonian-like disorder, severe gastrointestinal problems, cardiac abnormalities, pleuropulmonary signs and symptoms, fever of un-known origin, or even sudden death.

Table 17-1   Clinical Manifestations of Whipple's Disease

Major Symptoms		Major Signs		Laboratory, Pathology, and Radiology Findings
Weight loss	95%	BP <110/60	83%	Anemia
Diarrhea	78%	Lymphadenopathy	55%	Lymphopenia, elevated ESR
Arthralgias	65%	Fever	55%	Hypoalbuminemia
Abdominal pain	60%	Abdominal tenderness	54%	Malabsorption
		Edema	18%	Hypocholesterolemia, hypokalemia, hypocalcemia, prolonged prothrombin time, steatorrhea, abnormal d-xylose testing
		Splenomegaly	18%	Upper gastrointestinal series: coarsening of duodenal and jejunal folds with dilation
				Small bowel biopsy: clubbed villi; foamy macrophages containing PAS-positive bacilli
				PCR: sensitive and specific

BP = blood pressure; ESR = erythrocyte sedimentation rate; PAS = periodic acid-Schiff; PCR = polymerase chain reaction.

The joint manifestations of WD tend to be early features, are often migratory and non-deforming arthralgias and arthritis, and can be accompanied by sacroiliitis and spondylitis. A symmetrical rheumatoid arthritis–like presentation can also be seen in some patients. Synovial fluid is commonly inflammatory with greater than 10,000 leukocytes/µL, with a predominance of neutrophils and at times demonstrating PAS-positive macrophages. Routine bacterial cultures are negative. Synovial biopsies show a mild, nonspecific synovitis with hyperplasia of the synovial lining cells and increased vascularity.

Neurological manifestations can vary over time and may dominate the disorder in some patients. Abnormalities include personality disorders, alteration in consciousness, encephalopathy, clonic movements, spastic paresis, presenile dementia, posterior column disease, and microinfarcts in the brain.

Less common but prominent atypical features include granulomatous disease of the liver, pulmonary artery involvement with pulmonary hypertension, vitreous opacities and inflammatory eye disease, scurvy, gastrointestinal hemorrhage, and testicular and prostatic involvement. Because of the multisystem involvement of WD, a broad differential diagnosis needs to be considered (Table 17-2).

Table 17-2   Differential Diagnosis of Whipple's Disease

Disease	*Overlapping Clinical Features with Whipple's Disease*
Collagen vascular diseases	Arthritis and arthralgias, fever, pleuropericarditis, lymphadenopathy, CNS disease, anemia, hypoalbuminemia
Malignancy	Fever, weight loss, lymphadenopathy, splenomegaly
Addison's disease	Hypotension, fever, weakness, hyperpigmentation, electrolyte abnormalities
Sarcoidosis	Lymphadenopathy, fever, splenomegaly, CNS disease, arthralgias, anemia, anergy, abnormal LFT
Tuberculosis	Fever, lymphadenopathy, hepatosplenomegaly, pleuritis, CNS disease, arthralgias, anemia
Inflammatory bowel diseases	Abdominal symptoms, diarrhea, fever, abnormal LFT, arthralgias, sacroiliitis, anemia
Viral infections such as HIV, hepatitis B and C, parvovirus B19	Fever, weight loss, arthralgias, lymphadenopathy, abnormal LFT, anemia

CNS = central nervous system; LFT = liver function tests; HIV = human immunodeficiency virus.

Diagnosis

A typical clinical presentation is that of a patient with an apparent systemic inflammatory disorder that has eluded a specific or satisfying diagnosis (such as those in Table 17-2) or has not responded appropriately to various therapeutic interventions. The possibility of WD is then raised when abdominal symptoms or manifestations of malabsorption arise. Unfortunately, however, the onset of gastrointestinal features tends to be late in the disease, thereby delaying diagnosis. Confirmation of the diagnosis is made by endoscopic small bowel biopsy and the finding of the characteristic histological findings described above (7). The use of PCR testing has been invaluable to assess inconclusive or suspicious cases, to confirm the diagnosis, and to define disease activity or response to treatment (8,9).

Prognosis

The clinical course of WD is insidious and unpredictable. If unrecognized and left untreated, it is potentially fatal. In most patients, a therapeutic response can be seen in 2 to 4 weeks after the onset of antibiotic therapy, which is typically maintained for at least a year to reduce the risk of relapses (10). Even with long-term antibiotics, however, relapses can still occur, commonly months to years after discontinuation of therapy. Relapses may resemble the initial disease presentation or include new manifestations but usually respond just as readily to antibiotics that initially induced a remission (2). A small subset of patients, particularly those with central nervous system involvement, appears to be refractory to a broad range of antibiotics and has the worst prognosis (2,11).

Management

Because patients are often systemically ill, the Whipple's pathogen cannot be cultured, and its antibiotic sensitivities cannot be assessed, initial antibiotic therapy is usually broad-spectrum and empirical. Courses of single-agent antibiotics or combinations of antibiotics have varied both in duration and outcome (12). An appropriate regimen may include an initial 2-week course of intravenous benzylpenicillin (2-4 million U q4h) or ceftriaxone (2 g/d), with intravenous streptomycin (0.5-1 g bid), followed by a 1-year course of oral co-trimoxazole (160/800 mg bid) or cefixime (400 mg/d). Macrolides, chloramphenicol, and tetracyclines have also been used. In cases that are refractory to antibiotic therapy, concomitant alternative treatments such as IFN-γ have been employed with some success (6).

The PCR test for the *T. whippelii* 16S ribosomal RNA gene may eventually be helpful in monitoring the eradication or persistence of infection (9). When more widely available, PCR testing may ultimately provide a more rational approach to treatment decisions such as antibiotic selection and duration of treatment. At present, however, clinical signs and symptoms of active disease remain the guides to the course and length of antibiotic treatment.

REFERENCES

1. **Marth T, Strober W.** Whipple's disease. Semin Gastrointest Dis. 1996;7:41-8.

2. **Feurle GE, Marth T.** An evaluation of antimicrobial treatment for Whipple's disease: tetracycline versus trimethoprim-sulfamethoxazole. Dig Dis Sci. 1994;39:1642-8.

3. **Yardley JH, Hendrix TR.** Combined electron and light microscopy in Whipple's disease: demonstration of "bacillary bodies" in the intestine. Johns Hopkins Hosp Bull. 1961;109:80-98.

4. **Relman DA, Schmidt TM, MacDermott RP, Falco S.** Identification of the uncultured bacillus of Whipple's disease. New Engl J Med. 1992;237:293-301.

5. **Raolt D, Birg ML, LaScola B, et al.** Cultivation of the bacillus of Whipple's disease. N Engl J Med. 2000;342:620-5.

6. **Schneider T, Stallmach A, von Herbay A, et al.** Treatment of refractory Whipple's disease with interferon gamma. Ann Intern Med 1998;129:875-7.

7. **Geboes K, Ectors N, Heidbuchel H, et al.** Whipple's disease: the value of upper gastrointestinal endoscopy for the diagnosis and follow-up. Acta Gastroenterol Belg. 1992;55:209-19.

8. **Von Herbay A, Ditton HJ, Maiwald M.** Diagnostic application of a polymerase chain reaction assay for the Whipple's disease bacterium to intestinal biopsies. Gastroenterology. 1996;110:1735-43.

9. **Ramzan NN, Loftus E, Burgart LJ, et al.** Diagnosis and monitoring of Whipple's disease by polymerase chain reaction. Ann Intern Med. 1997;126:520-7.

10. **Keinath RD, Merrell DE, Vlietstra R, Dobbins WO 3rd.** Antibiotic treatment and relapse in Whipple's disease. Gastroenterology. 1985;88:1867-73.

11. **Fleming JL, Wiesner RH, Shorter RG.** Whipple's disease: clinical, biochemical and histopathological features and assessment of treatment of 29 patients. Mayo Clin Proc. 1988;63:539-51.

12. **Dobbins WO 3rd.** Whipple's Disease. Springfield, Ill: Charles C. Thomas; 1987.

SECTION VI

DEGENERATIVE DISEASES AND REGIONAL PAIN SYNDROMES

18

■ ■ ■

Osteoarthritis

Susan Goodman, MD

O steoarthritis (OA) is the most common form of arthritis and one of the most common reasons for physician visits. Per 100,000 person-years, the numbers of new cases of symptomatic OA of the hands, hips, and knees were 100, 88, and 240, respectively, in one study (1). The incidence of symptomatic OA increases with age until the age of 80 but then seems to stabilize thereafter. Although most people aged 65 and older will have radiographic evidence of OA, many people with abnormal radiographs have no complaints attributable to OA. OA typically progresses slowly over decades and years, generally with minimal inflammation, especially when compared with rheumatoid arthritis (Table 18-1). However, although OA is associated with older populations, it is no longer thought to be an inexorable consequence of aging, and it is known that the pathogenesis of this disorder involves complex interactions among genetic factors, environmental influences, and local changes in cartilage and bone biology.

Pathogenesis

OA represents an imbalance between articular cartilage degradation and repair, ultimately resulting in net degeneration of cartilage and hypertrophic changes of periarticular bone. Normal articular cartilage is a relatively acellular tissue composed of a small population of chondrocytes that are responsible for the synthesis and maintenance of the extracellular matrix that is composed largely of type II collagen and proteoglycans. Type II collagen is the primary collagen of articular cartilage and is responsible for maintaining the shape of the tissue. The proteoglycans are found primarily in large aggregates that are responsible for the compressive properties of articular cartilage. The best characterized form is aggrecan, which is composed of

Table 18-1   Distinguishing Features of Osteoarthritis and Rheumatoid Arthritis

	Osteoarthritis	Rheumatoid Arthritis
Synovial fluid analysis	Non-inflammatory (WBC < 1000/μL)	Inflammatory (WBC 1K-50K/μL)
Erosions	In rare variant forms	Common
Number of joints*	Mono-, pauci-, or polyarticular	Polyarticular
Distribution of joints	Asymmetric	Symmetric
Joints commonly affected	DIPs, PIPs, first CMCs, neck, lumbosacral spine, hips, knees, MTPs	PIPs, MCPs, wrists, elbows, shoulders, neck, hips, knees, ankles, MTPs
Joints usually spared	MCPs, elbows, shoulders, ankles	DIPs, lumbosacral spine
Systemic manifestations	Absent	Present
Rheumatoid factor	Negative	Positive in 80%

* Monoarticular (1 joint); pauciarticular (2-4 joints); polyarticular (5 or more joints).
WBC = white blood count; DIP = distal interphalangeal joints; PIP = proximal interphalangeal joints; CMC = carpometacarpal joints; MCP = metacarpophalangeal joints; MTP = metatarsophalangeal joints.

hundreds of molecules of the proteoglycans chondroitin sulfate and keratan sulfate around a hyaluronic acid core. Hyaluronic acid is also an important component of synovial fluid and has an essential lubricating role at the cartilage-on-synovium surface.

Mechanical stress and microtrauma induce the local production of proinflammatory cytokines such as interleukin-1 and tumor necrosis factor-alpha by synovial monocytes or chondrocytes. These cytokines modulate the activities of proteases such as stromelysin, eventually resulting in degradation of the extracellular matrix (2). The articular cartilage becomes softened, and if left unchecked, eventual progressive erosion of cartilage leads to denudation down to subchondral bone. Subsequently, microfractures of the subchondral bone caused by abnormal or excessive loading of the joint in the setting of cartilage loss accelerate the degenerative process.

There is increasing evidence of genetic influences in the susceptibility for the development of OA. Mutations of the type II collagen gene and other genes encoding specific protein constituents of cartilage have been linked to severe premature generalized OA. The genetic contribution to idiopathic late-onset OA is more complex. Marked racial differences in the development of hip OA have been described, with very low prevalence in southern Chinese and South African black populations. Studies in areas with limited emigration (such as Iceland) have demonstrated strong familial clustering of OA (3). Siblings of hip replacement patients had three times the risk of undergoing hip replacement for OA than did matched controls. Additionally, Heberden's nodes have long been recognized as having strong familial associations, and twin studies support a genetic link for hand and knee OA.

Environmental and acquired factors are also associated with OA (4). Obesity and trauma are the most significant and modifiable risk factors in the development of OA in the knee and hip. In addition, quadriceps muscle strength may influence the development or progression of knee OA. Quadriceps weakness has been demonstrated in patients with radiographic knee OA who have no history of knee pain, suggesting that quadriceps weakness may be a risk factor for knee OA and not the result of diminished weight-bearing on the affected limb due to discomfort. Some occupations, such as farming or mining, are associated with an increased incidence hip and knee OA. At particular risk are those who bend, kneel, or squat during the performance of their work, and obesity markedly increases this occupational risk. Recreational sports do not seem to cause an increase in knee OA. Longitudinal studies of recreational runners have not demonstrated an increase in radiographic incidence or progression of OA compared with age-matched controls. However, injury is an important cause of OA of the knee, and elite athletes subjected to high-impact sports injuries do have an increase in hip and knee disease. Meniscal injury and complete meniscectomy significantly increase the risk of subsequent OA of the knee.

Case Presentation

A 65-year-old woman presents with multiple joint complaints. Her symptoms had been intermittent for years but have become more persistent over the past 6 months, especially during the performance of daily activities. She has had pain in her right groin and knee, which is exacerbated by walking downstairs and has caused difficulty getting out of a low chair. She has had to give up jogging, which made these symptoms worse. Although she has never fallen, she perceives instability upon bearing weight on her right leg. She also complains of low back pain that often bothers her at the end of the day. She has had decreased ability to open jars and doorknobs because of discomfort at the base of her thumb and in her fingers. Acetaminophen offers only partial relief of her symptoms. Her history is otherwise unrevealing except for a 20-pound weight gain that she has attributed to immobility.

Physical examination reveals a painful and antalgic right leg limp. Cervical spine range of motion is limited on extension and lateral flexion. There are tender Heberden's and Bouchard's nodes overlying several proximal and distal interphalangeal joints, and basal joint pressure elicits moderate pain of the right first carpometacarpal joint. She has a slight dextroscoliosis of the thoracolumbar spine with diminished forward flexion. Hip motion is normal on the left, but diminished flexion and internal rotation of the right hip is present. Minimal crepitus of the left knee is present with a preserved flexion-extension arc. There is a varus deformity of, and marked crepitus in, the right knee, which was slightly warm and swollen with an obvious joint effusion.

Clinical Features

The clinical syndromes produced by OA vary with the joints affected. Gelling, a short-lived stiffness lasting no more than several minutes after extended inactivity, is common. With prolonged use or loading, affected joints become increasingly painful, reflecting the deranged architecture and/or mechanics of the diseased joint; rest will typically alleviate symptoms. However, in advanced cases of OA, even minimal movement may be intolerable. (In contrast, pain and stiffness associated with inflammatory disorders such as rheumatoid arthritis or the spondyloarthropathies characteristically worsen with immobility and improve with continued movement.) The quality of the pain may be variably described as dull, throbbing, achy, or sharp.

Symptoms of OA may also be positional because of encroachment onto adjacent structures; an example of this is spinal stenosis in which standing erect results in impingement of nearby nerve roots. Although joint swelling may be present at times, other signs of inflammation such as heat and redness are not prominent features of OA and when present should raise suspicion for concomitant diagnoses such as gout, pseudogout, or infection.

Osteoarthritis of the Spine

Patients with OA of the cervical spine report pain with neck motion or bending. Typically, the patient has pain and stiffness of the neck or back, which are worse after a full day's activities and for a short period upon awakening in the morning. Some patients may be awakened from sleep due to poor neck positioning during the night. Symptoms can arise from disc degeneration and from typical osteoarthritic changes in the diarthrodial apophyseal joints. The patient may complain of discomfort directly attributable to degeneration of the affected joints or of symptoms produced by nerve root or spinal cord compression by extruded intervertebral disc material, bony spurs arising from the apophyseal joints, or from slippage of the vertebral body (spondylolisthesis).

Low back or buttock pain with leg heaviness or calf cramps can result from spinal stenosis, which refers to a central narrowing of the spinal canal by the cumulative effects of disc degeneration, osteophyte encroachment, and ligmentum flavum hypertrophy of the lumbosacral spine. In this common clinical syndrome, symptoms are produced by activity such as walking and relieved by rest. These symptoms are frequently confused with those of lower extremity vascular claudication and are termed pseudoclaudication. Aside from the presence of distal pulses, one distinguishing feature between claudication and pseudoclaudication is that the latter can be often relieved by walking flexed forward with a "simian stance." This maximizes the potential space available for the spinal canal, thereby minimizing compression of neurological structures. Conversely, hyperextension of the back often aggravates symptoms in spinal stenosis.

Pain produced by OA of the spine has little correlation with the radiographic findings. Patients who have extensive X-ray abnormalities frequently have minimal symptoms, while a patient with a small but strategically located osteophyte may have profound radicular symptoms from nerve root compression.

It must be emphasized that not all back pain originates in the spine. Visceral pathology arising in the abdominal organs or vasculature can often present as back pain. (A full discussion of low back pain is presented in Chapter 27.)

Osteoarthritis of the Knee

OA of the knee frequently presents with pain in the medial aspect of the knee, although pain that is poorly localized is also common. The patient may have asymmetric deterioration of one of the three compartments of the knee (medial, lateral, or patellofemoral). When the medial compartment is disproportionately affected, a varus or bow-legged deformity results (Figure 18-1). "Knock knees" or a valgus deformity results when the lateral compartment is narrowed. Ligamentous instability contributes to and is exacerbated by these deformities. Patients with advanced OA of the knee frequently complain of instability, and falls may result from the affected knee buckling or giving way. The patient may be unable to walk up or down stairs with a normal alternating gait.

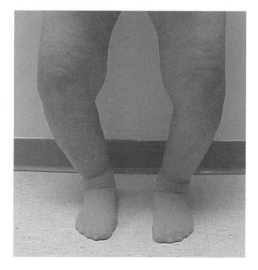

Figure 18-1 Severe narrowing of the medial compartment of both knees can result in a prominent varus or bow-legged deformity.

Mechanical factors play a significant role in knee OA (4). Weight gain increases the symptoms produced by OA, and OA of the knee is more frequent in obese women. It has been estimated that one pound of body weight is translated to five pounds of force for the hips and knees. Symptoms resulting from OA of weight-bearing joints improve with weight reduction. Quadriceps weakness contributes to knee pain and in fact may contribute to the development or progression of OA of the knee by increasing the force of impact and decreasing the stability of the knee.

Osteoarthritis of the Hip

OA of the hip typically produces pain in the groin, although symptoms are also commonly referred to the knee. Patients will frequently call pain in the lateral thigh "hip pain," when pain in the lateral thigh is actually more commonly caused by trochanteric bursitis or iliotibial band syndrome and may not indicate hip joint pathology. Pain in the buttock and anterior thigh usually develops in more advanced cases of hip arthritis and is rarely seen as an early manifestation of hip OA. As arthritis of the hip progresses, mobility is lost. The earliest deficit is usually seen in internal rotation with subsequent loss of motion in flexion and external rotation. Patient will note that they are unable to tie their shoelaces or cut their toenails. OA of the hip in younger patients is often secondary to various problems such as rheumatoid arthritis, osteonecrosis, hip dysplasia, trauma, or dislocation.

Osteoarthritis of the Hand

OA of the hand presents with pain and stiffness and loss of dexterity. Many patients with prominent bony nodules overlying the proximal and distal interphalangeal joints, known as Bouchard's and Heberden's nodes, respectively, have few complaints. Mucoid cysts that are similar to ganglion cysts may precede the emergence of these nodes (Figure 18-2). OA of the first

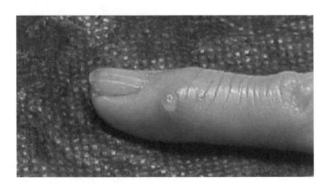

Figure 18-2   A thick gelatinous mucus can be expressed after puncture of a mucoid cyst of the distal interphalangeal joint.

carpometacarpal or basal joint is more likely to be symptomatic (Figure 18-3). Pain is noted with grip and grasp. Opening jars or turning door handles may be difficult. A "square hand" deformity can result when the first carpometacarpal joint becomes subluxed as a result of advanced arthritis.

Erosive Osteoarthritis

Erosive OA describes a syndrome of swelling and inflammation with a predilection for the proximal and distal interphalangeal joints, most commonly seen in perimenopausal women. The distribution of the affected joints, particularly involvement of the distal interphalangeal joints, helps to differentiate this from rheumatoid arthritis. Radiographic findings show both bony erosions and osteophyte formation.

Diagnosis

The diagnosis of OA can usually be made based solely on the history and physical examination, without extensive use of the clinical laboratory or radiological studies. Laboratory testing is probably most useful in identifying relative contraindications (such as renal or hepatic insufficiency) or toxicities to medications. OA is not a systemic inflammatory disease, and therefore a significantly elevated erythrocyte sedimentation rate or serum C-reactive protein should prompt a search for comorbidities or alternative diagnoses. Arthrocentesis is rarely necessary unless an alternative diagnosis is suspected (e.g., infection, crystalline arthritis) or unless debulking a swollen joint is symptomatically therapeutic. Synovial fluid in OA is usually clear or minimally turbid with fewer than 1000 leukocytes/mm^3.

Plain radiographs can reveal osteophytes at the margin of the affected joint, subchondral sclerosis of bone, cysts, and joint space narrowing

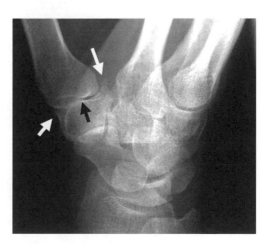

Figure 18-3 Plain radiography of osteoarthritic changes of the first carpometacarpal joint, demonstrating joint space narrowing (black arrow) and prominent osteophytes (white arrows).

(Figure 18-4). Plain radiographs are extremely accurate for the diagnosis of OA, but it should be emphasized that they should always be correlated with the patient's specific complaints. There is often a disparity between the degree of radiologic changes and the severity of symptoms. Other imaging studies such as magnetic resonance imaging are more appropriate when derangements of soft tissue structures such as ligaments, tendons, cartilage, and neurological structures are suspected.

On occasion, patients may have clinical pictures that are confusing. For example, although hip pathology classically presents as groin pain, groin discomfort may also result from radiculopathic pain secondary to lumbosacral OA. In such cases, symptomatic relief with fluoroscopy-guided hip joint injection with xylocaine can identify the hip joint as the source of discomfort.

Prognosis

Because OA is a chronic degenerative condition, early recognition and intervention are the most important factors in ensuring optimal outcomes. Modification of behaviors, activities, or comorbid conditions (e.g., obesity) that contribute to the development of OA is essential in the prevention or retardation of disease progression.

Although plain radiographs are the most common study used to evaluate and follow the course of OA, their overall usefulness is actually unclear because radiological findings do not universally correlate with symptoms. Nonetheless, it should not be surprising that rapid loss of joint space on radiographs is predictive of early surgical intervention (5). For example, a

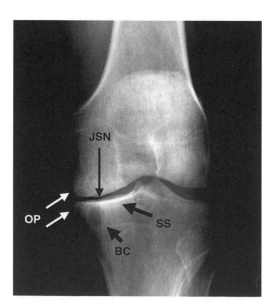

Figure 18-4 Radiographic hallmarks of osteoarthritis are demonstrated in this standing anteroposterior radiograph of the left knee: asymmetric joint space narrowing (JSN), osteophyte (OP) formation, subchondral sclerosis (SS), and bone cysts (BC).

15% to 20% loss of the joint space in the hip over a 4-year period was found to be a highly sensitive and specific predictor for an eventual total hip arthroplasty.

Management

Relief of pain and improved function with decreased disability are the primary goals of therapy for OA. Primary care physicians should feel comfortable managing all but the most difficult cases, at which point consultation with a rheumatologist, orthopedist, physiatrist, or pain management specialist may be warranted. Appropriate management of OA should integrate nonpharmacological, pharmacological, and surgical approaches (6,7).

Nonpharmacological Therapy

Nonpharmacological therapy is not adequately emphasized in the management of OA. Simple and inexpensive interventions as listed in Table 18-2 can have profoundly positive effects on the outcome of OA, especially when administered early in the course of illness. Patients who participate in programs that teach self-management techniques, such as those offered by the Arthritis Foundation, report improved quality of life and increased activity as well as decreased pain and physician visits. Patient education and support are important in reaching the endpoints of therapy. Early referral for supervised physical therapy and development of a home exercise program can enable more rapid recovery of function, amelioration of pain, and less reliance on analgesic medications.

Exercise programs should be directed towards specific areas affected by OA, and it must be emphasized to patients that such programs should be incorporated into their everyday routine. OA of the lumbosacral spine should be treated with exercises that emphasize stretching the thigh muscles in combination with strengthening the paraspinal and abdominal muscles. Flexion exercises are helpful in maintaining range of motion. Bed rest

---

Table 18-2   Nonpharmacological Therapy for Osteoarthritis

• Patient education	• Muscle-strengthening exercises
• Self-management programs	• Assistive ambulation devices
• Social support	• Assistive devices for activities of daily living
• Weight loss (if overweight)	• Patellar taping
• Aerobic conditioning regimen	• Appropriate footwear and insoles
• Range-of-motion exercises	• Occupational therapy

Modified from Hochberg MC, Altman RD, Brandt KD, et al. Arthritis Rheum. 1995;38:1535-40,1541-6.

will only lead to deconditioning and has no role in the treatment of chronic back pain due to OA.

Knee pain from OA or chondromalacia patella is best addressed by quadriceps-strengthening exercises that have been shown to decrease knee symptoms. Medial patellar taping may improve symptoms in patellofemoral arthritis. Physical modalities for maintaining or restoring hip motion include strengthening of the hip abductors and extensors and range-of-motion exercises aimed at maintaining at least 30 degrees of flexion and full extension. Additional physical modalities that can reduce OA pain in the lower extremities include wedged insoles and a cane held in the contralateral hand. General aerobic conditioning and weight loss are also of benefit for patients with OA of the weight-bearing joints. Each pound of body weight is reflected five-fold in the hip and knee. Walking speed as well as improvement in measures of general well-being were increased for patients in a comprehensive conditioning program over patients who simply performed range-of-motion exercises.

Hand OA should be treated with range of motion and grip-strengthening exercises. Patient education for techniques to protect joints is also extremely helpful because it enables patients to become more aware of how to prevent further trauma to affected joints. Joint protection techniques include splinting of the basal joint in a position of function, the use of assistive devices that increase the size of the tool handle rendering tasks easier to perform, and modifying habits that exacerbate symptoms.

Pharmacological Therapy

Table 18-3 lists pharmacological agents that are commonly used for the treatment of pain caused by OA. Although extremely useful in pain control, they should always be given in conjunction with nonpharmacological therapies.

Table 18-3   Pharmacological Therapy for Osteoarthritis

Oral agents
- Acetaminophen
- Nonacetylated salicylates
- NSAIDs*
- COX-2 inhibitor
- Analgesics
  (e.g., tramadol,
  low-potency opiates)

Intra-articular agents
- Glucocorticoids
- Hyaluronic acid

Topical agents
- Capsaicin
- Methylsalicylate
- NSAIDs

Putative disease-modifying agents
- Glucosamine/chondroitin sulfate

---

* Misoprostol, proton pump inhibitors, or histamine H_2-receptor blockers should be strongly considered for all patients receiving chronic NSAID therapy or in patients at high risk for gastrointestinal adverse effects.
Modified from Hochberg MC, Altman RD, Brandt KD, et al. Arthritis Rheum. 1995;38:1535-40,1541-6.

Pharmacological therapy for OA begins with simple analgesia. Acetaminophen should be first-line therapy for almost all patients. It is very well tolerated and has been proven to be effective in treating mild-to-moderate pain. More importantly, there are few side effects. Patients with liver disease may be at increased risk for hepatotoxicity, but this generally occurs only at supratherapeutic doses. However, alcohol use may enhance potential liver toxicity in patients at risk. Drug interactions are rare, but the half-life of warfarin can be prolonged, and the international normalized ratio (INR) may require more frequent monitoring.

Nonsteroidal Anti-Inflammatory Drugs and Cyclooxygenase-2 Inhibitors

Non-steroidal anti-inflammatory drugs (NSAIDs) and cyclooxygenase (COX)-2-selective inhibitors are very effective in treating pain and improving functional capacity in OA patients. Although preferred by many patients over acetaminophen, these drugs have more potential toxicities, particularly in this older population of patients with more frequent co-morbidities. Cardiovascular disease can lead to poor tolerance to the salt- and water-retaining properties shared by both the traditional NSAIDs and COX-2 inhibitors. Fluid retention can lead to the development or worsening of hypertension and congestive heart failure. Patients treated with angiotensin-converting enzyme inhibitors or diuretics are more likely to develop renal insufficiency from NSAIDs and COX-2 inhibitors, as are those patients whose serum creatinine is greater than 2.0 mg/dL at the onset of therapy. Renal function in these patients is highly dependent on prostaglandin-mediated vasodilation within the kidney, and this physiological process is inhibited by the NSAIDs and COX-2 inhibitors.

Nonselective NSAIDs have effects on platelet aggregation that can result in an increased risk of bleeding and bruising, particularly in patients taking warfarin or other anticoagulants. The COX-2 inhibitors and nonacetylated salicylates such as salsalate do not have an effect on platelet aggregation and can therefore be used concomitantly with warfarin. However, these drugs may affect warfarin protein binding and bioavailability, so the INR should be carefully monitored if these drugs are used concurrently.

Gastrointestinal toxicity is the most common reason for the discontinuation of traditional NSAID therapy, which may lead to gastric erosions, ulcers, and bleeding. The patients at highest risk have been well defined: those over the age of 65, those with a previous history of peptic ulcer or bleeding, those on chronic NSAID therapy, and those taking concomitant glucocorticoids or anticoagulants. After weighing the appropriate risks and benefits, patients who are treated with NSAIDs for the long-term should generally be treated with a gastroprotective agent as well. Misoprostol, proton pump inhibitors, and histamine H_2-receptor blockers have all been shown to decrease the risk of gastrointestinal events in NSAID-treated patients.

The popularity of selective COX-2 inhibitors stems from their lower incidence of upper gastrointestinal disease and frank ulcerations but are no more effective than traditional NSAIDs in therapeutic properties. Recent, controversial, and as yet unanswered questions have been raised about the effect of COX-2 inhibitors on inducing cardiovascular disease. At present, until the risk of cardiac events has been clarified, most recommendations favor concurrent low-dose aspirin therapy in patients at risk for coronary artery disease, even if the gastroprotective effects of COX-2 inhibitors are partially undermined.

Tramadol

Tramadol, a centrally acting mu-opioid receptor agonist, has been shown to be effective in controlling pain associated with OA and is particularly useful in patients with contraindications to NSAIDs or COX-2 inhibitors. Low-potency narcotics can also be used sparingly, but their utility is limited by their addiction potential.

Intra-Articular Glucocorticoids

Intra-articular glucocorticoids are effective in relieving pain and improving function in OA. The duration of this effect is unpredictable and may last from days to months. Aspiration of joint fluid, when present, increases the benefit. Resting the joint after injection is also is of benefit in prolonging the effect of the injection. Because there is a hypothetical concern about accelerating the breakdown of cartilage if injections are given too often, it is advised that they be given no more frequently than at 4- to 6-month intervals. When joints are injected using standard aseptic technique, there is very little risk of infection. Intra-articular injections have also been shown to be safe in individuals taking warfarin whose INRs are in the therapeutic range.

Hyaluronic Acid

As discussed above, hyaluronic acid is a major component of articular cartilage and synovial fluid and functions as both a shock absorber and a lubricant. The levels of hyaluronic acid in synovial fluid from OA patients are significantly reduced. Therapeutic preparations of hyaluronic acid are now available for intra-articular viscosupplementation therapy in the treatment of knee OA. Hyaluronic acid is given as a series of injections into the knee with a large bore needle after aspiration of an existing effusion. However, the turnover of injected hyaluronic acid in synovial fluid is rapid, and injected hyaluronic acid is cleared within days. These observations cast doubt on any benefit that might be ascribed to raising the level of intra-articular hyaluronic acid. A recent meta-analysis studied the efficacy of intra-articular hyaluronic acid injection by analyzing three large placebo-controlled trials (greater than 200 subjects). No significant benefit could be shown in the treatment group compared with the placebo injection group. Additional studies have documented a high dropout rate for hyaluronic acid injection patients and less benefit than with NSAIDs. However, these studies did not stratify patients to severity of OA, and so it is still possible that patients with milder disease may benefit from hyaluronic acid viscosupplementation. At best, intra-articular hyaluronic acid therapy may offer transient and marginal benefit (8).

Topical Agents

Topical preparations of capsaicin, methylsalicylate, and NSAIDs have been used for the relief of pain in OA. Capsaicin is derived from Tabasco-type pepper plants. It depletes substance P, a major pain mediator, from peripheral nerves. Topical capsaicin relieves pain in OA of the hand and knee. Up to 3 to 4 weeks of therapy may be required before an effect is observed, and the ointment must be applied 3 to 4 times daily. Although methylsalicylate and topical NSAIDs have long been in use, there are no controlled trials demonstrating their benefit. Toxicity of most topical analgesics is minimal as long as the user is careful not to introduce the drugs into the eyes through rubbing.

Glucosamine Sulfate and Chondroitin Sulfate

Wide use of glucosamine sulfate and chondroitin sulfate preparations in veterinary medicine and in human subjects throughout Europe, as well as an appealingly low-toxicity profile, has stimulated interest in these compounds in the United States. They have been shown to promote chondrocyte proteoglycan synthesis in vitro, suggesting a potential disease-modifying role in the clinical setting. However, a recent meta-analysis of 15 clinical trials using stringent study design and inclusion criteria suggests only modest pain relief from glucosamine sulfate and chondroitin sulfate in the treatment of OA symptoms (9). Large prospective double-blind placebo-controlled trials are underway; however, at present the hope for drugs that might affect the rate of cartilage breakdown or stimulate cartilage repair by chondrocytes and alter the evolution of OA remains unfulfilled.

Surgical Therapy

Total joint arthroplasty (TJA) is effective therapy for advanced OA of the knee, hip, and shoulder but is less commonly used in the elbow and ankle. Consideration of TJA is warranted in the presence of persistent pain and disability in a patient who demonstrates radiographic evidence of advanced joint damage. The outcome of surgery is highly dependent on the skill of the surgeon and diligent post-operative medical care and physical rehabilitation.

Total hip replacement (THR) surgery may be indicated for the patient who has persistent pain and limited function from severe OA of the hip. In a large study conducted at Hospital for Special Surgery, close to 90% of patients reported satisfaction with post-operative results after rehabilitation and recuperation (10). Using a pre-operative assessment in which four parameters (hip pain, walking, range of motion and muscle strength, and function) were scored on a scale of 0 to 10 (worst cumulative score of zero;

a normal cumulative score of 40), it was found that patients with the lowest pre-operative cumulative scores were most likely to be satisfied with the results of THR. Persistent pain, leg-length discrepancy, a new limp, dislocation, need for revision surgery, unhappiness with the incisional scar, and need for antibiotic prophylaxis were causes of dissatisfaction.

Severe daily pain, night pain, and loss of function are the most common reasons for recommending total knee replacement (TKR). Benefits anticipated from TKR include improved function, decreased pain, and improved quality of life. Multiple studies demonstrate good-to-excellent results in 80% to 90% of patients who undergo TKR (11). Age, weight, and co-morbidities such as vascular disease influence the decision to perform TKR.

TJA should be considered only in those patients who meet medical requirements for major surgery. Age, general health status, and goals of therapy should all be reviewed before this is recommended. Patient outcome is clearly better in those patients who have realistic goals and expectations and in those who have high motivation. Complications such as infection are increased in patients who require immunosuppressive therapy or in patients on renal dialysis. Thromboembolic complications are well recognized and challenging to prevent after lower extremity TJA and demand the effective use of prophylactic modalities. Patients at higher risk include those on estrogen therapy, those with known hypercoagulable states, or those with a history of previous thromboembolic disease. Cardiovascular disease can increase the risk of surgical complications. Severe peripheral vascular disease may preclude TJA.

Arthroscopic debridement of the knee for OA has been used in patients who are not felt to be candidates for TJA, but there are no studies demonstrating the efficacy of this procedure (12). In fact, a recent intermediate-sized prospective study that was randomized and placebo-controlled and compared arthroscopic debridement, arthroscopic lavage, and placebo in knee OA demonstrated no differences between the three groups in terms of pain relief or function at either 1 or 2 years (13). In a separate retrospective study of 14,391 arthroscopic knee debridements, 9.2% and 18.4% proceeded to TKR within 1 and 3 years, respectively, after arthroscopy (14).

REFERENCES

1. **Oliveria SA, Felson DT, Reed JI, et al.** Incidence of symptomatic hand, hip, and knee osteoarthritis among patients in a health maintenance organization. Arthritis Rheum. 1995;38:1134-41.

2. **Lotz, M.** Cytokines in cartilage injury and repair. Clin Orthop. 2001;391(Suppl): S108-15.

3. **Ingvarsson T, Stefansson SE, Hallgrimsdottir IB, et al.** The inheritance of hip osteoarthritis in Iceland. Arthritis Rheum. 2000;43:2785-92.

4. **Hunter DJ, Marsh L, Sambrook PN.** Knee osteoarthritis: the influence of environmental factors. Clin Exp Rheumatol. 2002;20:93-100.

5. **Maillefert JF, Gueguen A, Nguyen M, et al.** Relevant change in radiological progression in patients with hip osteoarthritis. I. Determination using predictive validity for total hip arthroplasty. Rheumatology. 2002;41:142-7.

6. **Hochberg MC, Altman RD, Brandt KD, et al.** Guidelines for the medical management of osteoarthritis. Part I. Osteoarthritis of the hip. American College of Rheumatology. Arthritis Rheum. 1995;38:1535-40.

7. **Hochberg MC, Altman RD, Brandt KD, et al.** Guidelines for the medical management of osteoarthritis. Part II. Osteoarthritis of the knee. American College of Rheumatology. Arthritis Rheum. 1995;38:1541-6.

8. **Felson DT, Anderson JJ.** Hyaluronate sodium injections for osteoarthritis: hope, hype, and hard truths. Arch Intern Med. 2002;162:245-7.

9. **McAlindon TE, LaValley MP, Gulin JP, Felson DT.** Glucosamine and chondroitin for treatment of osteoarthritis: a systematic quality assessment and meta-analysis. JAMA. 2000;283:1469-75.

10. **Mancuso CA, Salvati EA, Johanson NA, et al.** Patients' expectations and satisfaction with total hip arthroplasty. J Arthroplasty. 1997;12:387-96.

11. **Dieppe P, Basler HD, Chard J, et al.** Knee replacement surgery for osteoarthritis: effectiveness, practice variations, indications and possible determinants of utilization. Rheumatology. 1999;38:73-83.

12. **Bradley JD, Heilman DK, Katz BP, et al.** Tidal irrigation as treatment for knee osteoarthritis: a sham-controlled, randomized, double-blinded evaluation. Arthritis Rheum. 2002;46:100-8.

13. **Moseley JB, O'Malley K, Petersen NJ, et al.** A controlled trial of arthroscopic surgery for osteoarthritis of the knee. N Engl J Med. 2002;347:81-8.

14. **Wai EK, Kreder HJ, Williams JI.** Arthroscopic debridement of the knee for osteoarthritis in patients fifty years of age or older: utilization and outcomes in the Province of Ontario. J Bone Joint Surg Am. 2002;84-A:17-22.

19

■ ■ ■

Osteonecrosis

Mathias P.G. Bostrom, MD
Scott M. Cook, MD

O steonecrosis (ON) or avascular necrosis is a syndrome of focal bone injury caused by ischemia and death of local osteocytes, resulting in subsequent resorption of the subchondral bone. While any bone may be affected, involvement of the femoral head is the most clinically significant. If left untreated, collapse of the femoral head ensues, resulting in secondary osteoarthritis and potentially a completely compromised joint. The condition was first described by Alexander Munro in 1738. In the early 19th century, Jean Cruveilhier reported on deformities of femoral heads resulting from an interruption in blood flow. In the early part of the modern era, ON was aptly described as "coronary disease of the hip" by Chandler.

The true incidence of ON is unknown because many cases are probably diagnosed as osteoarthritis. It has been estimated that there are 10,000 to 20,000 new cases in the United States each year, and in large series of total hip replacements, ON accounts for approximately 10% of primary arthroplasties. The male-to-female ratio of ON is approximately 4:1. Given that the majority of patients who undergo total hip arthroplasty for ON are relatively young (average age, 40), most will eventually require a revision surgery at some point in their lifetime. Many of these patients will spend significant amounts of time disabled during the prime of their working lives, and so the economic impact of ON is significant.

Pathogenesis

Trauma is the most common identifiable etiology for ON, generally occurring after a femoral neck fracture or hip dislocation (1). The vascular supply to the subchondral bone in the femoral head is compromised either through direct disruption or a tamponade effect from increased intracapsular pressure. The reported incidence of ON after internal fixation of a displaced femoral neck fracture ranges from 16% to 22%. Osteonecrosis after hip dislocation occurs in 6% to 40% of cases and appears to be more common after posterior dislocations than anterior or when reduction is delayed for more than 12 hours.

Multiple atraumatic etiologies for ON have been identified (Table 19-1), but unlike trauma, where the cause-effect mechanism for ON is easily discerned, the pathogenesis of atraumatic ON has proven more difficult to elucidate. Dysbarism (symptom complex resulting from rapid decompression during underwater diving), corticosteroid use, excessive alcohol consumption, hemoglobinopathies, human immunodeficiency virus (HIV) infection, systemic lupus erythematosus (SLE), pregnancy, pancreatitis, and hyperuricemia have all been identified as causative factors. In some clinical series, more than half of the cases have no identifiable etiology, but it is of extreme interest that recent reports have shown that many of these idiopathic cases are associated with subclinical hypercoagulability (2).

With improved safety standards and formalized decompression schedules for commercial divers and tunnel workers, Caisson's disease or decompression sickness is mainly of historical interest. ON secondary to pressure-related illness does not occur at atmospheric pressures below 17 pounds per square inch or when diving at depths less than 30 meters.

Alcohol consumption is felt to be a major cause of ON in the United States. Two major epidemiological studies of ON showed that almost 40% of cases can be traced to alcohol use (3). There appears to be a clear dose-response relationship. Data from Japan have shown that individuals who consume more than 400 mL of alcohol per week were 9.8 times more likely

Table 19-1   Risk Factors for Development of Osteonecrosis

Trauma	Human immunodeficiency virus (HIV) infection
Corticosteroid use	
Ethanol abuse	Hyperuricemia
Tobacco and nicotine use	Radiation therapy
Systemic lupus erythematosus	Cancer chemotherapy
Vasculitides	Pregnancy
Hyperlipidemia	Osteomyelitis
Hypercoagulable states	Metabolic bone diseases
Pancreatitis	Dysbaria
Sickle cell anemia and other hemoglobinopathies	Gaucher's disease

to develop ON, and those who consumed more than 1000 mL of alcohol per week were at a 17.9-fold higher risk. The pathogenesis of alcohol-induced ON is probably multifactorial. The fatty liver, resulting from chronic alcohol use, release small fat emboli that can occlude the vasculature of the femoral head. Some have also suggested that lipids can accumulate in the osteocytes of the femoral head, eventually compressing the nuclei and causing cell death. Chronically elevated blood alcohol levels are also directly toxic to osteocytes and marrow cells.

Corticosteroid use accounts for a large portion of atraumatic ON. Rates range from 28% to 45%, and figures from major transplant centers are higher; corticosteroid use is the most important iatrogenic cause of ON (3). High-dose corticosteroid use leads to fatty changes in the liver, which in turn can result in systemic fat embolization (4). Corticosteroids also change lipid metabolism, resulting in the formation of large aggregates of coalesced lipoproteins that can obstruct the intraosseous microvasculature. Animal models have also shown that high doses of corticosteroids induce fatty marrow hypertrophy, with resultant increased intramedullary pressures and decreased blood flow (5). Patients exposed to high-dose corticosteroid therapy (even for brief periods of time) may be more likely to develop ON than those who receive chronic low-dose corticosteroids. In a 10-year prospective study of patients with asthma or inflammatory arthritis receiving chronic low-dose oral prednisone (average cumulative dosages of 2201 mg/yr in asthma patients and 1967 mg/yr in arthritis patients), no cases of ON developed in 142 hips that were followed (6). In contrast, high doses of corticosteroids have been correlated with the development of ON in multiple studies, and a daily prednisone dose of 20 mg or greater has been identified as a significant risk factor, particularly in patients with SLE (7). Chronic use of high-potency topical corticosteroids (e.g., clobetasol) has also been associated with the development of ON.

Sickle cell anemia, along with other hemoglobinopathies, are also known etiologies of ON. Sickling or stasis within the sinusoids and microvasculature of the femoral head leads to necrosis. The incidence of ON in patients with sickle cell anemia ranges from 3% to 41%.

Recent attention has been focused on HIV as a cause of ON. Rates of ON as high as 4.4% have been shown in cross-sectional studies of patients with HIV infection. HIV infection is associated with elevated levels of anticardiolipin antibodies, protein S deficiency, and the presence of anti-protein S antibodies, all of which may increase propensity for vascular thrombosis (8).

In addition to the hip, ON also occurs (although less frequently) in other joints such as the knee, ankle, and shoulder. ON in these joints can be equally disabling, especially in the weight-bearing joints. Osteonecrosis of the talus is typically associated with trauma, whereas ON of the knee is usually idiopathic.

The causes of ON are not completely understood, but they are probably multifactorial and result in a final common pathway in which vascular interruption, thrombotic occlusion, and extravascular compression lead to decreased blood flow, ischemia, and eventual osteocyte necrosis.

Case Presentation

A 29-year-old woman with a known history of mixed connective tissue disease (MCTD) is evaluated for right groin pain with weight-bearing. The patient initially presented 10 years ago with symmetric inflammatory polyarthritis of the hands, wrists, and knees, Raynaud's phenomenon, pleuritic chest pain, and positive serological tests for antinuclear and anti-ribonucleoprotein antibodies. She subsequently developed proximal muscle weakness and was diagnosed with an inflammatory myopathy based on elevated muscle enzymes and a characteristic muscle biopsy. Prednisone 40 mg daily followed by a slow taper over several months was prescribed, with resolution of the myopathy.

During the past 5 years, the patient was able to discontinue standing corticosteroid therapy but required brief courses of prednisone for intermittent exacerbations of polyarthritis and pleurisy. Two months ago, the patient began noticing pain in her right groin with prolonged weight bearing. Despite nonsteroidal anti-inflammatory medications, her groin pain progressed, and she began walking with an obvious limp. Notably, a review of systems revealed no hand, wrist, or knee arthritis, which had been characteristic of previous exacerbations of MCTD.

Physical examination was remarkable for a marked painful and antalgic gait favoring her right hip. Her vital signs were normal, as was the examination of her heart, lungs, and abdomen. There was some mild duskiness of the fingers but no tenderness or swelling of the small joints of the hands. Examination of the right groin showed nearly full passive range of motion with minimal discomfort.

Plain radiography of the right hip was normal with no evidence of erosions, sclerosis, or collapse. Radionuclide bone scanning, however, revealed increased vascularity and focal uptake in the right femoral head consistent with avascular necrosis; no abnormalities in the left hip were noted. Magnetic resonance imaging (MRI) demonstrated edema in both femoral heads, consistent with avascular necrosis.

The patient subsequently underwent bilateral core decompressions. Four years after the procedures, the patient remains pain-free, and repeated MRI has shown no progression of necrosis and no evidence of collapse.

Clinical Features

Signs and symptoms of ON can be variable and non-specific. Pain in the involved joints is the typical initial complaint, but it is not unusual that affected joints are asymptomatic and are discovered incidentally. The onset of symptoms may be abrupt or insidious. Pain is generally provoked by physical activities that stress the diseased joint but may also be present at rest. Loss of range of motion is normally not appreciable until significantly compromising structural changes occur (e.g., collapse of the femoral head or secondary osteoarthritis).

For ON of the hip, groin pain exacerbated by bearing weight is the most common initial presentation. Many patients also complain of radiating pain to the anterior thigh and knee, but buttock pain is much less common. When ON of one hip is diagnosed, it is important for the clinician to assess for contralateral hip disease because bilateral involvement occurs in up to 80% of cases (9). Asymptomatic contralateral hip involvement without initial x-ray evidence of ON has been shown to progress to femoral head collapse at a mean of 23 months if left untreated (10).

Other commonly affected joints include the shoulders, knees, and ankles. However, the natural progression of disease in these joints is not as rapid as in the hip, and patients can often maintain good long-term function with conservative care.

Diagnosis

Early diagnosis is essential for optimal outcomes. Therefore, the single most important diagnostic factor is maintaining a high level of suspicion, especially in patients with risk factors for developing ON.

Diagnostic testing is important not only for establishing the diagnosis of ON of the hip but also for guiding treatment approaches. Plain radiography is the study of first choice. If the plain X-ray films are diagnostic, no further testing for that joint is necessary. However, if the plain X-ray films are normal, the clinician should not be lulled into a false sense of security, particularly if the index of suspicion for ON is high (such as in a patient taking chronic corticosteroids). At this juncture when plain radiography is unrevealing or equivocal, further evaluation with radionuclide bone scanning and/or MRI is appropriate.

Uptake on radionuclide bone scanning reflects new bone formation or increased general metabolic activity at the site of necrotic bone. In the pre-collapse femoral head, the sensitivity of bone scanning approaches 80%, while the specificity is about 75% (11). Advantages to this technique include wide availability, relative low cost, and the ability to assess multiple areas of the body at once. One important disadvantage is that comparisons of radionuclide uptake are made to the contralateral joint, and so accurate assessment of bilateral disease can be limited.

The sensitivity and specificity of MRI for ON of the hip approaches 90% and 100%, respectively, even in the pre-collapse hip (12). A low-intensity focal defect at the anterosuperior aspect of the femoral head seen on T_1- and T_2-weighted imaging is the most common finding, observed in 96% of cases. Although expense and the ability to assess only one joint at a time are important drawbacks, MRI has become a regular part of the diagnostic and prognostic approach to ON.

Radiographic Staging

As diagnostic technology advances, so do classification systems for ON (Table 19-2). Ficat and Arlet first described a four-stage classification scheme based on standard radiographs (12). Normal radiographs are seen in stage I. In stage II, sclerosis and cyst formation can be seen. Stage III is defined by early signs of subchondral collapse or flattening of the femoral head. Stage IV consists of joint space narrowing, secondary degenerative changes, or frank collapse of the femoral head.

With the advent of radionuclide bone scanning and MRI, classification schemes have become more complex and descriptive. In 1995, Steinberg published a classification system that expanded Ficat's to seven stages (0 to VI), with the goal of enabling better evaluation of prognosis and disease progression that may have an impact on treatment options. A grading system indicating the area of femoral head involvement was also added.

Table 19-2   Classification Schemes for Osteonecrosis of the Femoral Head

Radiographic Characteristics	Ficat	Steinberg	ARCO*	ARCO and Steinberg Subdivisions
High index of suspicion for ON but normal plain radiographs, bone scan, and MRI		0	0	None
Normal plain radiographs but abnormal MRI	I	I	I	A:<15%[†] B:15%-30%[†] C:>30%[†]
Sclerotic and cystic changes on radiographs	II	II	II	
Subchondral collapse producing a crescent sign	III	III	III	A:<15%[‡] B:15%-30%[‡] C:>30%[‡]
Flattening of the femoral head		IV	IV	A:<15% or <2mm[‡] B:15%-30% or 2-4mm[‡] C:>30% or >4mm[‡]
Joint space narrowing with or without acetabular involvement	IV	V	V	
Advanced degenerative changes		VI	VI	None

ARCO = Association Research Circulation Osseous, ON = osteonecrosis, MRI = magnetic resonance imaging.
* Stages I-V are subdivided into medial, central or lateral based on location in the femoral head.
[†] As determined on MRI.
[‡] As determined on antero-posterior and lateral radiographs.

Stage 0 is defined by a high index of suspicion for ON but with normal plain radiographs, bone scan, and MRI. Stage I consists of normal radiographs but an abnormal MRI or bone scintigraphy (Fig. 19-1). Sclerotic and cystic changes on radiographs are seen in stage II. Subchondral collapse producing a crescent sign defines stage III (Figure 19-2). Stage IV consists of flattening of the femoral head. Stage V is joint narrowing with or without acetabular involvement. Advanced degenerative changes are seen in stage VI. Perhaps the most important contribution of the newer classification scheme is the addition of categories for quantifying the extent of femoral head involvement. Involvement is graded as A, B, or C, corresponding to <15%; 15% to 30%, and >30% of the femoral head, respectively. The inclusion of this system was based on the growing recognition that the size of the lesion has important prognostic and treatment implications (13).

More recently, the Association Research Circulation Osseous (ARCO) proposed a new classification, which incorporated aspects from the Ficat

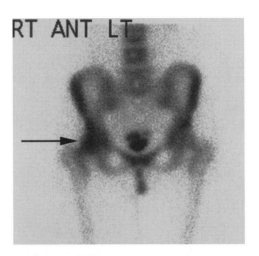

Figure 19-1 Delayed imaging using technetium-99m bone scanning shows increased uptake in the right femoral head (*arrow*) consistent with osteonecrosis. Note the asymmetry in uptake between the two hips.

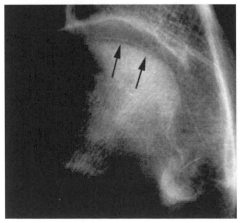

Figure 19-2 Plain radiograph demonstrating subchondral collapse/crescent sign (*arrows*) seen as a sliver of lucency below the cortex of the femoral head.

and Steinberg systems and added lesion location to the database (14). It is now recognized that medial lesions are not as likely to progress to collapse as superolateral lesions. At present, all three classifications are used, rendering interpretation of the literature difficult. However, most treatment decisions will be largely based on whether or not collapse of the femoral head has already occurred.

Arthroscopy

A recent study has examined correlation between radiography, MRI, and hip arthroscopy in the staging of ON and determined that arthroscopic findings, such as large flaps of loose articular cartilage, resulted in significant changes to treatment plans in 11 of 52 hips (15). The recommendation was made for hip arthroscopy to be considered in all hips with any radiographic evidence of flattening or depression of the femoral head.

Prognosis

Most series have reported dismal results when ON is followed clinically and treated conservatively with modified weight-bearing, anti-inflammatory agents, and analgesia, with failure rates ranging from 75% to 94%. Perhaps as imaging techniques improve and staging classifications become more uniform, diagnoses can be made earlier and more accurately, and better information will become available to help stratify patients into groups amenable to conservative therapy and those that will require early surgical intervention.

Management

All currently available treatments for ON have shown widely varying rates of success in the literature. These wide variances can be attributed to several factors: the true natural history of ON without treatment has not been fully investigated; there are no good animal models for atraumatic ON; the classification systems used in various studies are not uniform; and there are few comparisons between different treatment modalities.

Non-Surgical Therapy

No medication has been proven to alter the natural course of ON in rigorously designed large trials. Patients are routinely made non-weight-bearing or partial weight-bearing for an extended period of time for up to 6 months. However, it is unclear whether this alters the natural history of the disease. Similarly, no known studies have shown an effect on the natural history of osteonecrosis by eliminating or decreasing corticosteroid use.

Many idiopathic cases of ON are thought to be caused by hypercoagulability, and there have been several case reports of patients whose disease progression has stopped or reversed with the use of anticoagulation therapy such as with warfarin (16). However, large prospective studies are lacking, and the use of anticoagulants is not routine at this time. An intriguing recent study reported on the potential benefit of the bisphosphonate alendronate in the treatment of ON (17). Conceptually, the inhibitory effects on bone resorption by alendronate may stabilize and prevent progression of the osteonecrotic lesion. Fourteen patients with atraumatic ON were treated with alendronate (10 mg/day), plus calcium supplementation and vitamin D. Pain, range of motion, disability scores, and walking capacity were all highly significantly improved. Additionally, analgesic requirements were reduced considerably. Although promising, these results have yet to be validated in large, long-term prospective studies, and the benefit of bisphosphonate therapy in ON remains to be established.

Electrical stimulation therapy for ON has been of some interest, but results from clinical trials have been variable. Part of the confusion stems from the fact that there are varying methods for providing electrical stimulation: non-invasive pulsed electromagnetic-field stimulation; direct-current stimulation of the necrotic area through insertion of an electrode at the time of core decompression; and non-invasive direct-current stimulation by capacitive coupling after a core decompression.

Core Decompression

Core decompression is the least invasive of the surgical treatments for ON and involves removing a core of bone from the femoral head and neck (Figure 19-3). The procedure is thought to decrease the intramedullary pressure and improves perfusion to the femoral head. The surgery itself requires less than 30 minutes and can be performed on an outpatient basis, after which patients are required to protect the operated hip with toe-touch or partial (less than 25% weight) weight-bearing for 6 to 12 weeks. Multiple small studies examining the efficacy of core decompression versus nonoperative management have recently been summarized and analyzed in a meta-analysis (18). Satisfactory clinical results were reported in 63.5% of hips in 24 studies of core decompression versus 22.7% of hips treated nonoperatively in 21 studies. In pre-collapse hips, the rate of good results was 71% (core decompression) versus 34.5% (non-surgical therapy). Recent literature continues to provide evidence that core decompression is most efficacious for the early (pre-collapse) stages of ON. Utilizing the ARCO classification, 90% clinical and 96.7% MRI success rates at stage I and 44.4% good clinical and radiographic results at stage II have been reported. Reported rates of treatment failure and conversion to a total hip replacement are 44% for core decompression in the post-collapse hip.

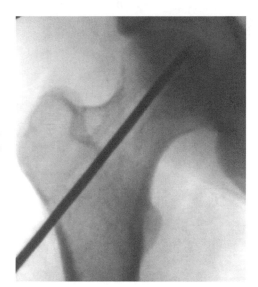

Figure 19-3   Intra-operative radiograph of a core decompression of the right femur.

Bone Grafting

Considerable controversy remains in the literature concerning bone grafting and the use of bone substituting materials in association with core decompression. As with core decompression, it appears that grafting works best when performed in patients before collapse of the femoral head. The rate of conversion to total hip arthroplasty after vascularized fibula grafting is 11% in pre-collapse hips and 23% to 29% in post-collapse hips. A unique method of providing autogenous bone graft directly to the area of necrosis through a trapdoor in the femoral head has shown some promise in the treatment of Ficat stage III ON of the hip with small- to medium-sized lesions.

Osteotomy

Osteotomy of the femoral neck or intertrochanteric region effectively moves the region of pathology away from the weight-bearing portion of the hip. In selected early stage cases, successful results have been shown in 80% at mid-term follow-up. However, conversion to hip arthroplasty occurs in 24% of patients after intertrochanteric osteotomy in the post-collapse hip.

Arthroplasty

As the ON progresses to collapse and then advanced osteoarthrosis, arthroplasty of some form becomes the only viable option. Because the majority of these patients are young, the perfect arthroplasty would provide complete pain relief while removing as little bone as possible and offering durability.

Before the advent of total hip arthroplasty, hemiarthroplasty (replacement of the femoral side) was offered to patients but was associated with a high rate of loosening and protrusion of the prosthesis into the pelvis (protrusio acetabuli).

Hemiresurfacing arthroplasty for ON, in which just the femoral head is covered with a prosthesis, has been shown to have limited durability. A recent study showed that joint survivorship for hemiresurfaced hips is 79%, 59%, and 45% at 5, 10, and 15 years, respectively. This procedure is postulated to preserve bone at risk, and subsequent conversion to a total hip arthroplasty is no more technically demanding than a primary total hip arthroplasty. The main reason for conversion to total joint replacement is pain, most likely due to wearing of the acetabular cartilage. Other techniques involving only partial resurfacing of the femoral surface are also being explored.

Total hip arthroplasty for the indication of ON has been less successful than when utilized in other diseases. It is generally accepted that this is because the patients are younger and have higher demands and functional expectations. Despite improvements in technique and implant design, few total hip replacements survive past 20 years without revision, and some recent reports continue to show that the results of total hip replacement for ON are inferior to those for other diagnoses. Yet, other studies are more optimistic, especially concerning the longevity of the bone-implant interface in cementless designs (19).

Osteonecrosis of Joints Other Than the Hip

Although the femoral head is the most clinically significant site of ON, ON may also occur in other joints such as the knee, the ankle, and the shoulder. However, ON in these joints tends to be much less progressive than in the hips, and patients can often remain functional for long periods. Appropriate interventions include minimizing risk factors (such as corticosteroid use) and maximally reducing mechanical loads on the affected joints. When the affected joints are irreparably compromised, surgery is indicated. Severe talar ON is often treated with fusion, while arthroplasty is utilized for advanced ON of the knee and shoulder.

Future Directions

Recent attention has focused on potential uses for bone growth and differentiation factors. Osteonecrosis is a disease process in which this technology could be useful. Investigators are looking at ways that synthetic compounds and autogenous spun marrow products can be introduced to the area of pathology to stimulate bone healing. Applicable results are slowed, however, by the lack of a good animal model for ON.

REFERENCES

1. **Bachiller FG, Caballer AP, Portal LF.** Avascular necrosis of the femoral head after femoral neck fracture. Clin Orthop. 2002;399:87-109.

2. **Berger CE, Kroner A, Stiegler H, et al.** Hypofibrinolysis, lipoprotein(a), and plasminogen activator inhibitor. Clin Orthop. 2002;397:342-9.

3. **Jacobs B.** Epidemiology of traumatic and nontraumatic osteonecrosis. Clin Orthop. 1978;130:51-67.

4. **Jones JP Jr, Engleman EP, Najarian JS.** Systemic fat embolism after renal homotransplantation and treatment with corticosteroids. N Engl J Med. 1965;273:1453-8.

5. **Wang GJ, Sweet DE, Reger SI, Thompson RC.** Fat-cell changes as a mechanism of avascular necrosis of the femoral head in cortisone-treated rabbits. J Bone Joint Surg Am. 1977;59:729-35.

6. **Colwell CW Jr, Robinson CA, Stevenson DD, et al.** Osteonecrosis of the femoral head in patients with inflammatory arthritis or asthma receiving corticosteroid therapy. Orthopedics. 1996;19:941-6.

7. **Zizic TM, Marcoux C, Hungerford DS, et al.** Corticosteroid therapy associated with ischemic necrosis of bone in systemic lupus erythematosus. Am J Med. 1985;79:596-604.

8. **Sorice M, Griggi T, Arcieri P, et al.** Protein S and HIV infection: the role of anticardiolipin and anti-protein S antibodies. Thromb Res. 1994;73:165-75.

9. **Ficat RP.** Idiopathic bone necrosis of the femoral head: early diagnosis and treatment. J Bone Joint Surg Br. 1985;67:3-9.

10. **Bradway JK, Morrey BF.** The natural history of the silent hip in bilateral atraumatic osteonecrosis. J Arthroplasty. 1993;8:383-7.

11. **Beltran J, Herman LJ, Burk JM, et al.** Femoral heand avascular necrosis: MAR imaging with clincopathologic and radionuclide correlation. Radiology. 1988;166:215-20.

12. **Ficat RP, Arlet J.** Ischemia and necroses of bone. Baltimore, MD: Williams and Wilkins; 1980.

13. **Steinberg ME, Hayken GD, Steinberg DR.** A quantitative system for staging avascular necrosis. J Bone Joint Surg. 1995;77:34-41.

14. International classification of avascular necrosis of the femoral head. ARCO (Association Research Circulation Osseous). Committee on Terminology and Classification. ARCO News. 1992;4:41-6.

15. **Ruch DS, Sekiya J, Dickson Schaefer W, et al.** The role of hip arthroscopy in the evaluation of avascular necrosis. Orthopedics. 2001;24:339-43.

16. **Glueck CJ, Freiberg RA, Fontaine RN, et al.** Hypofibrinolysis, thrombophilia, osteonecrosis. Clin Orthop. 2001;386:19-33.

17. **Agarwala S, Sule A, Pai BU, Joshi VR.** Alendronate in the treatment of avascular necrosis of the hip. Rheumatology. 2002;41:346-7.

18. **Mont MA, Carbone JJ, Fairbank AC.** Core decompression versus nonoperative management for osteonecrosis of the hip. Clin Orthop. 1996;324:169-78.

19. **Xenakis TA, Gelalis J, Koukoubis TA, et al.** Cementless hip arthroplasty in the treatment of patients with femoral head necrosis. Clin Orthop. 2001;386:93-9.

20

■ ■ ■

Fibromyalgia

Jessica R. Berman, MD

Lisa R. Sammaritano, MD

ibromyalgia syndrome (FMS) is a disorder of chronic widespread mus-culoskeletal pain without a clearly defined pathophysiology. It is esti-mated to affect approximately 2% of the United States population, and 80% of those affected are women. Fibromyalgia patients may constitute up to 10% of all patients seen in rheumatology practices and clinics. The mean age of onset is 45 years.

Because of the diffuse nature of the pain, criteria have been developed to aid in diagnosis. In epidemiological and clinical studies, the diagnosis is made when 11 out of 18 discretely defined bilateral symmetrical soft tissue "tender points" are symptomatic for longer than 3 months (Figure 20-1). In practice, however, these patients are often tender more diffusely and seem-ingly out of proportion to visible pathology. This dichotomy often causes skepticism on the part of the physician and a sense of being "branded" and misunderstood by the patient. Fibromyalgia is a clinical diagnosis, and be-cause there are no diagnostic tests that can definitively confirm or exclude FMS, treatment is often empiric, leading to physician and patient frustration because of the element of apparent uncertainty. It is important, therefore, to validate the patient's experience of pain, exclude other causative disor-ders, and approach these patients with an open mind and supportive manner. Current treatment is largely directed at symptomatic relief and maintaining function.

Pathogenesis

No single pathophysiological causative mechanism for the development of FMS has yet been consistently identified, although multiple associated

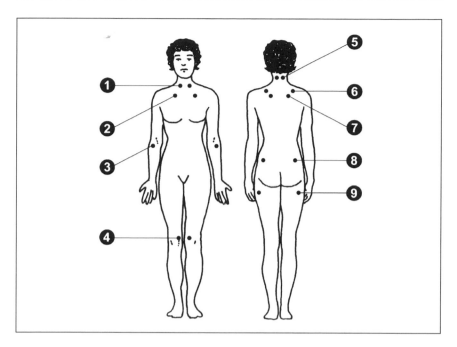

Figure 20-1 The 18 defining bilateral tender points of fibromyalgia: 1) low cervical at the anterior of the intertransverse spaces at C5-C7; 2) second costochondral junctions; 3) lateral epicondyles; 4) medial fat pads of the knee proximal to the joint line; 5) occiput; 6) trapezius; 7) supraspinatus above the medial edge of scapular spine; 8) gluteal; and 9) greater trochanters. A tender point is identified if the patient reports pain with digital palpation applying a force of about 4 kg, roughly enough pressure to blanche the distal tuft of the examiner's finger. (Illustration by Ms. Lisa Yee.)

physical and chemical abnormalities have been recognized. FMS is not felt to be an immunologically mediated or myopathic disorder. The most convincing evidence so far suggests that FMS is a multifactorial syndrome characterized by dysregulation in pain-processing mechanisms.

ABSENCE OF MUSCLE ABNORMALITIES
No pathological abnormality of muscle or soft tissue structures has been convincingly demonstrated in FMS. Although subtle changes in metabolism and blood flow to muscles have been described, these are most likely explained by general deconditioning. Assessment of muscle strength is complicated by pain and lack of voluntary effort, but, in general, electromyography has failed to convincingly demonstrate either muscle abnormality or neuromuscular dysfunction (1).

ABNORMAL PROCESSING OF PAIN
Multiple studies support the concept that the patient with FMS has an abnormal response to pain when compared with normal individuals. Studies

have attempted to sort out whether patients have lower pain thresholds, respond more quickly to thermal and pressure stimuli, or have a greater sensation of pain for a given noxious stimulus (hyperalgesia).

"Central sensitization" is the process by which neuronal pain pathways, initially transmitting signals to the brain from a clearly defined noxious source, later become constitutively activated in the absence of clear stimuli. This permits what is termed "non-nociceptive pain"; that is, pain elicited by stimulation of nerve fibers that normally relay non-painful sensations to the spinal cord. This is felt to be responsible for the high degree of hyperalgesia (exaggerated response to noxious stimulus) and allodynia (pain with normally non-noxious stimulus) commonly present in FMS patients. Several observations support this theory, although whether these are causative or secondary findings and whether, in any given patient, single or multiple factors predominate remain unclear:

- Positron emission tomography has identified abnormalities of regional cerebral blood flow in the thalamus and the caudate nucleus that are associated with low pain thresholds in patients with FMS (2).

- Substance P, an important mediator of pain, has been found to be elevated in the cerebrospinal fluid of FMS patients and could be one explanation for the amplification of pain perception (3).

- Activation of N-methyl-D-aspartate (NMDA) receptors, a phenomenon associated with chronic pain has been observed. Ketamine, which blocks NMDA receptors, temporarily relieves some FMS pain (4).

- Upregulation of peripheral opioid receptor expression has been reported, with higher than normal numbers of delta and kappa opiate receptors identified in the skin of some FMS patients, but how this relates to abnormal pain perception is unclear (5).

- Plasma levels of nociceptin, a neuropeptide involved in modulation of pain, may be altered in FMS, but precisely how these changes are regulated and how they modify pain perception have not been clarified (6).

- A relative deficiency of serotonin has been described. In addition to effects on pain, this may be of particular interest in understanding why depression is often seen concomitantly with FMS and has led to the use of selective serotonin uptake inhibitors as potential therapeutic agents (7).

- Electroencephalography studies have shown that alpha-wave intrusion into non-REM delta-wave sleep is present in those with FMS. This finding may explain why FMS patients often report that they wake up feeling they did not sleep soundly (8).

NEUROENDOCRINE ABNORMALITIES

Decreased nocturnal growth hormone secretion, decreased melatonin secretion, a blunted cortisol response to stress, and low levels of oxytocin have been described, but their clinical significance has not been explained.

ENVIRONMENTAL FACTORS

The possibility of environmental factors such as chemicals, viruses, or other exposures has been investigated, but no clear causative agents have been identified.

Case Presentation

Soon after a severe viral-like illness, a 30-year-old woman without a significant past medical history developed pain "all over" her body. She describes 6 months of moderately severe muscle and joint pain in her back, neck, arms and legs. Although the severity of her discomfort can vary daily, the pain is never completely gone and does not appear to be relieved or exacerbated by any specific activities. She usually awakens with some stiffness that improves as the day goes on. Although she reports some morning hand and finger pain, there has never been visible swelling, erythema, or warmth of any joint on repeated physical examinations. There has been no loss of range of motion in any joint. She has had no fever or weight loss, but persistent fatigue and problems with concentration have limited her function. Her sleep is unrefreshing because she is easily aroused. On review of systems, she notes several years of intermittent stomach bloating and episodes of alternating diarrhea and constipation, even though a complete gastroenterological evaluation has been unrevealing. Her laboratory tests are notably unremarkable, with a normal complete blood count, biochemical profile, erythrocyte sedimentation rate, and thyroid function tests, as well as negative serological tests for antinuclear antibodies (ANA) and rheumatoid factor (RF).

Clinical Features

Patients with FMS may report that they "hurt everywhere" and that their "muscles," "bones," and/or their "joints" hurt. Tenderness, however, is not usually confined to the joints but is often widespread, involving soft tissue and muscular areas, usually in a symmetrical fashion. The tenderness reported by the patient is often surprisingly severe and disproportionate to the patient's demeanor and general physical examination; it is not uncommon for it to be rated "10 out of 10" or "unbearable." Subjective swelling and morning stiffness are also reported. These patients also commonly have a constellation of associated symptoms that may include headache, dysphoria, disordered sleep, poor concentration, fatigue, memory disturbances, irritable bowel symptoms (particularly diarrhea alternating with constipation), and paresthesias. An increased prevalence of depression has been associated with FMS in patients followed at tertiary care centers but not in a community population of patients with FMS, suggesting a selection bias in specialty care facilities (9).

Diagnosis

An essential role for the primary care provider is to comfortably exclude other conditions. Tender points are by definition consistently found in individuals with FMS and are useful in both diagnosing and monitoring patients. The finding of tender points is part of the criteria established in 1990 for the diagnosis of fibromyalgia by the American College of Rheumatology. This definition requires chronic widespread pain lasting longer than 3 months in all four quadrants of the body and the finding of 11 out of 18 tender points. These include the following sites bilaterally: occipital, low cervical, trapezius, anterior second rib, supraspinatus, lateral epicondylar, gluteal, greater trochanteric, and medial fat pad of the knee (see Figure 20-1). It is important to note that these criteria were developed and established mainly as an epidemiological tool to assist in studying groups of patients. In practice, however, FMS patients may have only a few of these defined tender points, or may report tenderness in other areas or even diffusely throughout the body. In the absence of other physical findings, history, or objective data to suggest otherwise, diffuse body pain in areas outside the described tender points can be diagnosed clinically as FMS.

The physical examination of the patient with FMS is surprisingly reproducible with regard to the consistency of subjective tenderness reported by the patient on palpation of soft tissues. The joints have no evidence of limitation of motion, swelling, redness or warmth. Occasionally, passive or active movement of a specific joint will prompt the report of pain involving the entire limb. There is no muscle deformity or atrophy. Strength testing is usually difficult because of the patient's pain, but true weakness is not present in FMS. Because FMS can occasionally be confused with or be seen concomitantly with systemic inflammatory disorders such as rheumatoid arthritis (RA) and systemic lupus erythematosus (SLE), it is important for the physician to look carefully for the signs of inflammation such as joint swelling in order to distinguish symptoms attributable to the primary disorder from those related to secondary fibromyalgia.

Laboratory tests and radiological studies are characteristically normal in the patient with FMS. Unlike other rheumatological conditions such as RA and SLE, no serological marker has yet been identified in FMS. The ANA and RF are typically negative. Similarly, the complete blood count, serum chemistries (including muscle enzymes), thyroid function tests, urinalysis, and erythrocyte sedimentation rate are normal in FMS but are reasonable screening tests to exclude other possible rheumatic, infectious, endocrine, or malignant diseases. FMS is a clinical diagnosis and one of exclusion.

Prognosis

Most patients diagnosed with FMS tend to have a chronic course that is best managed with a combination of modalities. The majority of patients can expect to experience cycles of increased pain alternating with pain-free periods. Some patients will experience a complete remission of symptoms. When identified early, as many as a quarter of FMS patients in the community are reported to be in remission 2 years after diagnosis. Up to 90% of those followed at academic centers, however, are still symptomatic after 3 years. Most patients with FMS who want to work are able to do so, but a large proportion of patients will change or modify their jobs as a direct result of the FMS. Of those FMS patients who work outside the home, about 10% stop work entirely and become classified as disabled.

Management

Forging a trusting and understanding relationship with the patient is a crucial element in the treatment of FMS. Current therapy for FMS emphasizes the use of multidisciplinary modalities, coordinated by the primary care provider, or by a pain management specialist in more difficult cases. Studies showing the most favorable outcomes have advocated combinations of medications, physical activity, cognitive-behavioral therapy (CBT), and patient education (10). These studies primarily used aerobic exercise as physical activity and coping skills and relaxation training as CBT.

Pharmacological Therapy

The goal of pharmacological treatment of FMS is symptomatic pain relief. There are no "disease-modifying anti-rheumatic drugs" because FMS is not an inflammatory or immunological disorder. As such, systemic corticosteroids like prednisone have been shown to have no benefit in a double-blind crossover study and should not be used to treat FMS (11). Many patients will benefit from one or more medications that can be individually tailored to patient response. Traditionally, use of narcotic analgesics is discouraged because these are not felt to be effective and can have serious adverse consequences, most notably, addiction.

Antidepressants
Antidepressants are usually considered first-line therapy in treating FMS. Tricyclic antidepressants and selective serotonin reuptake inhibitors have

been shown to be helpful for reduction of pain and fatigue and improvement in sleep. Benefit is often seen as early as 1 week after initiating treatment and may be independent of any effect on depressive symptoms (12). In a recent randomized, double-blind, placebo-controlled trial, the 5-HT3-receptor antagonist tropisteron, given at 5 mg daily for a 10-day short-term course showed significant clinical benefit as evidenced by a decrease in the number of tender points and improved sleep (13). More rapid benefit may be seen with intravenous therapy, although there are no randomized trials of this therapy to date (14).

Neuroleptics
Neuroleptics such as gabapentin (up to 300-600 mg three times daily) may be useful in patients who do not respond to antidepressants. Use of the atypical neuroleptic olanzapine (5-20 mg/d) has been reportedly successful for patients refractory to other treatments (15). It has not yet been studied in randomized placebo-controlled trials and is currently not routinely used in FMS but deserves further study.

Nonsteroidal Anti-Inflammatory Drugs (NSAIDs)
Although no inflammatory component has been found for FMS, the NSAIDs do occasionally have modest benefit in reducing pain in patients with FMS. The doses used are generally similar to those used in other pain disorders. These medications generally are preferred to acetaminophen by FMS patients (16). In those patients with a history of peptic ulcer disease or gastrointestinal intolerance, however, acetaminophen or a cyclooxygenase-2 selective inhibitor may be preferable.

Muscle Relaxants
Muscle relaxants have been studied in FMS. Cyclobenzaprine (10 mg three times daily) has been shown in a short-term randomized, placebo-controlled trial to be effective (17). However, efficacy may wane over the ensuing 6 months. When started, muscle relaxants are best given before bedtime to minimize sedating side effects and to perhaps address concomitant sleep disturbances.

Tramadol
Tramadol is a mu-opioid receptor agonist that may have lower addictive potential than traditional narcotic drugs. It has been reported to be useful in FMS for patients who have had incomplete relief with the tricyclic antidepressants or have not tolerated other medications. In a double-blind crossover study, reduction in pain was demonstrated with tramadol (18). There are no double-blind, randomized placebo-controlled studies yet to validate this experience. Dosages of 50-100 mg up to four times a day can be prescribed. Often it is best to start at 50 mg twice a day and increase slowly until the patient's response can be gauged and sedating effects diminish.

Nonpharmacological Therapy

Non-medication-based approaches to treating FMS are considered an essential part of the overall therapeutic plan. Regular activity and physical therapy are of clear benefit and should be strongly encouraged in FMS patients.

Exercise

Regular exercise is considered essential in the treatment of FMS. Aerobic exercise several times a week has clear benefit. Although pain may limit initial efforts, patients should be encouraged to progress slowly through a program of increasing difficulty. The physical therapist can help to establish a home program for the patient. Patients who are conscientious and continue the exercises at home fare better. Short-term resumption of physical therapy during periods of increased symptoms seems to be beneficial; this may prevent deconditioning and provide supervised activity time.

Pool/Hydrotherapy

Pool/hydrotherapy was recently examined in a prospective randomized study of FMS patients and was shown to effect significant improvement in pain, disability, psychological distress, and quality of life (19). For those patients with access to a pool, this is often an effective addition to a regular exercise program.

Tender Point Injections

Tender point injections with lidocaine are sometimes administered in hopes of providing symptomatic relief. There is no evidence, however, that these are of any long-term benefit. The use of steroids in such injections is unlikely to be of benefit because of the lack of true focal inflammation in FMS.

Cognitive-Behavioral Therapy

CBT, including biofeedback, has been shown to be of proven benefit for patients with FMS. Many integrated approaches include the use of meditation and movement-exercise such as yoga and have been shown to be useful adjuncts in pain management in many disorders. Of note, many FMS patients have also benefited from psychological therapy, particularly those who clearly have depression as part of or as a result of their disorder.

Alternative and Complementary Treatments

There are a number of non-traditional approaches that have been advocated in the treatment of FMS. However, most have not been rigorously studied. For this reason, it is often difficult to recommend them with confidence to patients. While some individuals will actively pursue alternative therapies, it should be emphasized to patients that neither efficacy nor safety has been established for most of these options.

Acupuncture is increasingly accepted as having a role in the treatment of many pain syndromes, and there have been a number of small studies suggesting usefulness in FMS patients. A recent blinded, controlled trial of 70 FMS patients showed clearly that those receiving acupuncture improved in five out of eight outcome measures (20).

S-adenosyl methionine (SAMe) has been evaluated in several double-blind randomized controlled trials that have shown mixed results (21). Because of the lack of conclusive benefit and the known interactions with antidepressants and other drugs, patients who decide to use SAMe should exercise caution and notify their physicians that they are taking this supplement.

REFERENCES

1. **Simms RW.** Is there muscle pathology in fibromyalgia syndrome? Rheum Dis Clin North Am. 1996;22:245-66.

2. **Mountz JM, Bradley LA, Modell JG, et al.** Fibromyalgia in women: abnormalities of regional cerebral blood flow in the thalamus and the caudate nucleus are associated with low pain threshold levels. Arthritis Rheum. 1995;38:926-38.

3. **Russell IJ, Orr MD, Littman B, et al.** Elevated cerebrospinal fluid levels of substance P in patients with the fibromyalgia syndrome. Arthritis Rheum. 1994;37:1593-601.

4. **Graven-Nielsen T, Aspegren Kendall S, Henriksson KG, et al.** Ketamine reduces muscle pain, temporal summation, and referred pain in fibromyalgia patients. Pain. 2000;85:483-91.

5. **Salemi S, Kaeser L, Bradley LA, et al.** Expression of opioid receptor variants in skin and muscle tissues of fibromyalgia patients. Arthritis Rheum. 2000;43(Suppl):S173.

6. **Fasy T, Russell IJ, Xiao YM, Lambert PJ.** Nocistatin-binding and nociceptin-binding autoantibodies in a subset of fibromyalgia patients. Arthritis Rheum. 2001;44(Suppl):S69.

7. **Wolfe F, Russell IJ, Vipraio G, et al.** Serotonin levels, pain threshold, and fibromyalgia symptoms in the general population. J Rheumatol. 1997;24:555-9.

8. **Moldofsky H.** Sleep and fibrositis syndrome. Rheum Dis Clin North Am. 1989;15:91-103.

9. **Aaron LA, Bradley LA, Alarcon GS, et al.** Psychiatric diagnoses in patients with fibromyalgia are related to health care-seeking behavior rather than illness. Arthritis Rheum. 1996;39:436-45.

10. **Hadhazy VA, Ezzo J, Creamer P, Berman BM.** Mind-body therapies for the treatment of fibromyalgia: a systematic review. J Rheumatol. 2000;27:2911-8.

11. **Clark S, Tindall E, Bennett RM.** A double-blind crossover trial of prednisone versus placebo in the treatment of fibrositis. J Rheumatol. 1985;12:980-3.

12. **O'Malley PG, Balden E, Tomkins G, et al.** Treatment of fibromyalgia with antidepressants: a meta-analysis. J Gen Intern Med. 2000;15:659-66.

13. **Farber L, Stratz TH, Bruckle W, et al.** Short-term treatment of primary fibromyalgia with the 5-HT3-receptor antagonist tropisetron: results of a randomized, double-blind, placebo-controlled multicenter trial in 418 patients. Int J Clin Pharmacol Res. 2001;21:1-13.

14. **Muller W, Stratz T.** Results of the intravenous administration of tropisetron in fibromyalgia patients. Scand J Rheumatol. 2000;113(Suppl):59-62.

15. **Kiser RS, Cohen HM, Freedenfeld RN, et al.** Olanzapine for the treatment of fibromyalgia symptoms. J Pain Symptom Manage. 2001;22:704-8.

16. **Wolfe F, Zhao S, Lane N.** Preference for nonsteroidal antiinflammatory drugs over acetaminophen by rheumatic disease patients: a survey of 1,799 patients with osteoarthritis, rheumatoid arthritis and fibromyalgia. Arthritis Rheum. 2000;43:378-85.

17. **Carette S, Bell MJ, Reynolds WJ, et al.** Comparison of amitriptyline, cyclobenzaprine, and placebo in the treatment of fibromyalgia: a randomized, double-blind clinical trial. Arthritis Rheum. 1994;37:32-40.

18. **Biasi G, Manca S, Manganelli S, Marcolongo R.** Tramadol in the fibromyalgia syndrome: a controlled clinical trial versus placebo. Int J Clin Pharmacol Res. 1998;18:13-9.

19. **Mannerkorpi K, Nyberg B, Ahlmen M, Ekdahl C.** Pool exercise combined with an education program for patients with fibromyalgia syndrome: a prospective, randomized study. J Rheumatol. 2000;27:2473-81.

20. **Deluze C, Bosia L, Zirbs A, et al.** Electroaccupuncture in fibromyalgia: results of a controlled trial. BMJ. 1992;305:1249-52.

21. **Tavoni A, Vitali C, Bombardieri S, Pasero G.** Evaluation of S-adenosylmethionine in primary fibromyalgia: a double-blind crossover study. Am J Med. 1987; 83:107-10.

21

■ ■ ■

Complex Regional Pain Syndromes and Reflex Sympathetic Dystrophy

Seth A. Waldman, MD

Complex regional pain syndromes (CRPS) are a diverse group of diseases characterized by neuropathic pain and abnormalities in the sympathetic nervous system. The common features in these poorly understood syndromes led the International Association for the Study of Pain (IASP) to adopt a revised taxonomy, in which many of the previously used names (such as reflex sympathetic dystrophy [RSD], Sudeck's atrophy, causalgia, erythromelalgia, and shoulder-hand syndrome) were replaced with more inclusive and general descriptions (1). The hope of the IASP in revising the diagnostic criteria for CRPS in 1994 was that more productive research would result. The features of these diagnoses, however, continue to be described vaguely, and this has reduced the impact of the few randomized controlled investigations performed since that time (2).

CRPS are disorders that develop after a noxious event, in which resultant neuropathic pain (i.e., pain that coexists with other sensory abnormalities such as increased or decreased sensation) is associated with symptoms usually indicative of sympathetic nervous system dysfunction. These can include edema, regional blood flow changes (causing erythema or cyanosis), and abnormal sudomotor (sweat gland) activity. It is not yet clear whether the sympathetic nervous system dysfunction is causative of neuropathic pain, the result of neuropathic pain, or an unrelated epiphenomenon.

CRPS are subdivided into types I and II (Table 21-1). CRPS type I (formerly referred to as reflex sympathetic dystrophies [RSD]) is not limited to the distribution of a single peripheral nerve and is not associated with a specific nerve injury. CRPS type II occurs in conjunction with a known peripheral nerve injury and is primarily, but not necessarily, limited to the

---

Table 21-1   Diagnostic Criteria for Complex Regional Pain Syndromes

COMPLEX REGIONAL PAIN SYNDROME TYPE I (REFLEX SYMPATHETIC DYSTROPHY)

1. The presence of an initiating noxious event or a cause of immobilization.
2. Continuing pain, allodynia, or hyperalgesia, in which the pain is disproportionate to any inciting event.
3. Evidence at some time of edema, changes in skin blood flow, or abnormal sudomotor activity in the region of pain.
4. This diagnosis is excluded by the existence of other conditions that would otherwise account for the degree of pain and dysfunction.

Criteria 2-4 must be satisfied.

COMPLEX REGIONAL PAIN SYNDROME TYPE II (CAUSALGIA)

1. The presence of continuing pain, allodynia, or hyperalgesia after a nerve injury, not necessarily limited to the distribution of the injured nerve.
2. Evidence at some time of edema, changes in skin blood flow, or abnormal sudomotor activity in the region of pain.
3. This diagnosis is excluded by the existence of other conditions that would otherwise account for the degree of pain and dysfunction.

All three criteria must be satisfied.

Adapted from Merskey H, Bogduk N. Classification of chronic pain: descriptions of chronic pain syndromes and definitions of pain terms. 2nd ed. Seattle: Intl Assoc for the Study of Pain. 1994.

distribution of the damaged nerve. This chapter will focus on the features and management of CRPS type I.

Because of the subjective nature of pain symptoms and the frequent paucity of objective findings, there remains significant controversy over the exact nature of CRPS (3). Conditions that are generally appreciated to be painful may produce more or less suffering, depending on the context or meaning of the pain and the pre-morbid psychological state of the patient. Moreover, pain is often an expression of many forms of psychological suffering and may be a somatoform product of anxiety, depression, or post-traumatic stress disorder. Finally, issues of secondary gain (psychosocial and financial) are very real factors given the wide variation in the evidence and impact of symptoms. However, because real and measurable disability can result from the disuse of an affected extremity (whether caused by a somatoform or neurological illness), CRPS must be treated aggressively once diagnosed, regardless of our current level of understanding of this problem.

Pathogenesis

Neuropathic pain is a coup and contrecoup lesion, in which an injury causes distant secondary damage, which in turn exacerbates sensation at the site of the initial insult. It has been shown that peripheral nerve lesions cause cellular changes in the local nerve as well as in the central nervous system; therefore, painful peripheral neuropathy is a disease of both the peripheral and central nervous systems. The interaction between the peripheral and central nervous systems is dynamic and bi-directional and also involves conscious processing. Centrally, α-adrenoreceptor expression is increased, and the attendant acquired adrenoreceptor sensitivity is critical to the relationship between activation of the sympathetic nervous system and CRPS pain. Peripherally, the main problem is the development of ectopic activity in an injured primary afferent neuron (PAN). Injured PANs discharge spontaneously, thereby producing dysregulated sensation.

The sensations generated by such ectopic discharges can mimic any "normal" sensation; the primary difference is that these sensations can be continuous or evoked when the stimulus is minimal or not obvious. Ectopic discharges from injured PANs trigger changes locally and also in the CNS. This is due to regenerative sprouting, which can been demonstrated at the site of axonal damage and at the cell body of the neuron in the dorsal root ganglion.

Sprouting can be found in neurons that have sustained axonal injury and in their uninjured neighbors. The critical CNS changes seem to be due to changes in nerve cell bodies that receive unmyelinated C-fibers. C-fibers release glutamate as their neurotransmitter, and so neurons that receive their input have glutaminergic receptors, of which the N-methyl-D-aspartate (NMDA) subtype is particularly important. Increased spontaneous activity from the C-fibers generates more glutamate, which, via the NMDA receptor, evokes a change in the post-synaptic cell, such that it responds more strongly to all its inputs. Accordingly, NMDA receptor antagonists can suppress the development of neuropathic pain in animal models. This can be demonstrated to a limited extent in humans, but the therapeutic use of commonly available NMDA antagonists (e.g., dextromethorphan, ketamine, amantadine, and methadone) is limited by their potential adverse effects.

A focal inflammatory process in a nerve may also be involved in inciting neuropathic pain, even in the absence of frank neuronal injury (4). There is evidence from animal models that inflammatory processes that accompany nerve injury can produce neuropathic pain in the absence of structural damage (5). Involvement of the inflammatory response may be continuous or present only in the early phases of the illness. In an animal model, exposure of a peripheral nerve to tumor necrosis factor (TNF)-α, an important cytokine mediator of the inflammatory response, produces ectopic firing in A-delta- and C-fibers and resultant hyperalgesia. Similar findings can be seen with other pro-inflammatory cytokines. Intriguingly, neuropathic pain may sometimes be alleviated by immunomodulatory drugs, such as systemic corticosteroids, thalidomide (which blocks TNF-α), and cyclosporine.

Case Presentation

A 25-year-old woman with a past medical history of migraine headaches and exercise-induced asthma presents to the pain clinic with persistent and severe pain in her dominant hand. There is no personal or family history of abnormal pain response or psychiatric disease. She takes no medications and has no known allergies to medications; however, there are multiple food and environmental allergies. Her work history is excellent, and she intends to start graduate school in child psychology once her pain is under better control.

Two years ago, she was employed as a teacher's assistant at a school for emotionally disturbed children and was injured in the hand while restraining an aggressive student. The onset of pain was immediate, but no pathology other than localized swelling was found. She did not return to work because of persistent symptoms. After a 4-week period of treatment with nonsteroidal anti-inflammatory drugs (NSAIDs), ice compresses, and immobilizing compression dressings, physical therapy was prescribed to improve strength and range-of-motion. The pain did not improve but instead seemed to intensify, precipitating multiple surgical opinions. Numerous other NSAIDs were tried without effect. It was felt that there was a previously unrecognized ulnar collateral ligament tear, and surgical repair was performed approximately 1 year after the injury. Postoperatively, the patient seemed to improve, but after her splint was removed, she was unable to tolerate physical therapy and worsened steadily.

At the time of her initial pain clinic evaluation, the patient had been out of work since the injury and had lost her job. She was clinically depressed, with complaints of insomnia, hyperphagia, and loss of social contacts. There was a 25-pound weight gain. She was unable to use her dominant hand, even to write, and noticed that the pain, which was described as a "sickening" and "burning" sensation, had spread to the ipsilateral elbow. The affected hand and forearm were edematous, stiff, and dusky in color, although pulses were intact. Hygiene was neglected in the hand. By thermistor measurement, the temperature was two degrees cooler in the affected hand. Sensory examination showed allodynia (pain from innocuous stimuli) with cold-testing at involved areas. There was non-dermatomal hyperesthesia to light touch in the affected extremity to the elbow and anesthesia at the margins of the surgical wound (in the area of allodynia). Physical examination of the asymptomatic contralateral extremity was completely normal. Plain x-rays demonstrated osteopenia in the painful limb, and triple-phase bone scanning showed a diffuse increase in vascularity. Bone densitometry showed osteopenia in the affected hand.

Based on the history, physical changes in the affected limb (i.e., edema, discoloration, coolness, and sensory abnormalities), and radiological findings, CRPS type I was diagnosed. The goals of pain control and recovery of functions were established with the patient. Controlled-release oxycodone 20 mg every 12 hours and gabapentin 300 mg three times daily were prescribed and offered partial relief of pain, enabling the patient to begin some passive physical therapy aimed at increasing mobilization. Intermittent stellate ganglion nerve blockades with bupivicaine were also administered, and the patient was subsequently able to tolerate more aggressive physical therapy. Over the course of the next several months, the patient was able to gradually recover a significant amount of function in her painful limb. Although she still continued to require chronic gabapentin therapy, she was able to reduce analgesic requirements and no longer needed sympathetic nerve blockades.

Clinical Features

Patients with CRPS type I present with a clinical picture of protracted pain usually occurring after a specific inciting event. Although by convention this is referred to as a "noxious" event, otherwise benign events, such as ligamentous sprain and immobilization, can also be causative; sometimes, no history of injury can be elicited. There does not appear to be a relation between the degree, duration, or recalcitrance of the condition to the severity of the initiating event. Although the extremities are most commonly affected in CRPS type I, axial, facial, visceral, and urogenital syndromes of neuropathic pain and autonomic dysfunction can also occur.

Common to other neuropathic pain syndromes, CRPS type I is characterized by pain that coexists anatomically with other sensory abnormalities such as hypoesthesia (decreased sensation), anesthesia (lack of sensation), or dysesthesia (a spontaneous abnormal sensation such as formication, the perceived feeling of crawling ants on the skin). What distinguishes a patient with CRPS is the presence of abnormalities referable to the autonomic nervous system. These signs, which can change in presence or prominence throughout the duration of the disease, include changes in skin perfusion, temperature, edema, sudomotor changes, trophic changes of the skin and its appendages, and motor abnormalities (such as weakness, spasm, and tremor).

Of the autonomic changes, vasomotor instability is often prominent. Such changes in blood flow can result in abnormal coloration, including mottling, cyanosis, and erythema. The sensory perception of changing temperature is a common symptom, but objective signs of temperature asymmetry by thermistor are found in less than half of patients who meet other criteria for CRPS.

Motor abnormalities are uncommon but increase in frequency as a secondary process in the setting of prolonged illness and disuse. Overall, approximately 40% of patients develop some weakness, and up to 5% may even develop tremor and dystonia (6).

Diagnosis

It is important to keep an appropriate level of suspicion when faced with an unusual pain syndrome and considering the diagnosis of CRPS type I. Although the history and physical examination remain the primary means of evaluating CRPS type I, various objective diagnostic tests have been applied to patients with this syndrome in both clinical practice and research. These include assessments of bone mineralization, blood flow, vasomotor instability, sudomotor function and response to sympathetic nervous system blockade. It is important to reiterate that although documentation of sympathetic nervous system pathology assists in making a diagnosis, it does not infer causation.

Psychological evaluation and testing are critical to identifying the presence of psychopathological factors that may modify the symptoms or response to treatment.

Bone mineralization can be affected by both increased vascular flow and disuse of the affected extremity, and in severe cases, osteopenia can be found on plain x-ray and densitometry.

Abnormalities of blood flow and vasomotor instability are best evaluated with triple-phase nuclear bone scanning, thermometry, and laser Doppler flow. Bone scanning, which can reveal diffuse uptake in the late phase reflecting the increase in vascularity seen in active CRPS type I, is probably the most accessible test in common clinical practice. Temperature asymmetry of greater than 2.2 degrees centigrade by thermistor has been shown to be a specific finding for the presence of CRPS (7), but thermometry is typically reserved for research purposes at this time.

Sudomotor function, although not commonly assessed in clinical practice, can be evaluated by measurement of resting sweat output and quantitative sudomotor axon reflexes (QSART). The most common abnormalities are reductions in both indices. The rate of reduction in the QSART correlates with the rate of skin temperature changes.

Response to sympathetic nervous system blockade either by systemic medications (such as intravenous phentolamine) or regional anesthetic techniques (such as stellate ganglion or lumbar sympathetic nerve blockade) can reinforce the clinical diagnosis of CRPS, and, particularly in acute cases, be useful simultaneously as treatment modalities. Significant rates of placebo responses and of false-positive results due to inadvertent somatic (i.e., nonsympathetic) blockade limit the specificity of these procedures. Although blinded administration of intravenous phentolamine may reduce the likelihood of placebo response, the effective dose has not been determined.

Prognosis

Given the very real potential for chronic disability, the possibility of neuropathic pain should always be considered when the intensity, quality, or duration of pain does not have a ready explanation or is inconsistent with the clinical picture. Although evidence from randomized, controlled trials does not yet exist, it is the experience of most pain physicians that neuropathic pain, particularly CRPS type I, is more effectively treated with early intervention. This may be because the pathological alterations within the central nervous system have not yet become permanent and can still be prevented. As in any chronic illness, recognition of the impending development of common secondary diseases (such as depression and disuse atrophy) allows us to attenuate their effects.

Unfortunately, despite the steadily increasing volume of controlled studies evaluating the effectiveness of therapies for CRPS, long-term prognoses remains poor, particularly when the diagnosis or intervention is delayed. It is hoped that with better understanding of the conscious processing of pain, more will be learned about the dynamic processes that modulate the expression of CRPS symptoms and the vast individual variability of perturbations to the sensory, autonomic, motor, and central nervous systems. Until that time, early recognition and supportive intervention will remain the basis of therapy for these disorders.

Management

A thorough search for an underlying condition must always be undertaken, not only to rule out other diseases (such as vascular occlusion, fracture, and central neuropathic pain), but also to ensure that a reparable cause of pain is not left untreated. The primary mode of treatment is to combine analgesia, rehabilitation, and psychological therapy in order to reduce pain as much as is practically possible so that normal mechanical function can be re-established (Figure 21-1). Coordinated treatment has been shown to be effective in randomized controlled trials of physical therapy combined with cognitive-behavioral therapy (CBT), reserving invasive sympathetic blockade for recurrent symptoms (8). A multidisciplinary team providing pain management, rehabilitation, and psychological specialists is often required for optimal therapy.

Analgesic regimens can include medication, anesthetic (reversible or ablative) blockade, and, in refractory cases, neuro-augmentative procedures (e.g., dorsal column stimulation and intrathecal medication infusion pump placement).

Pharmacological Therapy

Developing a medication regimen for CRPS type I often requires polypharmacy in order to take advantage of the multiple neuroreceptor types involved in pain transmission and modulation. The involvement of a pain specialist is important to optimize therapy and to minimize adverse effects

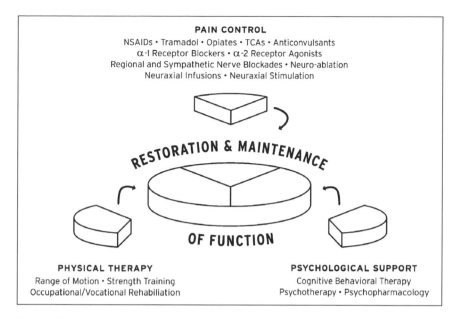

PAIN CONTROL
NSAIDs • Tramadol • Opiates • TCAs • Anticonvulsants
α-1 Receptor Blockers • α-2 Receptor Agonists
Regional and Sympathetic Nerve Blockades • Neuro-ablation
Neuraxial Infusions • Neuraxial Stimulation

RESTORATION & MAINTENANCE

OF FUNCTION

PHYSICAL THERAPY
Range of Motion • Strength Training
Occupational/Vocational Rehabiliation

PSYCHOLOGICAL SUPPORT
Cognitive Behavioral Therapy
Psychotherapy • Psychopharmacology

Figure 21-1 Approach to the management of complex regional pain syndromes. NSAIDs = nonsteroidal anti-inflammatory drugs; TCAs = tricyclic antidepressant drugs. (Illustration by Ms. Lisa Yee.)

of medications. General agents for neuropathic pain include common analgesics such as NSAIDs, tramadol, and opioid analgesics. In CRPS, when opiates are needed, it is preferable to use long-acting rather than short-acting preparations because of the chronicity of the illness. Short-acting agents, by definition, require the patient to experience pain before redosing. Furthermore, the behavioral aspects of self-medication and rapid fluctuations in serum drug level potentiate dependence and tolerance to opiates to a greater extent than would occur with a time-released agent.

There is good randomized controlled evidence that some antidepressant drugs (e.g., amitriptyline, nortryptyline) and anticonvulsant medications (e.g., gabapentin, carbamazepine) are effective treatments for some types of neuropathic pain (9-11). Current practice includes the broad use of these medications for the treatment of CRPS, with widely reported but largely anecdotal success. Further studies will be needed before it is possible to justify their use in an evidence-based fashion. Modulation of the autonomic nervous system with systemic α_1-receptor blockade (e.g., terazosin or phenoxybenzamine) or α_2-agonists (e.g., clonidine) is similarly part of common practice but as yet is also not supported by randomized clinical trials (12).

Systemic or locally injected corticosteroids have not been demonstrated to have an appreciable effect in a randomized, controlled study. However, there is anecdotal support for their use, particularly in the initial stages of CRPS (13).

Anesthetic Blockade

Regional anesthetic blockade of the sympathetic chain (e.g., lumbar sympathetic and cervico-thoracic or stellate ganglion block) has been employed for many years in the treatment of CRPS (14). Their primary role is to provide analgesia for rehabilitation and restoration of normal function. There is wide variability in practice with regard to the technique and frequency of administration, and while short-term efficacy is widely reported, determining long-term effectiveness will require further rigorously designed studies. In practice, however, for many patients, physical therapy is not possible without aggressive anesthetic blockade.

Neuro-ablation of the sympathetic chain has become less commonly utilized because of the increasing number of alternative therapies. In patients who experience a reproducible and definite but short-lived effect of local anesthetic sympathetic blockade, chemical, surgical or radio-frequency sympathectomy has been offered (15). However, these procedures are complicated by the risk of permanent side effects, the possibility of recurrent symptoms caused by central progression of the disease, or enhanced symptoms due to increased central pain sensitivity caused by surgical injury to peripheral nerves and resultant loss of afferent input.

Neuro-augmentation procedures, specifically dorsal column or peripheral nerve stimulation and intrathecal infusion pump placement, have emerged as potentially useful, albeit invasive, treatments for refractory neuropathic pain (16). These have the advantages of being reversible (compared with ablative techniques) and can be evaluated during a trial period before implantation.

Dorsal column stimulation has a central effect and therefore may be useful whether or not there has been a response to sympathetic blockade. Temporary (or if effective, permanent) electrodes are implanted percutaneously in the epidural space overlying the dorsal column in the affected region of the spinal cord. An implanted generator, operating in much the same way as a cardiac pacemaker, can then provide continuous stimulation. There is evidence from randomized controlled trials that dorsal column stimulation in conjunction with physical rehabilitation is of benefit in CRPS (17).

Neuraxial infusions of clonidine for pain due to CRPS have been validated in controlled trials (18). The most common use of intrathecal infusion, to deliver concentrated opioids (e.g., morphine) and local anesthetics (e.g., bupivicaine) to the CSF, allows the use of these medications in doses that could not otherwise be delivered because of side-effects resulting from systemic distribution.

Physical Rehabilitation and Psychological Support

Physical rehabilitation focuses on the maintenance of normal body mechanics to preserve range of motion and strength, as well as desensitization of the hyperalgesic areas. Occupational therapy is useful for treating specific functional loss, such as writing or work-related activities.

Psychological support is crucial in the treatment of CRPS, particularly in cases of protracted illness or when treatment has been delayed. CBT can help patients to correct maladaptive patterns of behavior that commonly occur in response to the limitations that often result from chronic pain. In CBT, the patient is trained to recognize how these behaviors worsen their symptoms and to better cope with attendant discomfort, thereby allowing them to interrupt this vicious cycle. Patients who develop other distinct psychiatric illness such as depression and anxiety may benefit from more specific ongoing treatment. Although there is no good evidence of an "RSD personality," pre-existing psychiatric illness does further impair patients' ability to cope with chronic pain and places them at increased risk for disability. Personality disorders, addiction, depression, and anxiety disorders can make treatment difficult, particularly in the patient who is unaware of their presence.

REFERENCES

1. **Merskey H, Bogduk N.** Classification of Chronic Pain: Descriptions of Chronic Pain Syndromes and Definitions of Pain Terms, 2nd ed. Seattle: International Association for the Study of Pain; 1994.

2. **van de Beek WJ, Schwartzman RJ, van Nes SI, Delhaas EM, van Hilten JJ.** Diagnostic criteria used in studies of reflex sympathetic dystrophy. Neurology. 2002;58:522-6.

3. **Ochoa JL.** Truths, errors, and lies around "reflex sympathetic dystrophy" and complex regional pain syndrome". J Neurol. 1999;246:875-9.

4. **Sorkin LS, Xiao WH, Wagner R, Myers RR.** Tumour necrosis factor-alpha induces ectopic activity in nociceptive primary afferent fibers. Neuroscience. 1997;81:255-62.

5. **Maves TJ, Pechman PS, Gebhart GF, Meller ST.** Possible chemical contribution from chromic gut sutures produces disorders of pain sensation like those seen in man. Pain. 1993;54:57-69.

6. **Low PA, Wilson PR, Sandroni P, et al.** Clinical characteristics of patients with reflex sympathetic dystrophy (sympathetically maintained pain) in the USA. In: Janig W, Stanton-Hicks M, eds. Reflex Sympathetic Dystrophy: A Reappraisal (Progress in Pain Research and Management, vol. 6). Seattle: International Association for the Study of Pain; 1996:49-66.

7. **Wasner G, Schattschneider J, Baron R.** Skin temperature side differences: a diagnostic tool for CRPS? Pain. 2002;98:19-26.

8. **Lee BH, Scharff L, Sethna NF, et al.** Physical therapy and cognitive-behavioral treatment for complex regional pain syndromes. J Pediatr. 2002;141:135-40.

9. **Kingery WS.** A critical review of controlled clinical trials for peripheral neuropathic pain and complex regional pain syndromes. Pain. 1997;73:123-39.

10. **Mellick GA, Mellick LB.** Reflex sympathetic dystrophy treated with gabapentin. Arch Phys Med Rehabil. 1997;78:98-105.

11. **Backonja MM.** Anticonvulsants (antineuroleptics) for neuropathic pain syndromes. Clin J Pain. 2000;16(2 Suppl):S67-72.

12. **Perez RS, Kwakkel G, Zuurmond WW, de Lange JJ.** Treatment of reflex sympathetic dystrophy (CRPS type 1): a research synthesis of 21 randomized clinical trials. J Pain Symptom Manage. 2001;21:511-26.

13. **Christensen K, Jensen EM, Noer I.** The reflex dystrophy syndrome response to treatment with systemic corticosteroids. Acta Chir Scand. 1982;148:653-5.

14. **Gibbons JJ, Wilson PR, Lamer TJ, Elliott BA.** Interscalene blocks for chronic upper extremity pain. Clin J Pain. 1992;8:264-9.

15. **Bandyk DF, Johnson BL, Kirkpatrick AF, et al.** Surgical sympathectomy for reflex sympathetic dystrophy syndromes. J Vasc Surg. 2002;35:269-77.

16. **Calvillo O, Racz G, Didie J, Smith K.** Neuroaugmentation in the treatment of complex regional pain syndrome of the upper extremity. Acta Orthop Belg. 1998; 64:57-63.

17. **Marchand S, Bushnell MC, Molina-Negro P, et al.** The effects of dorsal column stimulation on measures of clinical and experimental pain in man. Pain. 1991;45: 249-57.

18. **Rauck RL, Eisenach JC, Jackson K, et al.** Epidural clonidine treatment for refractory reflex sympathetic dystrophy. Anesthesiology. 1993;79:1163-9.

22

■　■　■

Crystalline Arthritic Diseases

Theodore R. Fields, MD

I n the crystal-induced arthritic disorders, crystal precipitation results in the phagocytosis of the relevant crystal and the subsequent inflammatory process leading to clinical disease. Table 22-1 reviews the clinically relevant crystal-induced diseases with their associated crystals and methods of identification.

Various factors, including increases in crystal size, rapid fluxes in systemic urate or calcium concentration, and local trauma, can increase the likelihood of crystal precipitation. Neutrophils play a key role in crystal-induced inflammation. For example, animals that are depleted of neutrophils have a defective inflammatory response to urate crystals. Many inflammatory mediators such as interleukin (IL)-1, tumor necrosis factor (TNF)-α, and prostaglandin E2 are synthesized locally and stimulate the further recruitment of inflammatory cells. Crystals in the synovial fluid become coated with immunoglobulins. Although this may initially promote phagocytosis of the crystals and fuel the inflammatory process, the removal of inciting crystals eventually accounts for the self-limited nature of most disease flares.

Crystal-related arthritis is common and can often be surprisingly more challenging diagnostically and therapeutically than would appear on the surface. Hasselbacher noted that on hospital rounds he "nearly came to the conclusion that all gout is difficult gout." Hospitalized patients with possible crystal arthritis provide additional challenges, and a strong familiarity with the natural history of crystal arthritis, along with a full appreciation of the benefits and risks of the various treatment options will serve the clinician well.

Gout

Pathogenesis

Gout is a common inflammatory arthritis triggered by monosodium urate (MSU) crystals deposited within joints. The prevalence of gout is 5 to 28 per

Table 22-1   Crystalline Disease Identification

Disease	Crystal and Method of Identification
Gout	Monosodium urate: needle-shaped, negatively birefringent crystals within neutrophils under polarized light microscopy
Pseudogout	Calcium pyrophosphate: variably shaped, classically rhomboid, positively birefringent crystals within neutrophils under polarized light microscopy, or positive alizarin red S staining
Hydroxyapatite deposition disease (e.g., calcific peri-arthritis, Milwaukee shoulder)	Calcium hydroxyapatite (a form of basic calcium phosphate): seen under electron microscopy and confirmed by X-ray diffraction
Arthritis in renal failure (unusual cause)	Calcium oxalate: pleiomorphic but characteristically bipyramidal or envelope-shaped; easily confused with CPPD if characteristic shapes not seen

1000 men and 1 to 6 per 1000 women. In some patients, it includes the extra-articular deposition of MSU in the form of tophi and the propensity to develop urate kidney stones.

Uric acid is the end-product of the metabolic breakdown of purines, the last step of which is the conversion of xanthine to uric acid by xanthine oxidase. Supersaturation of MSU crystals results in their precipitation in joints. The major risk factor for supersaturation is hyperuricemia. In some hyperuricemic patients, there may be a genetic basis to urate overproduction or renal undersecretion. Excretion of over 800 mg per day of urate in the 24-hour urine on a standard diet identifies urate overproducers. There are also many secondary causes of hyperuricemia, including renal insufficiency, drug effects, lead toxicity, and tumor lysis (Figure 22-1).

A number of factors can disproportionately increase local urate levels above the systemic concentrations (1). Dependent joints such as the first metatarsophalangeal (MTP) joint may, with recumbency, have preferential resorption of water, resulting in higher intra-articular urate concentrations. This may explain the frequent nighttime onset of gouty attacks. MSU crystals are less soluble at lower temperatures, perhaps accounting for the propensity of gouty attacks to occur in the feet where the body temperature is the coolest. Rapid changes in serum urate concentration, as with the beginning of urate-lowering therapy, may also paradoxically precipitate exacerbations.

Local injury may also influence crystal deposition. Joints with prior trauma or intrinsic mechanical derangements such as osteoarthritis-associated Bouchard's and Heberden's nodes are more prone to gouty attacks, suggesting that local structural factors, such as proteoglycan loss, may increase vulnerability to crystal-induced inflammation. Similarly, infectious

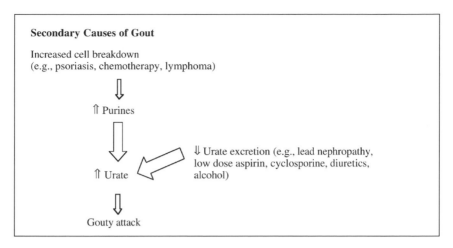

Secondary Causes of Gout

Increased cell breakdown
(e.g., psoriasis, chemotherapy, lymphoma)

⇓

⇑ Purines

⇓   ⇐ ⇓ Urate excretion (e.g., lead nephropathy,
            low dose aspirin, cyclosporine, diuretics,
⇑ Urate   alcohol)

⇓

Gouty attack

Figure 22-1   The secondary causes of gout can affect concentrations of uric acid by increasing its production or decreasing its excretion.

arthritis may cause "strip-mining" of uric acid crystals within the joint and precipitate exacerbations of gout. Concomitant joint infection should always be considered in any flare of crystalline arthritis, particularly when there are signs of systemic inflammation such as a prominent fever or peripheral leukocytosis.

Case Presentation 1

A 56-year-old man presented with an acutely painful, red, hot, and swollen right ankle. He had a past medical history of end-stage renal disease secondary to diabetes mellitus and underwent a cadaveric renal transplantation 1 year ago, after which he was placed on prednisone and cyclosporine. Although he had no history of gout prior to his transplant, he has subsequently had recurrent attacks of gout documented by synovial fluid analysis and has developed multiple tophi. His serum creatinine and uric acid concentrations are 2.1 mg/dL and 11.5 mg/dL, respectively. He has a recent history of a bleeding duodenal ulcer.

Different treatment options for the acute gouty flare were considered. Renal insufficiency and active peptic ulcer disease precluded the use of nonsteroidal anti-inflammatory drugs (NSAIDs). Systemic corticosteroids were less than optimal because of diabetes. Although not absolutely contraindicated, colchicine carried significant risks in the setting of renal disease. For the acute exacerbation, then, arthrocentesis followed by an intra-articular injection of methylprednisolone 60 mg was performed with resolution of the gouty exacerbation. Synovial fluid analysis under polarizing microscopy revealed many polymorphonuclear leukocytes with intracellular needle-shaped negatively birefringent crystals.

Because of the presence of tophi and the recurrent flares, prophylactic hypouricemic therapy with daily allopurinol 100 mg was started 1 month after the resolution of the recent attack and gradually increased to 200 mg daily in order to lower the serum urate concentration to below 6.0 mg/dL. The patient's gouty flares became much less frequent, and his tophi became smaller.

This case illustrates many issues commonly encountered in the management of gout. Patients very frequently are taking medications (e.g., warfarin) or have comorbidities such as hypertension, peptic ulcer disease, diabetes, or renal insufficiency that are relative or absolute contraindications to NSAIDs, corticosteroids, or colchicine in the management of a gouty flare. Bearing in mind that acute gouty arthritis is generally a self-limited condition, occasional patients with many comorbidities may actually be best managed with simple analgesics alone. Comorbid states also help determine whether preventive therapy is indicated and, if so, which prophylactic agents may be appropriate.

Clinical Features

Gouty flares often develop acutely without provocation during the night and are characterized by severe pain, heat, edema, erythema, and exquisite tenderness. Low-grade fever may accompany the attacks but rarely goes above 38°C. (High fever should raise suspicion for infection.) The first MTP joint is the most common area for a gout attack ("podagra"), although first MTP joint inflammation can also occur in many other conditions such as osteoarthritis, rheumatoid arthritis, and psoriatic arthritis. Other joints commonly involved in gout are the mid-tarsal joints, the ankles, the knees, and the olecranon bursae. Shoulders and hips are extremely rare areas for gouty attack. Attacks tend to be discrete and self-limited (lasting several days) in the early phase of the disease, with a normal joint examination between attacks. Flares may be recurrent. In late phases, chronic gouty arthritis can occur. Hospitalized patients are particularly prone to gouty attacks, often polyarticular. Deposition in non-articular tissues such as skin or kidney results in tophi and uric acid stone formation, respectively.

Diagnosis

Crystal Analysis
The definitive diagnosis of an acute gouty arthritis is made by the visualization of uric acid crystals within neutrophils as defined by polarizng microscopy of synovial fluid or in a pathological specimen, and it is strongly advised that crystal examination be performed whenever possible. Moreover, it has recently been shown that patients with negative crystal analysis during a single episode of gout may demonstrate gouty crystals during subsequent attacks, justifying repeated attempts at this important diagnostic

procedure in questionable cases (2). In cases where it is particularly important to make the diagnosis of gout but the patient is seen between arthritic flares, MSU crystals can also been found in synovial fluid of asymptomatic joints. Many patients erroneously carry the diagnosis of gout for years without crystal diagnosis and may inappropriately receive prophylactic therapy with allopurinol or colchicine.

In cases where crystals cannot be identified or a specimen cannot be obtained, a presumptive diagnosis of gout can be made if 6 of 12 minor diagnostic criteria established by a subcommittee of the American Rheumatism Association are met (Table 22-2) (3).

Urine Studies

A 24-hour measurement of urate excretion is helpful in the management of gout when a patient is being considered for therapy to lower serum uric acid levels, and there is a choice between a uricosuric agent (e.g., probenecid) or a xanthine oxidase inhibitor (e.g., allopurinol). If the decision to treat with allopurinol is already made, a 24-hour urate determination may not be needed. Excretion of over 800 mg of uric acid in a 24-hour period indicates overexcretion of urate and identifies patients that may benefit

---

Table 22-2   Criteria for the Diagnosis of Gout

Major Criteria   Either of these is definitive for the diagnosis of gout:

- Crystal documentation in joint fluid or tophus
- Crystal identification in pathologic specimen

Minor Criteria   Major criteria are always preferred, but the diagnosis can be made if 6 of the following 12 criteria are present:

1. More than one discrete arthritic attack
2. Maximal inflammation within 24 hours
3. Episode of monoarticular arthritis
4. Joint erythema
5. First metatarso-phalangeal joint (MTP) with swelling or pain
6. Unilateral inflammation of the MTP
7. Unilateral inflammation of a tarsal joint
8. Possible tophus
9. Hyperuricemia
10. Asymmetric swelling in a joint on x-ray
11. X-ray showing subcortical cysts without erosion
12. Negative bacterial culture in an inflamed joint

Modified from Wallace SL, Robinson H, Masi AT, et al. Preliminary criteria for the classification of the acute arthritis of primary gout. Arthritis Rheum. 1977;20:895-900; with permission.

from treatment with allopurinol. True urate overexcretors will be very likely be detected with a single 24-hour urine study.

Despite greater convenience for the patient, the usefulness of spot one-time urine studies has been questioned. Spot urinary uric acid to creatinine ratio has been recently described as an inadequate proxy for 24-hour urate excretion (4). Instead, Simkin has recommended using the following spot urine formulation as an initial screening test: *urinary urate* × (*plasma creatinine/urinary creatinine*) (5). If this value is greater than 0.6 mg/dL, then 24-hour urate excretion should be measured for further evaluation. Nevertheless, the role of spot urine studies remains to be determined.

Prognosis

In most cases of acute gout, the response to appropriate therapy and overall prognosis are generally quite good. However, as illustrated in the case presented above, management of acute gout can be complicated if, as often is the case, the patient has comorbid conditions that are absolute or relative contraindications to available treatment choices. Nevertheless, it should be emphasized that acute gout is generally self-limited even when untreated, and so the clinician may rely on purely analgesic agents only (narcotics, if necessary) if left no other options.

Repeated episodes of gout are more likely in patients with severe hyperuricemia and can result in chronic secondary mechanical joint changes that can become symptomatic even without the inflammatory aspects of gout. The recurrence rate, without preventive measures, is 62% in 1 year and 93% in 10 years.

Before the advent of effective hypouricemic therapies, tophi formation occurred in over 70% of patients after 20 years; the average time for the appearance of the first visible tophus was more than 11 years (6). With the availability of urate-lowering agents, about 55% of patients develop visible tophi after 20 years (7).

The severity of hyperuricemia is directly related to the risk of developing nephrolithiasis. The yearly incidences of uric acid kidney stones in normal controls, in asymptomatic hyperuricemic individuals, and in gouty patients are 0.1%, 0.3%, and 0.9%, respectively (8). In some long-term studies, as many as 20% to 40% of patients with gout develop uric acid kidney stones (9).

Management

The appropriate management of gout depends on the stage of disease at which the patient is seen: 1) asymptomatic hyperuricemia, 2) acute gout attacks, 3) intercritical gout (between attacks), or 4) chronic, often tophaceous gout. Special issues also arise when the patient has a history of, or is at high risk for, uric acid renal stones.

ASYMPTOMATIC HYPERURICEMIA

The current consensus is that uric acid levels less than 12.0 mg/dL, in the absence of gouty arthritis, tophi, or kidney stone, do *not* need to be treated (10). Recent evidence does not favor serum uric acid concentrations as a direct marker for coronary artery disease (11), even though elevated serum urate levels are associated with known coronary risk factors such as hypertension and obesity. Certainly, there is no evidence that reducing serum urate concentrations in any way reduces coronary risk. In patients with very high serum urate levels (e.g., >12.0 mg/dL), 24-hour urinary urate excretion should be measured. If greater than 800 mg, many rheumatologists recommend using allopurinol to lower the risk of kidney stone formation.

ACUTE GOUT ATTACKS

Table 22-3 summarizes the short-term options for the management of acute gout. An important general principle is that the more quickly therapy is instituted, the more likely it is to be effective.

Nonsteroidal anti-inflammatory drugs (NSAIDs) are the mainstay in the treatment of acute gouty arthritis. Indomethacin (25-50 mg tid) has traditionally been the drug of choice, but naproxen and other NSAIDs are equally effective. Anecdotal data suggest that cyclooxygenase-2 (COX-2) inhibitors have equal benefit. NSAIDs are generally well-tolerated for the short duration needed to treat acute gout. Many patients who learn to recognize the earliest symptoms of an attack can often abort a gouty flare by immediately instituting NSAID therapy.

Intra-articular injection with local corticosteroids (e.g., methylprednisolone acetate 20-80 mg, depending on the size of the joint) is extremely effective in treating acute gout, particularly in patients with monoarticular involvement or in those who fail to respond adequately to NSAIDs. It is a reasonable first-line approach when contraindications to NSAIDs exist and septic arthritis is reasonably excluded.

Brief courses of systemic corticosteroids (e.g., oral prednisone 20-40 mg daily with a rapid taper) or adrenocorticotropic hormone (intramuscular ACTH 25-40 U every 8 hours for up to two days) may be used for patients with multiple joint involvement, especially when there are contraindications to the use of NSAIDs (12). Short-term systemic corticosteroids and ACTH appear to be well tolerated in most patients, although patients with

---

Table 22-3   Management Options for Acute Gout

- Traditional and cyclooxygenase-2 selective nonsteroidal anti-inflammatory drugs (NSAIDs)
- Local corticosteroid injection
- Systemic corticosteroids or adrenocorticotropic hormone
- Oral or intravenous colchicine

---

uncontrolled diabetes mellitus or poorly compensated congestive heart failure may not be appropriate patients for their use. ACTH should not be used in patients already on chronic steroid therapy because the adrenal response may be insufficient.

Oral colchicine may be used for acute gout attacks in select circumstances. Colchicine decreases granulocyte migration to the joint by inhibiting a urate crystal-associated glycoprotein chemotactic factor. Peak concentrations of colchicine occur in 30 to 120 minutes after an oral dose. For acute flares, oral colchicine 0.6 mg is administered hourly until the patient achieves relief or develops diarrhea, whichever comes first. Because colchicine is cleared by the kidneys, it carries increased toxicities in patients with renal insufficiency and is not the optimal agent for the treatment of acute gout in these individuals. Because of the high incidence of adverse gastrointestinal effects, oral colchicine for acute gout is now prescribed much less frequently and is generally used only for those patients with a history of successful response and good tolerance to this treatment. However, because only a few arthritides other than those induced by crystals respond to colchicine, its use can sometimes be of diagnostic value.

Potential bone marrow toxicity limits the use of intravenous colchicine for acute gout. However, in patients with contraindications to both NSAIDs and corticosteroids (e.g., a diabetic patient with peptic ulcer disease), intravenous colchicine offers a useful option and has the added benefit of diagnostic specificity. For example, a response to intravenous colchicine can support the diagnosis of gout or other crystalline arthritides. Patients with renal insufficiency or chronic use of oral colchicine are most at risk for bone marrow suppression from intravenous colchicine, and so extreme caution and reduced dosages must be used in these individuals if colchicine is to be used at all. Moreover, oral colchicine should be avoided for at least 1 week after the administration of intravenous colchicine. Intravenous colchicine is also contraindicated in patients with neutropenia and significant hepatic disease. When given to patients with normal renal and hepatic function, an intravenous loading dose of colchicine 2.0 mg is administered followed by 0.5 mg boluses every 8 hours as necessary up to a maximum cumulative dose of 4 mg. In patients with even mild renal or hepatic insufficiency, the loading dose should be no more than 1.0 mg and the maximum cumulative dose not more than 2.0 mg. Intravenous colchicine is very irritating to the skin, and care needs to be taken to prevent extravasation. Colchicine is not removed with hemodialysis.

INTERCRITICAL GOUT

Table 22-4 summarizes the options for the management of intercritical gout, which is defined as the asymptomatic periods between exacerbations. All patients should be counseled on dietary adjustments. Prophylactic therapy may also be considered in appropriate candidates. In patients that are treated with agents to lower serum uric acid levels, significant reduction in

---

Table 22-4   Management Options for Intercritical Gout

- Dietary adjustments (e.g., avoidance of alcohol, roe, meat gravies, yeasty breads, and shellfish)
- Adjustment of medications that raise serum uric acid concentrations
- Colchicine
- Uricosurics: probenecid or sulfinpyrazone
- Xanthine oxidase inhibitors: allopurinol or oxypurinol
- Experimental regimens (urate oxidase, benzbromarone)

---

the frequency of attacks can generally be obtained within 12 to 18 months. However, the frequency of attacks within the first 6 months of hypouricemic therapy may actually increase if concomitant colchicine therapy is not prescribed. Nevertheless, identifying and treating patients for whom prophylactic therapy is appropriate can be challenging.

After a single attack of gout, most authorities will not recommend prophylactic therapy, unless the patient meets criteria for treatment with allopurinol (Table 22-5). However, when gouty attacks become frequent (e.g., more than four attacks yearly) or more refractory to treatment, prophylactic therapy should be considered. Options include chronic colchicine or hypouricemic agents (uricosurics, xanthine oxidase inhibitors). The clinician should nevertheless be aware that agents that lower serum uric acid levels, allopurinol and the uricosurics, may exacerbate gouty flares if started too soon after an acute attack and should not be started for at least 2-3 weeks after resolution of symptoms. Once started, treatment to lower serum urate levels generally needs to be continued for life.

CHRONIC AND TOPHACEOUS GOUT

The options described for intercritical gout also apply to this group of more severe gout patients. Colchicine has no role in treating tophi because it is not a hypouricemic agent, although it still may be used to minimize the frequency or severity of inflammatory joint exacerbations. Some of these cases will require even more aggressive lowering of serum urate levels, often to 5.0 mg/dL or less, in order to see significant shrinkage of tophi. Occasional patients will require surgical removal of severe tophi in order to prevent secondary infection or encroachment onto adjacent structures such as tendons.

Dietary Adjustments

Dietary adjustments are important but often not sufficient in the management of intercritical gout. Modifications are made to reduce the intake of purines, which are the metabolic precursors to uric acid. Foods that have high purine content include roe, meat gravies, yeasty breads, and shellfish. Alcohol decreases urate excretion and should be avoided. Beer is particularly problematic because of its high yeast content. Diuretics, cyclosporine, and

---

Table 22-5   Indications for Allopurinol Therapy

---

1. Recurrent gout (e.g., >4 attacks per year) in a patient refractory to colchicine prophylaxis with creatinine clearance <80 mL/min (and thus not a candidate for uricosuric therapy)
2. Hyperuricemia with kidney stones (urate or calcium-containing) or urate excretion >800 mg/24h associated with gouty arthritis
3. Failure of uricosurics to maintain serum urate levels to <6.0 mg/dL (in a patient with colchicine-refractory gout)
4. Allergy or intolerance to uricosuric agents (in a patient with colchicine-refractory gout)
5. Tophaceous gout
6. Prophylaxis against acute urate nephropathy in patient on cancer chemotherapy

---

low-dose salicylates are common medications that can cause hyperuricemia, and adjustments of these medications should be considered if possible.

Colchicine Prophylaxis

Chronic oral colchicine therapy has no effect on serum urate levels but decreases the frequency of gouty attacks and their severity by reducing the inflammatory response to MUS crystals. In patients with normal kidney and liver function, the usual dose is 0.6 mg once or twice daily. The interval should be extended to every other day in patients with underlying mild renal or hepatic insufficiency. Colchicine can cause diarrhea in some patients even at these dosages, and chronic use in patients with even mild renal insufficiency has been reported to rarely cause a neuromyopathy with proximal muscle weakness and elevated serum muscle enzyme levels. Patients with moderate-to-severe renal (creatinine clearance <50 mL/min) or hepatic insufficiency should not receive chronic colchicine.

Hypouricemic Agents

Hypouricemic agents (uricosuric agents, xanthine oxidase inhibitors) are used to lower urate serum levels to levels <6.0 mg/dL when prophylactic therapy with colchicine is inadequate or not tolerated. By decreasing the overall uric acid load in the body, the frequency of gouty flares can be reduced and the formation of tophi retarded or reversed. Allopurinol, a xanthine oxidase inhibitor, is the most widely prescribed hypouricemic agent and is generally considered to be first-line therapy when lowering uric acid levels is desired. Unfortunately, adverse reactions are common, and uricosuric drugs may be more appropriate in some patients. Colchicine is often given concurrently with the onset of hypouricemic therapy for three to six months to reduce the risk of treatment-induced gouty flares.

Uricosuric Agents

Because of their relative safety, uricosuric agents are good options in the patient with recurrent gouty attacks despite colchicine prophylaxis and a creatinine clearance greater than 80 mL/min. Probenecid (250-1000 mg bid) and sulfinpyrazone (50 mg bid to 100 mg qid) are the available uricosurics in the United States. Probenecid is much less effective if the creatinine clearance is less than 80 mL/min, while sulfinpyrazone can still be effective at slightly lower creatinine clearances. (Benzbromarone, currently only available outside the United States, is a more effective uricosuric than probenecid and sulfinpyrazone, is efficacious with creatinine clearances less than 20 mL/min, and appears to be well-tolerated [13].)

A 24-hour urine determination for uric acid excretion is needed before uricosuric therapy because patients with urinary urate excretion greater than 600-800 mg/24 h are already at increased risk for renal stone development and therefore would not be good candidates for uricosurics, which increase this propensity. Aside from nephrolithiasis, other adverse effects associated with probenecid include skin rashes, gastrointestinal intolerance, and significant drug interactions notably with penicillin. Also, salicylates antagonize the uricosuric activity of both probenecid and sulfinpyrazone. Sulfinpyrazone appears to cause more gastrointestinal upset than probenecid. If tophi are present, allopurinol is preferred over uricosurics. Patients taking uricosurics must also maintain sufficient hydration to reduce the risk of renal calculi. The effects of dose adjustments of these agents on serum urate concentrations are detectable within 1 or 2 weeks. Dosing is typically adjusted to maintain serum uric acid levels below 6.0 mg/dL.

Xanthine Oxidase Inhibitors

Allopurinol and oxypurinol reduce uric acid production by inhibiting xanthine oxidase, the enzyme that catalyzes the conversion of xanthine to uric acid. Allopurinol (starting dosages 100-400 mg qd) is the most commonly used long-term prophylactic agent for patients with gout. The dosage of allopurinol is adjusted to maintain serum uric acid levels below 6.0 mg/dL. The effects of dosage adjustments can be seen after 1 week. In a few patients, a lower serum uric acid concentration may be required to control symptoms and appropriate dosage increase is indicated.

Although quite effective for the vast majority of gout patients, allopurinol can have significant potential toxicity. Liver function test abnormalities can occur, as can leukopenia, a maculopapular skin rash and cutaneous vasculitis. The rare but feared allopurinol hypersensitivity syndrome presents with fever, liver function test abnormalities, and leukopenia, and can be fatal. In view of these toxicities, it is important to be sure that all patients placed on allopurinol have clear and definitive indications for its use (see Table 22-5). It is common to find patients with osteoarthritis and asymptomatic hyperuricemia inappropriately treated with chronic allopurinol therapy. Studies have demonstrated that a majority of cases of allopurinol hypersensitivity syndrome occurred in patients without indications for allopurinol therapy (14). Allopurinol needs to be used very cautiously and at decreased dosages in patients with renal insufficiency (15). Although allopurinol has a half-life of 30 minutes to 3 hours, its major metabolite, oxypurinol, has a half-life of 14 to 28 hours. Because azathioprine is a purine normally metabolized by xanthine oxidase, allopurinol markedly increases serum levels of azathioprine. Thus, in patients taking concomitant azathioprine, the dosage of azathioprine should be reduced to 25% of the original dosage or an alternative agent should be used. Allopurinol also prolongs the half-life of warfarin and increases the risk of rash from ampicillin. A recent study suggested that chronic use of allopurinol for longer than 3 years or after a cumulative dose of more than 400 g was associated with mildly increased risk of cataract extraction.

A significant number of patients with clear indications for allopurinol develop rashes or frank cutaneous vasculitis due to the drug. Because cutaneous manifestations can at times be quite severe with allopurinol, it is generally not advisable to rechallenge with the full dose of the drug in these individuals. In patients who clearly need a xanthine oxidase inhibitor, one alternative agent is oxypurinol, which is the natural metabolically active breakdown product of allopurinol. This drug is available directly from Burroughs Wellcome. Unfortunately, the cross-reactivity rate between oxypurinol and allopurinol is still 50%, and so many patients will risk a recurrence of their allergic reaction (16). Because there are few options to allopurinol and because the medication can be of unique therapeutic value for many patients, desensitization regimens are sometimes necessary. Desensitization regimens should be conducted with the guidance of an experienced allergist or rheumatologist.

In one oral regimen for patients with pruritic maculopapular rashes (but not more serious reactions to allopurinol such as leukopenia, liver disease, and toxic epidermal necrolysis, or the catastrophic allopurinol hypersensitivity syndrome), minute dosages of allopurinol (as little as 10 µg) can be administered initially (17). The dosage can then be escalated every 3 days with appropriate reductions made in the event of recurrent cutaneous reactions. Oral desensitization may be successful in more than 75% of patients with minor cutaneous reactions to allopurinol. Intravenous desensitization can be reserved for oral regimen failures but require hospitalization, ideally under observation in an intensive care unit (18). Patients who have undergone either desensitization regimen need to be followed closely because hypersensitivity symptoms can return at a later date or as dosages are increased.

In the future, urate oxidase, an investigational intravenous agent that promotes urate breakdown, may show promise but is not currently available in the United States (19).

Urate Nephrolithiasis

Patients with gout should be encouraged to maintain high fluid intake to reduce their risk of nephrolithiasis. Urate nephrolithiasis occurs in the approximately 20% of gout patients who are overproducers of urate and therefore have hyperuricosuria. Kidney stones in these patients can be purely uric acid, or urate can be the "nidus" which allows a calcium oxalate stone to form around it. Gout patients with history of renal stones or those with >800 mg of 24-hour urinary urate excretion, should be treated with allopurinol to simultaneously lower both serum and urinary urate. Uricosuric agents increase the risk of kidney stones and are not appropriate in this setting. Gout patients with a history of kidney stones will benefit from alkalinization of the urine, especially early in allopurinol therapy. Supplemental alkali such as potassium citrate, 1 to 3 mmol/kg of body weight daily administered in four divided doses, or acetazolamide 250 to 500 mg at bedtime can be used to raise urine pH to 6.0 or greater.

Patient Communication
Because of the complexity of the "short-term" and "long-term" approaches to gout therapy, it is important to make sure patients understand the overall principles of gout therapy. Urate crystals have been likened to unlit matches as a way to explain the different arms of management. When a gouty flare occurs, the matches have been "lit," and drugs such as NSAIDs, colchicine, or corticosteroids are required to "put them out." For the long-term, however, the total number of "matches" can be reduced with allopurinol or uricosurics, or they can be made "damp" with colchicine thereby reducing their likelihood of becoming "lit."

Pseudogout: Calcium Pyrophosphate Deposition Disease

Pathogenesis

Pseudogout is an inflammatory arthritis triggered by calcium pyrophosphate dihydrate (CPPD) crystals deposited within joints. The likelihood of CPPD crystal formation is affected by multiple factors including trauma, mechanical derangements of the joint, and local pH and ion concentrations (e.g., calcium, inorganic pyrophosphate, iron). Exacerbations of pseudogout can occur when there are significant changes in calcium concentrations as occurs commonly after the onset of diuretic therapy or parathyroidectomy. As with gout, pseudogout attacks can also follow local trauma or infection, which is thought to result in "enzymatic strip-mining" and release of CPPD crystals within the affected joint. Pseudogout flares have also been reported to follow intra-articular injection of hyaluronic acid preparations used in treatment of osteoarthritis (20).

Case Presentation 2

A 64-year-old woman presents 4 days after developing acute pain, swelling, and erythema of the right knee and a low-grade fever of 38°C. There has been no history of recent trauma or infections. She has had several years of pain in the right knee with prolonged weight-bearing that had been treated success-fully as "arthritis" with small doses of ibuprofen but did not take any med-ications during the acute illness. She had a mild leukocytosis of 12,500/µL and an erythrocyte sedimentation rate of 42 mm/h, but laboratory testing was otherwise normal. X-rays of the right knee showed mild osteoarthritis changes and calcifications of the medial and lateral menisci consistent with chondrocalcinosis. Next, 40 cc of cloudy fluid were aspirated from the knee, showing many neutrophils with no organisms on Gram staining. There were 34,000 leukocytes/µL, with 80% neutrophils by cell count. Positively bire-fringent rhomboid crystals consistent with calcium pyrophosphate were seen within many neutrophils on polarized light microscopy, and the diagnosis of acute pseudogout was made. She was prescribed ibuprofen 400 mg every 6 hours for 2 days, at which time she had only a partial improvement. The cultures from the arthrocentesis by this time were negative, and the knee was reaspirated and injected with methylprednisolone acetate 60 mg. She had a complete resolution of her acute arthritis after several days. Although she continued to have occasional flares of pseudogout about once a year, they were easily controlled with prompt treatment with ibuprofen.

Clinical Manifestations

Acute pseudogout most commonly presents as a monoarticular arthritis in an elderly person, often involving a knee, ankle, shoulder, or wrist. First MTP joint involvement with pseudogout has been reported but is infre-quent. The degree of inflammation can be as intense as that seen with acute gout. When less inflammatory, it may present as a "pseudo-osteoarthritis." Oligoarticular and polyarticular presentations can also occur; a "pseudo-rheumatoid arthritis" presentation occurs in about 5% of cases.

Diagnosis

As with gout, the diagnosis of pseudogout by crystal identification is defin-itive and is the preferred means of diagnosis. Calcium pyrophosphate crys-tals within neutrophils are visualized by polarized light microscopy (see Table 22-1). When crystal examination is not revealing or not available, other criteria may be used to help make a diagnosis of pseudogout (Table 22-6). X-rays of involved joints normally show chondrocalcinosis, calcifica-tions within the articular cartilage or meniscus (Figure 22-2). However, as many as 20% of elderly patients have these radiological findings without a clinical history of pseudogout.

Because pseudogout and osteoarthritis often appear in the same individ-ual, it is useful to be able to identify features in a patient with osteoarthritis that suggest the presence of pseudogout. Clues to differentiating osteoarthritis from pseudogout are given in Table 22-7.

Table 22-6   Criteria for the Diagnosis of Pseudogout

Definitive diagnosis
- Acute arthritis, with intracellular calcium pyrophosphate crystals documented in joint fluid

Probable diagnosis
- Acute inflammatory arthritis, with typical calcifications (chondrocalcinosis) on X-ray

Features *suggesting*, although not diagnostic of, pseudogout include:
- Preferential involvement of the patellofemoral joint over the medial and lateral compartments of the knee joint
- Chronic inflammatory arthritis, especially of the knees, wrists, shoulders or metacarpophalangeal joints, with acute exacerbations and remissions

---

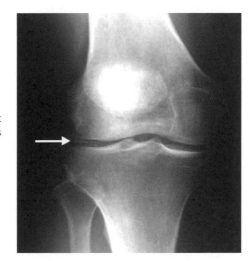

Figure 22-2   Radiograph of the right knee demonstrating chondrocalcinosis of the menisci (*arrow*).

The diagnosis of pseudogout should also lead to an investigation for secondary causes (Table 22-8), even though the arthritic complications may not always remit after treatment of the underlying diseases. For example, parathyroidectomy for the treatment of primary hyperparathyroidism does not appear to reverse X-ray findings of CPPD deposition (23). Nonetheless, early identification of secondary causes such as hemochromatosis may prevent other complications of the underlying illness. In the past, it had been felt that diabetes mellitus was associated with pseudogout, but this connection has not held up to more careful scrutiny. Although rare, familial cases of pseudogout have been reported and can be quite striking. The appropriate evaluation of a patient with no specific clues to any secondary cause should include serum calcium, uric acid, magnesium, ferritin, iron saturation, and liver function tests.

Table 22-7   Differentiation of Pseudogout from Osteoarthritis

---

Pseudogout tends to have the following features:

- Involvement of sites that are not typical for osteoarthritis such as wrist, metacarpophalangeal joints, elbow, or shoulder
- Joint space narrowing localized to the radiocarpal or patellofemoral joint
- Severe subchondral cyst formation
- Severe joint degeneration with subchondral bony collapse and fragmentation
- Tendon calcification

Table 22-8   Possible Secondary Causes of Pseudogout

Association	*Comment/Reference*
Hyperparathyroidism	Most common association
Hypermagnesemia and hypomagnesemia	Rare but well-documented (21)
Hemochromatosis	Important association
Hyperthyroidism and hypothyroidism	Recent data have disputed these associations (22)
Gouty arthritis	MSU and CPPD crystals have been frequently noted to co-exist, especially in the setting of chronic renal insufficiency

MSU= monosodium urate; CPPD = calcium pyrophosphate dihydrate.

Prognosis

The only measures of treatment success are the decreased incidence and severity of flares. Although no treatment has been documented to alter the natural history of disease, it is reasonable to hypothesize that decreasing the frequency of inflammatory episodes will reduce the risk of irreversible joint damage. Pseudogout is more difficult to treat prophylactically than gout because no drug has been clearly shown to prevent local calcification. The patients who continue to get pseudogout attacks despite preventive measures can often be managed only by recurrent courses of NSAIDs, local corticosteroid injections, or systemic corticosteroids. Fortunately, most attacks of pseudogout can be controlled with relative ease, so that even the recurrent need for treatment may only require fairly short exposures to medications.

Management

The management of pseudogout is generally divided into 1) treatment of acute attacks, 2) prophylaxis against recurrent flares, and 3) management of chronic disease. At present, there are no effective ways to remove calcium deposits from joints.

ACUTE PSEUDOGOUT ATTACKS

Even when CPPD crystals are identified during an episode of acute inflammatory arthritis, it is always important to exclude septic arthritis. Joint infection may dislodge CPPD crystals via a "strip-mining" effect, precipitating a pseudogout flare. Accordingly, synovial fluid specimens should always be examined not only for crystal analysis but also for Gram staining and microbial cultures. Although large-scale clinical evidence is often lacking, treatment for pseudogout attacks is generally similar to that for gouty arthritis (see Table 22-3). One difference is that it has been noted anecdotally that a reasonable percentage of pseudogout attacks will resolve after joint aspiration alone, and so arthrocentesis alone can be potentially therapeutic.

PROPHYLACTIC THERAPY

Colchicine prophylaxis, as with gout, does appear to reduce the frequency and severity of pseudogout attacks. The administration of colchicine (0.6 mg once or twice daily in patients with normal kidney function) and necessary precautions are as for intercritical gout. One small study and several case reports have suggested that hydroxychloroquine may have some benefit in preventing flares (24). No treatment has been shown to remove CPPD deposits from cartilage.

CHRONIC PSEUDOGOUT

Some patients may develop accelerated osteoarthritis because of recurrent inflammation from pseudogout. Such patients benefit from physical therapy and other adjunct therapies for osteoarthritic problems. Others may eventually require total joint replacement. A small group of pseudogout patients have chronic painful inflammatory arthritis and may need NSAIDs on a continual basis.

Calcium Hydroxyapatite: Basic Calcium Phosphate Deposition Disease

Pathogenesis

Inflammatory arthritis and periarthritis (e.g., tendinitis) may be induced by calcium hydroxyapatite crystals in and around joints (25). Joints with previous injuries or damage appear to be particularly at risk. Periarticular structures (e.g, tendons, bursae) appear to be more prone than in gout or pseudogout. Hydroxyapatite crystals are part of a broader class of basic calcium phosphate (BCP) crystals. As opposed to the extensive knowledge of urate deposition disorders and the growing understanding of CPPD arthritis (i.e., pseudogout), less is known of the pathophysiology of hydroxyapatite deposition and disease. The increased calcium content of osteoarthritic cartilage and other injured musculoskeletal tissue relative to normal tissue may predispose to hydroxyapatite precipitation, but the exact pathogenic mechanisms are not known.

Clinical Manifestations

Hydroxyapatite crystal deposition is associated with periarthritic syndromes, particularly calcific periarthritis and tendinitis of the shoulder. Other joints that are commonly involved include the hips, knees, and fingers. The elderly and patients with underlying chronic or end-stage renal disease are more often affected. Hydroxyapatite crystal deposition may co-exist with pseudogout and, like CPPD disease, has a tendency to affect sites with osteoarthritis or other mechanical derangement.

Milwaukee shoulder is a chronic syndrome, more commonly affecting elderly women, in which hydroxyapatite deposition is associated with instability of the shoulder joint, marked loss of the structural integrity of the humeral head, calcifications of the surrounding soft tissues, and rotator cuff tears. Pseudopodagra (i.e., first metacarpophalangeal joint involvement) has been reported in young women with hydroxyapatite deposition disease (26).

Diagnosis

The diagnosis is normally based on the clinical picture alone with support from the physical examination (e.g., periarthritis) and X-ray evaluation (e.g., periarticular calcifications). Synovial fluid tends to be less inflammatory than in gout or pseudogout; leukocyte counts of less than 2000 cells/μL are typical. Although crystal identification is desired, BCP crystals are small and are not birefringent, rendering them difficult to identify by readily available means. The crystals are best visualized by electron microscopy, and confirmation may require examination by X-ray diffraction. "Clumps" of small crystals can sometimes be seen on polarized light microscopy, but these are non-specific and not diagnostically definitive.

Prognosis

Hydroxyapatite deposition tends to cause intermittent episodes of articular and periarticular inflammation. Although generally well controlled with appropriate therapy, rare individuals may develop a chronic destructive arthropathy. No prophylactic regimens have been shown to be effective, other than phosphate reduction in renal failure. Surgical intervention in Milwaukee shoulder can significantly improve function.

Management

Like other crystalline disorders, management of hydroxyapatite crystal disease is directed towards 1) treating acute attacks, 2) prophylaxis against future flares, and 3) control of chronic disease.

ACUTE ATTACKS OF HYDROXYAPATITE CRYSTAL DEPOSITION

Acute attacks are handled similarly to gout and pseudogout attacks (see Table 22-3), although the use of NSAIDs and colchicine may require more caution since many patients will have chronic renal insufficiency or end-stage renal disease.

PROPHYLAXIS OF HYDROXYAPATITE-RELATED ARTHRITIS

In patients with chronic renal failure, control of phosphate levels may help control attacks. In patients without chronic renal failure, no specific prophylactic regimens have been described. In calcific periarthritis of the shoulder, some authorities believe that mechanical disruption of deposits with a needle, even without aspiration or steroid injection, helps to prevent further attacks.

CHRONIC HYDROXYAPATITE ARTHRITIS AND PERIARTHRITIS

Conservative treatment of Milwaukee shoulder has generally not been successful. Acromioplasty with rotator cuff repair and total shoulder replacement have been used in this condition.

Calcium Oxalate Disease

Calcium oxalate-related arthritis is rare and tends to occur in the setting of renal failure (27). It can present as acute monoarthritis or oligoarthritis, often involving the knees, elbows, or ankles. The crystals can be identified in synovial fluid (see Table 22-1), and X-ray can show peri-articular and soft-tissue calcification. On occasion, there can be a chronic polyarthritis, with prominent tenosynovitis. The management of acute exacerbations is like that for other crystalline arthritides, but chronic disease tends to be less responsive to colchicine than gout or pseudogout.

REFERENCES

1. **Simkin PA.** The pathogenesis of podagra. Ann Intern Med. 1977;86:230-3.
2. **Mader R.** Repeated synovial fluid analysis may be needed to find crystals in gout. Clin Rheumatol. 1998;17:549-50.
3. **Wallace SL, Robinson H, Masi AT, et al.** Preliminary criteria for the classification of the acute arthritis of primary gout. Arthritis Rheum. 1977;20:895-900.
4. **Moriwaki Y, Yamamoto T, Takahashi S, et al.** Spot urine uric acid to creatinine ratio used in the estimation of uric acid excretion in primary gout. J Rheumatol. 2001;28:1306-10.
5. **Simkin PA.** When, why, and how should we quantify the excretion rate of urinary uric acid? J Rheumatol. 2001;28:1207-10.
6. **Hench PS.** The diagnosis of gout and gouty arthritis. J Lab Clin Med. 1936;22:48-55.
7. **Yu TF.** Diversity of clinical features in gouty arthritis. Semin Arthritis Rheum. 1984; 13:360-8.

8. **Fessel JW.** Renal outcomes of gout and hyperuricemia. Am J Med. 1979;67:74-82.

9. **Yu TF, Gutman AB.** Uric acid nephrolithiasis in gout: predisposing factors. Ann Intern Med. 1967;67:1133-48.

10. **Liang MH, Fries JF.** Asymptomatic hyperuricemia: the case for conservative management. Ann Intern Med. 1978;88:666-70.

11. **Gelber AC, Klag MJ, Mead LA, et al.** Gout and risk for subsequent coronary heart disease. The Meharry-Hopkins Study. Arch Intern Med. 1997;157:1436-40.

12. **Ritter J, Kerr LD, Valeriano-Marcet J, Spiera H.** ACTH revisitied: effective treatment for acute crystal induced synovitis in patients with multiple medical problems. J Rheumatol. 1994;21:696-9.

13. **Zurcher RM, Bock HA, Thiel G.** Excellent uricosuric efficacy of benzbromarone in cyclosporine-A-treated renal transplant patients: a prospective study. Nephrol Dial Transplant. 1994;9:548-51.

14. **Singer JZ, Wallace SL.** The allopurinol hypersensitivity syndrome: unnecessary morbidity and mortality. Arthritis Rheum. 1986;29:82-7.

15. **Hande KR, Noone RM, Stone WJ.** Severe allopurinol toxicity: description and guidelines for prevention in patients with renal insufficiency. Am J Med. 1984;76: 47-56.

16. **Lockard O Jr, Harmon C, Nolph K, Irvin W.** Allergic reaction to allopurinol with cross-reactivity to oxypurinol. Ann Intern Med. 1976;85:333-5.

17. **Fam AG, Dunne SM, Iazzetta J, Paton TW.** Efficacy and safety of desensitization to allopurinol following cutaneous reactions. Arthritis Rheum. 2001;44:231-8.

18. **Walz-LeBlanc BA, Reynolds WJ, MacFadden DK.** Allopurinol sensitivity in a patient with chronic tophaceous gout: success of intravenous desensitization after failure of oral desensitization. Arthritis Rheum. 1991;34:1329-31.

19. **Ippoliti G, Negri M, Campana C, Vigano M.** Urate oxidase in hyperuricemic heart transplant recipients treated with azathioprine. Transplantation. 1997;63:1370-1.

20. **Disla E, Infante R, Fahmy A, et al.** Recurrent acute calcium pyrophosphate dihydrate arthritis following intraarticular hyaluronate injection. Arthritis Rheum. 1999;42:1302-3.

21. **Resnick D, Rausch JM.** Hypomagnesemia with chondrocalcinosis. J Can Assoc Radiol. 1984;35:214-6.

22. **Chaisson CE, McAlindon TE, Felson DT, et al.** Lack of association between thyroid status and chondrocalcinosis or osteoarthritis. The Framingham Osteoarthritis Study. J Rheumatol. 1996;23:711-5.

23. **Van Geertruyden J, Kinnaert P, Frederic N, et al.** Effect of parathyroid surgery on cartilage calcification. World J Surg. 1986;10:111-5.

24. **Rothschild B, Yakubov LE.** Prospective 6-month, double-blind trial of hydroxychloroquine treatment of CPDD. Compr Ther. 1997;23:327-31.

25. **Schumacher HR, Smolyo AP, Tse RL, Maurer K.** Arthritis associated with apatite crystals. Ann Intern Med. 1977;87:411-6.

26. **Fam AG, Rubenstein J.** Hydroxyapatite pseudopodagra: a syndrome of young women. Arthritis Rheum. 1989;32:741-7.

27. **Rosenthal A, Ryan LM, McCarty DJ.** Arthritis associated with calcium oxalate crystals in an anephric patient treated with peritoneal dialysis. JAMA. 1988;260: 1280-2.

23

Metabolic Bone Diseases: Osteoporosis and Paget's Disease

Linda A. Russell, MD

Osteoporosis

Osteoporosis is a chronic progressive disorder that is defined by the presence of low bone mass, micro-architectural deterioration, bone fragility, and increased susceptibility to fracture. Osteoporosis differs from osteomalacia in that mineralization of osteoid is normal.

Roughly 25 million Americans are estimated to have osteoporosis. It is commonly encountered in the primary care setting, and the primary care provider should keep well informed as to current management issues and options; referral to a rheumatologist, endocrinologist, or other metabolic bone disease specialist is required only in severe or refractory cases. Nonetheless, despite its prevalence, osteoporosis is grossly underdiagnosed and undertreated. The overall burden placed by osteoporosis onto affected individuals and onto society can be greatly relieved with greater awareness and attention to this condition.

The impact of osteoporosis on public health is enormous (Table 23-1). In the United States, an estimated 1.5 million fractures per year are attributed to low bone mass. The majority of fractures are vertebral, which are often asymptomatic and noted incidentally on X-ray. Annually, there are about 700,000 vertebral fractures, 300,000 hip fractures, and 250,000 wrist fractures. Despite advances in the management of hip fractures, mortality within the first year after a hip fracture remains in excess of 15% to 20%. This impressive figure probably reflects not only the direct clinical consequences of hip fractures but also underlying co-morbidities that predispose patients to fractures. Fewer than one third of patients are ultimately restored to their premorbid functional status. Some estimates indicate that short-term costs associated with a new hip fracture exceed $40,000.

Table 23-1   Societal Impact of Osteoporosis in the United States

- 10 million individuals have osteoporosis.

- 18 million individuals have low bone mass.

- Direct financial expenditures for treatment of osteoporotic fractures are $10 to $15 billion annually.

- There are 700,000 spine fractures, 300,000 hip fractures, 250,000 wrist fractures and 300,000 other fractures annually.

- Mortality within the first year after a hip fracture is in excess of 15% to 20%.

Humans reach their peak bone mass in the third and fourth decade. Thereafter, men lose bone density at a slow steady pace (0.3% to 0.5% per year) throughout their lives. Women lose density at the same pace until menopause, when they begin to lose 2% to 5% per year for approximately 5 years, and then resume a rate of loss comparable to that in men.

Pathogenesis

In normal physiology, there is a tight coupling of bone formation by osteoblasts and resorption by osteoclasts. Through young adulthood, bone density increases because osteoblastic bone formation exceeds osteoclastic bone resorption. However, after the age of 40, pits created by osteoclasts within bone are inadequately filled in by osteoblasts, resulting in net loss of bone density due to bone resorption exceeding bone formation. In the healthy individual, trabecular bone is more affected than cortical bone due to its greater surface area. Because vertebral bodies are predominantly composed of trabecular bone, bone loss is often more readily apparent in the spine than in long bones. The actual dimensions of the trabeculae decrease, and more importantly, trabecular struts lose their connectivity. (There are a few exceptions to this pattern—e.g., in hyperparathyroidism, bone loss may be greater in cortical bone.)

Risk Factors and Etiology

Low bone mass and a prior fragility fracture are the most reliable predictors of fracture risk (1). It is estimated that one of every two Caucasian women will experience an osteoporotic fracture at some point in her life. The lifetime risk of hip fracture in white women is similar to the combined risk of breast, endometrial, and ovarian cancer. The risk for men is lower but, as for women, increases with age. Under World Health Organization (WHO) criteria, it is estimated that 15% of all Caucasian women in the United States and 35% of all women over the age of 65 years have osteoporosis. Most studies suggest that Caucasian and Asian women are more affected than African-American women. Regardless of epidemiologic data, however, all men and women of any ethnicity can be at risk for the development for osteoporosis, and patients should be considered individually, independently of sex and ethnicity.

Many risk factors for the development of osteoporosis have been identified. Some are modifiable, such as cigarette smoking, low calcium intake, lack of weight-bearing exercise, certain medications (e.g., corticosteroids), alcoholism, and poor general health and nutrition. Non-modifiable factors include a family history of osteoporosis or insufficiency fracture, Caucasian or East Asian race, advanced age, and female sex.

Maintaining an adequate intake of calcium and vitamin D throughout life is necessary to achieve and sustain peak bone mass. Hyperparathyroidism, due to a hyperfunctioning adenoma or a glandular response to an inadequate absorption or increased excretion of calcium, has a negative effect on calcium balance and promotes bone resorption. Hyperthyroidism also promotes bone resorption. Both estrogen and testosterone help achieve and maintain peak bone mass. Lack of mechanical load and its bone-stimulating effects will result in decreased bone mass, and any state leading to reduced activity will cause this. However, it should be emphasized that exercise resulting in amenorrhea will have a negative impact on bone density, as has been shown in elite long-distance runners. For the non-elite athlete, exercise seems to maintain but does not increase bone density.

Many drugs contribute to bone loss (Table 23-2), and the combined effect of exposure to these substances in the setting of hormonal abnormality or immobilization can lead to a more profound bone mass deficiency. The most common cause of drug-induced bone loss is corticosteroids. Corticosteroids inhibit osteoblast development and cause hypercalciuria and decreased calcium absorption in the intestine. This results in secondary hyperparathyroidism and increased bone resorption. Other drugs commonly implicated in bone loss include heparin, phenytoin, and excessive thyroid replacement.

Table 23-2   Medicines and Agents Associated with Bone Loss

• Corticosteroids	• Excessive alcohol
• Adrenocorticotropin	• Excessive thyroxine
• Gonadotropin-releasing hormone antagonists	• Cytotoxic drugs (e.g., cyclosporine, methotrexate)
• Heparin	• Aluminum toxicity
• Lithium	• Tamoxifen (premenopausal use)
• Phenytoin	• Aromatase inhibitors
• Tobacco	

Case Presentation

A 65-year-old Caucasian female who entered menopause two years ago is evaluated for possible osteoporosis. The evaluation was prompted by a recently recognized height loss in the setting of six months of corticosteroid therapy for polymyalgia rheumatica. She had been in good health and has never had a known fracture or a bone densitometry study. She has taken daily multivitamins containing vitamin D and calcium supplements sporadically for years and also occasionally drinks calcium-fortified juices. She reports that her deceased mother had a "hump" on her back. The physical examination is generally unremarkable, although she is 5 feet 6 inches in height and recalls being two inches taller in college.

A dual-energy X-ray absorptiometry (DEXA) scan revealed a T-score of -1.8 and a Z-score of -0.62 in the lumbar spine and a T-score of -1.4 and a Z-score of -0.41 in the femoral neck. The urine N-telopeptide (NTX) was elevated at 70 bone collagen equivalents (BCE)/nM creatinine.

Calcium supplementation (1500 mg/d in 3 divided doses) with vitamin D_3 800 IU daily was recommended. Because of the presence of osteopenia, the family history, and the continued need for corticosteroid treatment, the patient was also started on weekly oral alendronate 70 mg. Three months later, the urine NTX had fallen to 35 BCE/nM creatinine.

The patient continued on this regimen over the next eighteen months without increases in the urine NTX and was able to wean completely off of prednisone without recurrence of polymyalgia rheumatica. A repeated DEXA at this juncture showed improved T-scores of -1.5 and -1.2 in the lumbar spine and femoral neck, respectively.

Clinical Features

Until there is a symptomatic fracture, osteoporosis is usually clinically silent and is recognized only after screening bone densitometry studies are obtained. Plain radiograph findings are unreliable and non-quantitative and should not be used in the evaluation of the presence or extent of osteoporosis. If bone loss is suggested on plain X-ray, there may already be a 30% or more loss of bone density.

Unfortunately, the first recognized sign of osteoporosis is all too often a fragility fracture, a fracture sustained from minimal or no trauma. Examples include a rib fracture after a cough or a vertebral fracture sustained after opening a window. The most common areas of insufficiency fractures include the vertebral bodies, the hips, the wrists, the ribs, the ankles, and the feet. Other clinical features that can alert a health care provider to low bone mass include a thoracic kyphosis and significant loss of height; loss of more than two inches in height warrants an evaluation.

Clinicians should be aware of the presentation of common fragility fractures. Interestingly, more than 65% of vertebral fractures are asymptomatic.

These fractures may be noted incidentally on a chest X-ray. When a vertebral fracture is symptomatic, pain at the involved site is sudden in onset, can be exquisite, and often radiates in a band-like distribution anteriorly. In general, the pain gradually subsides over the course of 6 to 8 weeks. Vertebral fractures and anterior wedging of the vertebral bodies contribute to the kyphosis often seen in patients with severe osteoporosis (Fig. 23-1). Consequently, multiplanar mechanical changes due to such fractures can predispose to significant degenerative joint and disc disease in the spine.

Patients with a wrist fracture have point tenderness at the site of the fracture with associated overlying soft tissue swelling and pain with wrist motion. A fracture of the distal radius (Colles fracture) is the most common wrist fracture and can usually be diagnosed by plain radiography. However, if the X-ray appears normal and clinical suspicion remains high, a stress fracture should still be considered and, if desired, can be documented by a nuclear bone scan.

Ninety percent of hip fractures result from falls. A fall to the side increases the risk of fracturing the hip six-fold, while a fall on or near the hip increases the risk of hip fracture by twenty-fold. Twenty-five to 30% of all falls are side falls. Most patients are immediately aware that an injury has occurred. Patients note pain in the groin and thigh and lack the power to stand. Many tell of hearing a "crack." The involved leg is shortened and externally rotated. However, in many ways, an occult stress fracture of the hip is more important to recognize than is a frank fracture, because early diagnosis can significantly reduce morbidity. Patients with occult stress fractures of the hip may be able to ambulate despite discomfort in the pelvic

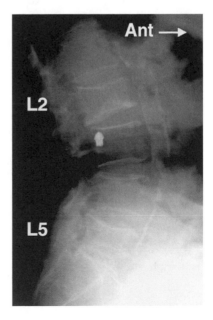

Figure 23-1 Plain radiograph (lateral view) of the lumbosacral spine showing compression fractures of L2 and L5 resulting in wedge deformities of the vertebral bodies. The metallic object overlying L3 is an artifact; Ant = anterior.

area, groin, buttock, or thigh. Continued weight-bearing may result in complete fracture of the compromised hip. The clinician must maintain a high level of suspicion, especially in patients suspected of severe osteoporosis, and obtain the appropriate imaging studies.

Diagnosis

Bone mass can be determined by a number of methods, the most common of which is dual-energy X-ray absorptiometry (DEXA), currently considered to be the gold standard. A bone mineral density (BMD) measurement should be considered for anyone deemed at risk for osteoporosis. The Bone Mass Measurement Act of 1998 details justifications for obtaining BMD and approves testing for estrogen-deficient women at risk for osteoporosis (Table 23-3). Other indications include a vertebral abnormality suggestive of fracture, systemic corticosteroid therapy (more than 3 months of 7.5 mg/day or greater of prednisone or equivalent), hyperparathyroidism, and monitoring during an FDA-approved treatment for osteoporosis.

The National Osteoporosis Foundation (NOF) recommends obtaining a bone density measurement on any patient with a fragility fracture. Consideration should also be given to women with an early menopause and anyone with a medical condition or using a drug known to predispose to osteoporosis. As technologies become more accessible and precise, BMD testing should become a more standard component of routine preventive health care.

Dual-Energy X-ray Absorptiometry (DEXA)
DEXA should be used for diagnosis and for monitoring the effects of treatment. With DEXA, the amount of mineralized tissue within a section of bone is measured and expressed in grams per centimeter squared. Axial DEXA, considered the gold standard for measuring BMD, has a precision of ±3%. Although any area of the body can be assessed, lumbar spine and hip measurements are the most commonly obtained because they are felt to be highly predictive of vertebral and hip fracture risks. Each individual

---

Table 23-3   Bone Mass Measurement Act of 1998

Obtain baseline BMD in
- Estrogen-deficient women at risk for osteoporosis
- Individuals with insufficiency fractures or suspected low bone mass by X-ray
- Individuals receiving corticosteroid therapy (more than 3 months of 7.5 mg/d or greater of prednisone or equivalent)
- Individuals with hyperparathyroidism

Obtain follow-up BMD
- Biyearly when monitoring patients on an FDA-approved therapy for low bone mass
- Yearly when monitoring patients with hyperparathyroidism or receiving corticosteroids

testing facility should perform frequent precision studies as outlined by the International Society for Clinical Densitometry, which recommends that both equipment and technicians are regularly evaluated.

Densitometers made by Hologic, Lunar, and Norland are the most commonly used in the United States. Currently, it is not possible to directly compare data obtained from densitometers made by two different manufacturers. Therefore optimal monitoring requires that serial studies be obtained on the same machine (or at least with the same manufacturer) to gain meaningful data to follow the clinical course of the patient.

Newer software permits a lateral view of the spine, which is helpful for the evaluation of vertebral fractures. Osteoarthritis and compression fractures can falsely elevate the BMD in the spine due to their increased bone density; an astute technician will eliminate data taken from vertebral bodies that might add artifact to measurements. Relative contraindications to spine DEXA include recent nuclear medicine tests and gastrointestinal contrast studies; it is advisable to wait 72 hours after the former and 2 weeks after the latter before obtaining a DEXA.

The results of DEXA yield two scores: the Z-score and the T-score (Fig. 23-2). The Z-score represents the number of standard deviations (SD) the measured bone density deviates from those of sex- and age-matched

Figure 23-2 Results of dual-energy X-ray absorptiometry of the lumbar spine (L1-L3) in a 74-year-old woman. Data from L4 had been excluded from analysis due to obvious degenerative changes that would falsely elevate bone density readings. The shaded areas in the graph depict the mean bone mineral density (±2 SD) as a function of age in a reference cohort of women. The darkly shaded region represents Z-scores from 0 to +2; the lightly shaded area represents Z-scores from 0 to -2. Although the patient has a bone mineral density that is close to average for her age (i.e., a Z-score of -0.24), she is nonetheless osteoporotic with a T-score of -2.57.

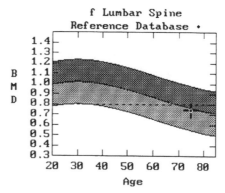

f Lumbar Spine
Reference Database •

BMD(L1-L3) = 0.735 g/cm^2

Region	BMD	T(30.0)		Z	
L1	0.673	-2.29	73%	-0.17	97%
L2	0.707	-2.91	69%	-0.56	92%
L3	0.808	-2.51	75%	-0.03	100%
N/A					
L1-L3	0.735	-2.57	72%	-0.24	97%

• Age and sex matched
T = peak BMD matched
Z = age matched   TK   10/25/91

healthy controls. In contrast, the T-score is the number of SD the measured bone density deviates from that of young healthy sex-matched individuals who are deemed to be at peak bone density.

The World Health Organization (WHO) has established criteria for the diagnosis of osteoporosis (Table 23-4). Individuals within one SD of peak bone density or better (T-score > -1.0) are considered to have normal bone density. If the bone density is between one and 2.5 SD below peak bone density (T-score = -1.0 to -2.5), osteopenia is diagnosed; if the bone density is 2.5 SD or more below peak bone density (T-score < -2.5), osteoporosis is diagnosed. In addition, individuals with T-scores of less than -2.5 *and* with a history of a fragility fracture (i.e., a fracture that occurs in the setting of minimal trauma), severe osteoporosis is diagnosed.

As reviewed below, there are several other methods available for the evaluation of bone density, but it should be appreciated that the most experience is with axial DEXA, on which the WHO criteria for the diagnosis of osteoporosis are based. All other methods must be compared with axial DEXA.

Other Modalities for the Assessment of Bone Density

DEXA and quantitative ultrasonography can measure BMD in peripheral areas such as the wrist or the heel. Because these are portable techniques, they can be used in populations not easily transported (e.g., group home or nursing home residents) and accordingly have been considered for screening purposes. However, diagnostic criteria have not been well established for these methods, and correlation with axial DEXA has not been standardized. In general, these techniques can be helpful when they identify osteoporosis, but a baseline axial DEXA should still be obtained so that response to treatment can be monitored. Moreover, even if these methods reveal normal measurements, a standard DEXA study should be obtained if the clinical suspicion for osteoporosis is high.

Axial quantitative computed tomography (CT) can be used in patients who weigh too much for the DEXA table (usually over 250 lb) or who have significant spinal degenerative arthritis that makes DEXA inaccurate. CT

Table 23-4   World Health Organization Definitions of Osteopenia and Osteoporosis

Normal	BMD within 1 SD of a "young normal" individual or better (T-score > –1)
Osteopenia	BMD between 1 and 2.5 SD below that of a "young normal" (T-score between –1 and –2.5)
Osteoporosis	BMD 2.5 SD or more below that of a "young normal" (T-score < 2.5)
Severe osteoporosis	T-score < –2.5 with previous insufficiency/fragility fractures

BMD = bone mineral density; SD = standard deviation.

may also provide more data on bone quality than DEXA; this information may be valuable in the research setting.

Markers of Bone Activity

Bone density measurements provide information about current skeletal mass but do not provide information about bone quality or its metabolic activity. This is extremely important because bone is a dynamic tissue in a constant state of flux involving osteoblasts and osteoclasts that respectively form and break down bone matrix continually. Markers of bone *formation* include osteocalcin, bone alkaline phosphatase, and the N- and C-terminal propeptides of type I collagen. Markers of bone *resorption* include urine and serum N-telopeptide (NTX), urine C-telopeptide, pyridinoline, and deoxypyridinoline. The most commonly used marker to assess bone turnover is the urine N-telopeptide, although the serum N-telopeptide is becoming increasingly available. In addition to osteoporosis, markedly elevated bone markers can be seen in other conditions characterized by bone resorption, such as hyperthyroidism, hyperparathyroidism, Paget's disease, hypercalcemia of malignancy, multiple myeloma, and bone metastatic disease.

Many studies have shown that levels of various bone markers have predictive value for BMD measurements in osteoporosis (2). For example, a 1 SD increase in urine NTX above that of a healthy premenopausal woman is associated with a 1.5-to 2.5-fold increase in bone loss over the next year. In a practical sense, in most commercial assays, a urine NTX value above 50 BCE/nM creatinine is suggestive of ongoing bone loss. One surrogate goal in the treatment or prevention of osteoporosis is to institute therapy that will lower the urine NTX value to the range seen in healthy premenopausal women (<45 BCE/nM).

Bone markers also predict fracture risk. Independently of absolute bone density, states of high bone turnover (i.e., increased osteoclast and osteoblast activity), as reflected in elevations in markers of bone activity, are associated with increased risk of fracture. The EPIDOS study found that each SD increase in C-telopeptide or free deoxypyridinoline level is associated with a 1.3- or 1.4-fold increase in hip fracture over a mean follow-up time of 22 months (3).

Markers are commonly used to monitor ongoing osteoporosis therapy. Within 3 to 6 months of the initiation of a successful treatment plan, bone marker values should improve. This has been demonstrated for hormone replacement therapy, bisphosphonates, calcitonin, and the selective estrogen receptor modulators. If a reduction in bone marker is not observed, the practitioner should reassess patient adherence, consider other diagnoses leading to bone loss, and/or consider a change in therapy.

There are limitations to the use of bone markers in clinical practice. There is a circadian rhythm to bone resorption, which is greater at night. To maximize reliability and optimize standardization, urine NTX specimens should be taken from the second voided urine of the day. Blood in the urine will interfere with testing. Although somewhat prohibitive secondary to cost, an average of several samples would be most representative of true bone turnover. Increasingly used automated assays for urine NTX should also improve testing. Serum testing, which is also becoming more commonly available, will eliminate inaccuracies due to correction for creatinine in urine samples and also allow measurement in patients with renal failure.

Synthesizing Laboratory Data

The BMD measurement and bone marker values provide useful information about a patient's bone health but may not provide all the needed information. If the patient has had a fragility fracture but the bone density value appears normal, the clinician must consider causes of impaired bone quality and causes for osteomalacia should be sought (Table 23-5). If a patient has multiple unexplained fragility fractures and a cause is not obvious, a bone biopsy may be indicated and can provide information about bone turnover. Tetracycline-labeling (i.e., an oral load of tetracycline) can aid the pathologist in making the diagnosis. Bone biopsy is rarely required, however, because the diagnosis can often be made based on clinical and non-invasive means.

If the Z-score (age-matched) is more than 1.0 SD below expected, secondary causes of osteoporosis should be considered (Table 23-6). Diseases commonly encountered include vitamin D deficiency, hyperthyroidism, hyperparathyroidism, malabsorption states, inflammatory diseases, Cushing's disease/syndrome, bone marrow processes such as multiple myeloma or storage diseases, Marfan's syndrome, alcoholism, liver disease, and estrogen/testosterone deficiency. Many studies have documented that vitamin D deficiency is quite common among the elderly, who tend to be exposed to less sunlight. Appropriate testing, as guided by the clinical setting, may include

- Calcium
- Phosphorus
- Alkaline phosphatase
- 25-hydroxy-vitamin D
- Thyroid function tests
- Intact parathyroid hormone
- Anti-gliadin antibody
- Anti-endomysial antibody
- Anti-tissue transglutaminase antibody
- Serum and urine immunoelectrophoresis
- 24-hour urine for calcium
- Dexamethasone suppression assay
- Follicular stimulating hormone
- Luteinizing hormone
- Testosterone

Recognition and treatment of underlying causes of osteoporosis are essential to the development of an optimal treatment plan.

Prognosis and Disease Outcomes

A loss of one SD from peak bone mass in the spine is associated with a two-fold increased risk of vertebral fracture, and a loss of one SD from peak

Table 23-5   Causes of Osteomalacia

Abnormalities of vitamin D metabolism
- Vitamin D deficiency
- Liver disease
- Renal disease
- 1-α-hydroxylase deficiency
- Vitamin D resistance

Hypophosphatemia
- Renal disease
- Antacid abuse

Toxins
- Fluoride
- Etidronate
- Aluminum

Others
- Acidosis
- Hypophosphatasia
- Oncogenic osteomalacia

Table 23-6   Disorders Associated with Osteoporosis

Endocrine disorders
- Acromegaly
- Cushing's disease/syndrome
- Eating disorders
- Gonadal insufficiency
- Hyperparathyroidism
- Hyperprolactinemia
- Hyperthyroidism or excessive thyroid replacement
- Type 1 diabetes mellitus

Gastrointestinal disease
- Celiac disease
- Gastrectomy
- Inflammatory bowel disease
- Jejunoileal bypass
- Malabsorption states
- Pancreatic insufficiency
- Parenteral nutrition

Marrow-related disorders
- Amyloid
- Hemochromatosis
- Hemophilia
- Leukemia
- Lymphoma

Marrow-related disorders (cont'd)
- Mastocytosis
- Multiple myeloma
- Sarcoidosis
- Sickle cell anemia
- Thalassemia

Organ transplantation

Rheumatologic disorders
- Ankylosing spondylitis and spondyloarthropathies
- Rheumatoid arthritis

Multiple sclerosis

Chronic obstructive pulmonary disease

Scoliosis

Marfan's syndrome

Congenital porphyria

Homocystinuria

Genetic disorders
- Hypophosphastasia
- Osteogenesis imperfecta

bone mass in the hip is associated with a 2.5-fold increased risk of hip fracture. Moreover, other data indicate that states of high bone turnover are also associated with higher fracture risks. This may, in part, explain why even modest increases in bone density may result in substantially lower fracture risks.

Needless to say, fragility fractures, especially of the hip, carry significant morbidity and mortality. The mortality rate in the first year after a hip fracture exceeds 15% to 20%. This is felt to represent the various disease states that predispose the patient to the fracture as well as complications directly resulting from the fracture itself. Vertebral fractures can result in severe pain, subject the patient to adverse effects of analgesic and anti-inflammatory medications, and result in substantial cardiopulmonary, gastrointestinal, neurologic, and orthopedic problems due to severe postural changes.

Despite the increasing awareness of osteoporosis, many studies have demonstrated that practitioners are not diagnosing and treating osteoporosis appropriately. In a recent study of postmenopausal ambulatory care female patients, almost half were unrecognized as having low bone density. More distressing is that even among patients with known insufficiency fractures, few are being evaluated or given appropriate therapy. An audit of patients with an incident fracture attending a tertiary teaching hospital revealed that only 32% subsequently had a BMD test and only 39% were offered treatment for osteoporosis. Given the high risk of a second insufficiency fracture after a first, these practices are unacceptable.

Management

General principles for the management of osteoporosis are summarized in Table 23-7. Emphasis is placed on early identification of patients at risk and a multifaceted approach to prevention and treatment of osteoporosis and reduction of fracture risks.

Calcium and Vitamin D Supplementation
All patients with bone loss or a potential for bone loss should receive adequate daily intake of calcium and vitamin D. Both the National Institutes of Health (NIH) and the NOF have published guidelines. If the diet does not provide sufficient quantity, supplements should be prescribed. In general, adults at risk for bone loss should obtain 1500 mg of calcium and 600 IU of

---

Table 23-7   Principles in the Prevention and Treatment of Osteoporosis

- Counsel all patients on the risk factors for osteoporosis.

- Advise patients on appropriate calcium and vitamin D intake.

- Evaluate bone density in patients deemed at risk (Table 23-6).

- Devise an appropriate weight-bearing/strengthening exercise program.

- If possible, discontinue any medications that may contribute to osteoporosis (Table 23-2).

- Prescribe pharmacologic therapy when indicated
   - Anti-resorptive agents: bisphosphonates, estrogens, selective estrogen receptor modulators, calcitonin
   - Anabolic agent: teriparatide

vitamin D_3 per day. Calcium and vitamin D_3 reduce bone resorption and mineralize osteoid, thereby increasing bone mass. In certain groups, this translates into decreased fracture rates. For example, in nursing home populations, the incidence of hip fracture is reduced with supplementation with calcium and vitamin D (4). However, because of rapid bone resorption around menopause, calcium and vitamin D supplementation alone cannot prevent net bone loss in women who are perimenopausal. In patients taking corticosteroids, supplemental calcium and vitamin D help slow the loss of bone density. However, the ability of calcium and vitamin D to maintain or increase bone density in either postmenopausal women or in patients on corticosteroids is limited, and concurrent anti-resorptive therapy is usually necessary for optimal care.

The two most widely available forms of calcium are calcium carbonate and calcium citrate, both of which are acceptable agents. Limited evidence suggests that calcium citrate is better absorbed, can be taken with or without meals, and may be a more judicious choice in patients with achlorhydria, nephrolithiasis, or constipation. There are many sources of vitamin D. Multivitamin tablets usually contain 400 IU of vitamin D_3, and vitamin D_3 can now be found in many calcium supplements as well. For patients with significant vitamin D deficiency, other forms of vitamin D such as cholecalciferol and calcitriol may be appropriate.

Lifestyle Modifications

Patients should be counseled on a multi-disciplinary approach to the management of osteoporosis and the prevention of fractures. The clinician should be involved in facilitating appropriate lifestyle modifications such as cessation of smoking and avoidance of excessive alcohol consumption. Vision should be monitored, and corrective eyewear prescribed when needed. Patients should be instructed in weight-bearing and muscle-strengthening exercises. Rigid hip protectors disperse the force from trauma to the trochanter and, if worn properly, have been shown to reduce the risk of hip fractures by as much as 50% and should be offered to any individual with osteoporosis deemed at risk for falls.

Malnutrition is present in many elderly patients who sustain hip fractures and may indeed be an important contributing factor to gait disturbances and bone fragility predisposing to falls and fractures. The NHANES I follow-up study data demonstrated that weight loss from a maximum reported body weight in women aged 50 to 64 years and 65 to 74 years increased the relative risks of hip fracture to 2.54 and 2.04, respectively. Thin women were at particular risk. Therefore, to ensure optimal recovery after a fracture, nutritional status should be addressed. Aggressive protein supplementation after repair of hip fractures results in weight gain, shorter hospitalizations, and fewer postoperative complications.

Fall prevention should be a focus of the health care team. Many elderly patients are reluctant to use assistive devices, and so their importance should be emphasized. Ensuring that the living environment is safe (e.g., installation of night lights, use of non-slip footwear, removal of loose rugs or wiring) is also crucial.

Finally, patients that have had fractures may begin to feel socially isolated because they fear leaving home. Progressive thoracic kyphosis and slow recovery after a spinal fracture make independent community ambulation more difficult. Physical rehabilitation after a fracture is essential to prevent further comorbidities and to hasten the return to normal function. Moreover, emphasis must be placed on addressing psychosocial issues such as treating possible depression and re-establishing independence. Modalities such as Tai Chi can help improve balance and strength as well as promote psychological well-being.

Pharmacological Therapy

Theoretically, bone density can be increased by either promoting bone formation by osteoblasts or inhibiting bone resorption by osteoclasts.

Agents for stimulating bone growth are limited. Teriparatide, recently approved by the FDA as the first available agent for the treatment of osteoporosis that acts by stimulating trabecular bone formation, is an important addition to the existing therapeutic options. Although sodium fluoride has long been known to increase bone formation, the quality of the newly formed bone with dosages used in available studies was found to be poor and in fact led to an increase in fracture rate. Investigations assessing the effects of different dosing regimens of sodium fluoride are in progress. Studies on the use of anabolic steroids in osteoporosis have demonstrated intolerable virilizing effects.

In contrast, many anti-resorptive therapies are now available, notably bisphosphonates, estrogen, raloxifene, and calcitonin. Many authorities recommend the addition of anti-resorptive therapy if the T-score is -1.5 or worse with major risk factors for fracture or -2.0 or worse without risk factors. Decisions about treatment must be made based on the individual's bone density and associated medical conditions. Factors to consider include menopausal status, degree of active bone turnover, concomitant medical illnesses, use of medications contributing to bone loss, and the patient's level of activity. If the patient is at risk for imminent bone loss, such as with the initiation of corticosteroid therapy, anti-resorptive therapy may be considered regardless of the results of bone densitometry. It is well established that the use of corticosteroids is associated with rapid bone loss during the first three months of therapy. The American College of Rheumatology has suggested that patients who are anticipated to require daily doses of prednisone of 5 mg or more for at least 3 months should be given prophylactic therapy against loss of bone mass (5). Some clinicians, in fact, are very aggressive and advocate developing a plan to combat osteoporosis as soon as the decision is made to use corticosteroids for more than 2 weeks. If a patient has already had an insufficiency fracture, anti-resorptive therapy should also be strongly considered. Moreover, if the T-score is worse than -2.5, combination therapy can be recommended; for example, the combination of alendronate and estrogen has been shown to produce larger increases in BMD than by either agent alone.

BISPHOSPHONATES

Bisphosphonates adhere to bone and inhibit osteoclast activity. Etidronate, a first-generation bisphosphonate, was shown to increase BMD and reduce vertebral fracture rate but has been associated with osteomalacia. This is less of a concern for the newer bisphosphonates, alendronate and risedronate. There is now nearly a decade of post-marketing data on the use of alendronate.

Alendronate has been shown to increase hip BMD by 5% and spine BMD by 8% at three years and to decrease the incidence of hip fractures by 51% and vertebral fractures by 47% (6). Its major adverse effect is esophageal irritation, occurring perhaps in up to 30% of patients, even though pre-marketing data suggest no increased incidence compared with placebo. Over a 3-year period, risedronate-treated patients had a BMD increase of 5.4% in the lumbar spine and 1.6% in the femoral neck, and the rates of new vertebral and non-vertebral fractures were reduced by 41% and 39% respectively (7). There are no convincing data that these two agents differ in efficacy, although there is some suggestion that risedronate may be less irritating to the esophagus. Both agents have been shown to prevent corticosteroid-associated bone loss.

Alendronate 5 mg daily can be given for the prevention of osteoporosis and 10 mg daily for the treatment of osteoporosis. Recent studies have revealed that weekly dosing (35 mg for prevention and 70 mg for treatment of osteoporosis) appears comparable to daily dosing both with respect to efficacy and safety. Risedronate is available in 5 mg tablets for daily dosing and a 35 mg tablet for weekly dosing for the prevention and treatment of osteoporosis. In general, both agents are effective, safe, and well tolerated.

The use of bisphosphonates in women of childbearing age has not been well studied, and the benefit of their use in this population should be weighed against the potential risks. Specifically, because the terminal elimination half-lives of these agents are exceedingly long (at least 10 years for alendronate), it is not clear whether slow leeching from maternal bone can affect fetal development. In contrast, bisphosphonates are often an excellent choice for the treatment of men with osteoporosis of all ages (8).

Although not FDA-approved for the treatment of osteoporosis, intravenous pamidronate administered over several hours has been fairly well studied for this application. In many studies, pamidronate 30 mg IV every 3 months significantly increases BMD and decreases fracture rate. Flu-like symptoms in the 48 hours after the infusion are common but can be prevented with diphenhydramine and acetaminophen. Intravenous zolendric acid, currently approved for the treatment of hypercalcemia of malignancy, is also being studied for the treatment of osteoporosis. Compared with pamidronate, the administration of zolendric acid requires a shorter infusion time (45 min) and less frequent dosing (yearly).

ESTROGEN

Estrogens bind to specific receptors within osteoclasts, resulting in altered expression of many genes and ultimately in the inhibition of bone resorptive activities. The effect of hormone replacement therapy (HRT) on bone health has not been studied with the same methodological rigor as have the bisphosphonates. Conjugated equine estrogen in the form of Premarin 0.625 mg daily has been studied in the treatment and prevention of osteoporosis and appears to increase bone mass by about 2% per year. In non-randomized studies, Premarin has been shown to decrease fracture rates at all sites by 50%. It is unclear whether a 0.3 mg dosage has an equivalent effect. The best prospective data comes from the Women's Health Initiative Randomized Controlled Trial in which 5 fewer hip fractures per 10,000 person-years were observed in women randomized to conjugated equine estrogen 0.625 mg/d plus medroxyprogesterone acetate 2.5 mg/d (9). The patients were followed for a mean of 5.2 years.

The use of estrogen for the treatment of low bone mass must be weighed against the potential risks of estrogen supplementation in each individual patient. The Women's Health Initiative also found that there were 7 more coronary artery disease events, 8 more strokes, 8 more pulmonary emboli, and 8 more invasive breast cancers per 10,000 person-years among women taking estrogen/progesterone when compared with those taking placebo. Importantly, the mortality rates in the two groups were not significantly different. At present, however, given the availability of alternative medications, estrogen is beginning to fall out favor for management of osteoporosis in most women.

SELECTIVE ESTROGEN RECEPTOR MODULATORS (SERMS)

SERMs are a new class of agents that includes raloxifene, which has been approved for the prevention and treatment of osteoporosis. The effect of SERMs on osteoclasts is similar to that of natural estrogens. Over three years, raloxifene 60 mg daily increases BMD in the spine by 3% and decreases the incidence of vertebral fractures by 40% (10). No benefit has yet been demonstrated in reducing hip fractures. SERMs appear to reduce the risk of breast cancer, and studies with raloxifene have not shown an increased risk of uterine cancer. The benefit on lipids is favorable. However, SERMs can precipitate postmenopausal symptoms, and there is an increased risk of thrombosis.

CALCITONIN

Calcitonin is available in a nasal spray. The daily dose is 200 IU, alternating nostrils each day. Of currently available options, it is the least effective antiresorptive agent. It is indicated for patients who cannot or prefer not to take other, more effective agents. One study demonstrated possible increase in spine BMD and reduction in vertebral fractures. No benefit has been noted in the hip. Limited data suggest that it may reduce pain associated with fracture. Side effects are minimal, including nasal irritation and minor epistaxis which occurs in 2% of patients. Calcitonin is also available as a subcutaneous injection (100 IU daily), but this form has fallen out of favor with the availability of the nasal preparation.

Teriparatide

Teriparatide, a recombinant polypeptide identical to the biologically active 34-residue amino-terminus of human parathyroid hormone (hPTH), has been recently approved for the treatment of osteoporosis in postmenopausal women and in hypogonadal men. hPTH stimulates both bone formation and resorption. Although continuous dosing leads to net bone loss, intermittent dosing results in net bone formation. Moreover, the quality of the new bone appears to be normal. The approved dose of teriparatide is 20 µg/d given subcutaneously for two years.

Over a median follow-up period of 21 months, postmenopausal women with prior vertebral fractures treated with teriparatide had increased BMD in the lumbar spine and femoral neck as compared to a loss of BMD in matched controls that received placebo (11). This was associated with a relative risk of 0.33 for a new vertebral fracture and a relative risk of 0.46 for a new non-vertebral fracture in patients treated with teriparatide. Smaller studies suggest teriparatide may be more effective than even bisphosphonates in improving BMD and reducing fracture rates in postmenopausal women with osteoporosis (12). Teriparatide has also been shown to improve vertebral and femoral neck BMD in osteoporotic men, but data on fracture rates are lacking (13).

One area of great interest is the prospect of combining the bone forming properties of teriparatide with the effects of antiresorptive agents, especially since the benefits of teriparatide are reversible with discontinuation of the drug. A small 3-year study has demonstrated that teriparatide given to women already receiving estrogen replacements resulted in increased spine and hip BMD compared with women receiving estrogen alone. The increased BMD remained stable even after teriparatide had been discontinued for one year. In another study of postmenopausal osteoporotic women, alendronate therapy given *sequentially* after a year of native hPTH treatment not only maintained hPTH improvement in spine BMD but actually increased it further, suggesting a synergistic beneficial effect to sequential therapy with hPTH followed by bisphosphonates (14). However, *simultaneous* administration of alendronate appears to diminish the clinical benefit of PTH, indicating that at least some bisphosphonates may interfere with the bone-forming properties of teriparatide when given concurrently. Ongoing studies evaluating combination therapies are in process.

In clinical trials, teriparatide demonstrates a good safety profile, but it may not be appropriate for patients with various causes of osteomalacia and those with hyperparathyroidism. The most common complaints associated with teriparatide were headache, nausea, dizziness, leg cramps, and injection site reactions (erythema and swelling). Mild hypercalcemia and hypercalciuria have also been noted, particularly with higher dosages. In young developing rats, there appears to be an increased incidence of osteosarcoma with long-term high-dose teriparatide, but this has not been demonstrated in human trials at therapeutic doses. Teriparatide should not be prescribed to patients with metabolic bone disorders other than osteoporosis (such as Paget's disese), prior radiation to the skeleton, or pre-existing hypercalcemia or to children and young adults with open epiphyses.

Corticosteroid-Induced Osteoporosis

Corticosteroids pose the greatest risk for drug-related osteoporosis and warrants special attention. Bone loss is greatest during the first three months after the start of corticosteroid therapy. There is no dosage of corticosteroid that does not adversely affect the balance between osteoblasts and osteoclasts: the greater the exposure to corticosteroids, the greater is the risk of bone resorption. However, the American College of Rheumatology has developed recommendations for the prevention and treatment of corticosteroid-induced osteoporosis (5). If a patient is expected to be taking more than 5 mg/d of prednisone (or equivalent) for more than 3 months, then a plan should be implemented to evaluate and treat potential bone loss. Similarly, patients exposed to frequent high dose pulses (e.g., corticosteroid dose packs for asthma exacerbations) should be considered at risk and managed accordingly.

Corticosteroid dosages should be the lowest possible necessary to control the disease process at hand in order to minimize adverse bone effects. Steroid-sparing agents should always be considered to minimize exposure to corticosteroids. All patients should have a baseline BMD study obtained early in the course of chronic corticosteroid therapy and every year thereafter. As for all individuals at risk for osteoporosis, weight-bearing activities and adequate calcium and vitamin D intake should be emphasized, and lifestyle risk factors that adversely affect bone should be identified and modified.

If the patient is osteopenic or osteoporotic, pharmacologic therapy should be immediately recommended. Alendronate and risendronate have been shown to prevent bone loss in patients receiving corticosteroids. Teriparatide has also been shown to prevent bone loss in corticosteroid-induced osteoporosis (15). Hormone replacement therapy can increase spine BMD by 3% to 4% in patients with rheumatoid arthritis taking corticosteroids (16). Thiazide diuretics reduce hypercalciuria associated with corticosteroid use; loop diuretics, on the other hand, promote hypercalciuria. This should be taken into account if diuretic use is required.

Patients treated with corticosteroids with normal initial BMD should still obtain yearly DEXA, but ACR and NOF guidelines do not generally recommend medications beyond calcium and vitamin D supplementation unless patients become osteopenic with continued corticosteroids use. Some clinicians nonetheless advocate bisphosphonate prophylaxis against osteoporosis if the daily dose of corticosteroids exceeds prednisone 15 mg (or equivalent), even in patients with normal BMD.

Male Osteoporosis

Increasing attention is being given to male osteoporosis. There are no strict recommendations on when to obtain a baseline BMD measurement in men. If a male patient has any risk factors for osteoporosis, then a baseline DEXA should be obtained. As testing becomes more available and less expensive, it may be reasonable to obtain a baseline BMD on all men at 70 years of age. If low bone mass is documented, possible secondary causes should be evaluated. Hypogonadism may be present in up to 30% of men with osteoporosis, and hormone replacement therapy may be indicated. Men being treated for prostate cancer with orchiectomy or gonadotropin releasing hormone inhibitors are at great risk for osteoporosis. These patients should have a baseline BMD, and the use of bisphosphonates or teriparatide, known to improve hip and spine BMD in men, should be strongly considered. Unfortunately, studies to date have been either too small or too brief to provide data on the risk of fractures with these medications in men.

Osteoporosis in Premenopausal Women

The use of bisphosphonates in women before conception has not been well studied. There are theoretical concerns about the effects of bisphosphonates on a developing fetus. Appropriate calcium and vitamin D supplementation should be emphasized. The importance of menstruation and adequate estrogen levels must be evaluated, and estrogen replacement may be indicated if a deficiency is identified. Calcitonin can be given safely, although it is only marginally efficacious. Teriparatide may also prove to be a very useful alternative for treatment of low bone mass in a premenopausal woman planning possible future conception.

Surgical Approaches

Several techniques have recently become available to treat vertebral fractures. In addition to causing severe pain, vertebral fractures have profound effects on posture, overall mobility, and cardiopulmonary function, resulting in marked morbidity. Vertebroplasty involves injecting cement directly into fractures within the vertebral bodies and has been shown to decrease pain, increase mobility, and improve spine stability. There is no effect on fracture risk reduction or deformities. Kyphoplasty involves injecting polymethyl methacrylate (with barium sulfate for visualization) under low pressure into the involved vertebral body. The fracture may be reduced, and pain relief is rapid. The procedure is well tolerated. Large randomized studies comparing these procedures to conservative management are planned.

Early surgical treatment of hip fractures has been shown to reduce morbidity and mortality. In one study of patients over the age of 80 with hip fractures, surgical repair performed within 24 hours was associated with one-year mortality rate of 0%, while the mortality rate was 25% when surgery is delayed for more than 72 hours. Surgical options include open reduction with internal fixation, hemiarthroplasty, and total arthroplasty. Diligent perioperative medical management is crucial in determining the ultimate outcome of surgery. Prevention of infectious complications, prophylaxis against thromboembolic disease, nutritional support, physical rehabilitation, and prevention of recurrences are essential aspects in the care of these patients (17).

Disease Monitoring

Serial DEXA scans every one or two years should be used to monitor response to therapy. For most postmenopausal women on appropriate therapy, two-year follow-up is adequate. For patients with known secondary causes of osteoporosis (e.g., corticosteroid use, hyperparathyroidism), one-year follow-up is appropriate. In patients with normal bone density or mild osteopenia, serial DEXA scans every two years will enable the practitioner to decide if and when to begin therapy.

If a patient appears to have a loss of bone density despite apparently appropriate therapy, further investigation is indicated to identify mitigating factors. Previously unrecognized or newly developed secondary causes of osteoporosis, lack of patient compliance to therapy, and technical difficulties with scanners may all obscure clinical monitoring.

The urine NTX can be helpful in monitoring therapy. A decrease in the urine NTX three months after the initiation of an antiresorptive regiment is an encouraging indication that therapy is effective. At present, peripheral bone density modalities are not considered to be reliable for the monitoring of therapy.

Paget's Disease

Paget's disease or osteitis deformans is a focal disorder of bone remodeling. There is accelerated focal remodeling of bone such that excessive bone formation and resorption result in structurally abnormal bone. The process can involve single or multiple bones and is driven by dysregulated bone resorption leading to a compensatory increase in osteoblast activity. The newly formed bone is structurally disorganized, resulting in an overall decrease in bone strength and an increase in susceptibility to bowing and fractures. The abnormal bone is characterized by a high level of vascularity and an excess of connective tissue in the marrow.

Clinical Features

The most commonly involved bones in Paget's disease are the pelvis, vertebrae, skull, femur, and tibia. Patients may present with bone pain and deformity, although quite often the lesion is noted incidentally on plain radiography (Fig. 23-3) or following evaluation of an elevated serum alkaline phosphatase. Mechanical complications of deformed bone generally account for symptoms. The skull can become enlarged and compress cranial nerves, most notably the eighth cranial nerve, leading to hearing loss. Pain in the lower extremities can result from bowing of the long bones, involvement of joints, or gait disturbances.

Rarely, involved bone can transform into an osteosarcoma, which is poorly responsive to chemotherapy.

Diagnosis

Diagnosis of Paget's disease can by made by X-ray in most instances, but a whole-body bone scan is helpful in assessing the full extent of the disease. Markers of bone formation and bone resorption are elevated. The serum alkaline phosphatase is considered an indicator of disease activity. Serial X-rays in patients with lytic lesions in weight-bearing bones are helpful to document healing.

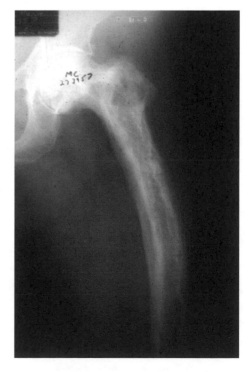

Figure 23-3 Plain radiograph showing cortical thickening, expansion, and mixed areas of osteolysis and sclerosis in the proximal left femur of patient with Paget's disease. Also characteristic is the bowing deformity of the bone and the concentric joint space narrowing of the hip.

Management

Treatment for Paget's disease is usually indicated for symptomatic patients and for patients with extensive disease and associated elevated metabolic rate. Because of increased vascularity, patients having elective surgery on involved bones (e.g., total hip replacement in a patient with pelvic or femoral involvement) should be treated first to minimize intra-operative blood loss. Rarely, Paget's disease can be complicated by hypercalcemia, another indication for therapy. Finally, therapy should be considered in patients with sites of involvement that may cause complicating secondary problems (e.g., skull and long bones of the lower extremities).

The bisphosphonates are effective inhibitors of bone resorption and consequently are the treatment of choice for Paget's disease (18). Six different bisphosphonates are currently available. Intravenous agents include pamidronate and zolendric acid, and etidronate, tiludronate, alendronate, and risedronate are available for oral therapy. Both alendronate (40 mg daily for 6 months) and risedronate (30 mg daily for 2-3 months) have been shown to normalize the biochemical indices for bone turnover in patients with moderate-to-severe Paget's disease. Etidronate and tiludronate are less potent and therefore now used infrequently. For patients who cannot tolerate oral bisphosphonates, intravenous pamidronate (60-90 mg every 3 months) or zolendric acid (4 mg once a year) can be given (19,20). Calcium and vitamin D should be supplemented during bisphosphonate therapy.

Subcutaneous salmon calcitonin (starting at 50-150 U daily) is an older therapy that has become less frequently used since the advent of bisphosphonate therapy. Daily doses can be administered for 1 to 3 months before tapering as dictated by the clinical response.

It can take 2 to 3 months after the onset of therapy to see biochemical improvement. The serum alkaline phosphatase is useful for assessing response to treatment and for monitoring relapses.

REFERENCES

1. **Lindsay R, Silverman SL, Cooper C, et al.** Risk of new vertebral fracture in the year following a fracture. JAMA. 2001;285:320-3.
2. **Miller PD, Baran DT, Bilezikian JP, et al.** Practical clinical application of biochemical markers of bone turnover: consensus of an expert panel. J Clin Densitom. 1999;2:323-42.
3. **Garnero P, Hausherr E, Chapuy MC, et al.** Markers of bone resorption predict hip fracture in elderly women. The EPIDOS Prospective Study. J Bone Miner Res. 1996;11:1531-8.
4. **Chapuy MC, Arlot ME, Duboeuf F, et al.** Vitamin D_3 and calcium to prevent hip fractures in elderly women. N Engl J Med. 1992;327:1637-42.
5. Recommendations for the prevention and treatment of glucocorticoid-induced osteoporosis; 2001 update. American College of Rheumatology Ad Hoc Committee on Glucocorticoid-Induced Osteoporosis. Arthritis Rheum. 2001;44:1496-1503.

6. **Liberman UA, Weiss SR, Broll J, et al.** Effect of oral alendronate on bone mineral density and the incidence of fractures in postmenopausal osteoporotic women. The Alendronate Phase III Osteoporosis Treatment Study Group. N Engl J Med. 1995; 333:1437-43.

7. **Harris ST, Watts NB, Genant HK, et al.** Effects of risedronate treatment on vertebral and nonvertebral fractures in women with postmenopausal osteoporosis: a randomized controlled trial. Vertebral Efficacy with Risendronate Therapy (VERT) Study Group. JAMA. 1999;282:1344-52.

8. **Orwoll E, Etttinger M, Weiss S, et al.** Alendronate for the treatment of osteoporosis in men. N Engl J Med. 2000;343:604-10.

9. **Rossouw JE, Anderson GL, Prentice RL, et al.** Risks and benefits of estrogen plus progestin in healthy postmenopausal women: principal results from the Women's Health Initiative randomized controlled trial. JAMA. 2002;288:321-33.

10. **Ettinger B, Black DM, Mitlak BH, et al.** Reduction of vertebral fracture risk in postmenopausal women with osteoporosis treated with raloxifene: results from a 3-year randomized clinical trial. Multiple Outcomes of Raloxifene (MORE) Investigators. JAMA. 1999;282:637-45.

11. **Neer RM, Arnaud CD, Zanchetta JR, et al.** Effect of parathyroid hormone (1-34) on fractures and bone mineral density in postmenopausal women with osteoporosis. N Engl J Med. 2001;344:1434-41.

12. **Body JJ, Gaich GA, Scheele WH, et al.** A randomized double-blind trial to compare the efficacy of teriparatide [recombinant human parathyroid hormone (1-340)] with alendronate in postmenopausal women with osteoporosis. J Clin Endocrinol Metab. 2002;87:4528-35.

13. **Kurland ES, Cosman F, McMahon DJ, et al.** Parathyroid hormone as a therapy for idiopathic osteoporosis in men: effects on bone mineral density and bone markers. J Clin Endocrinol Metab. 2000;85:3029-76.

14. **Rittmaster RS, Bolognese M, Ettinger MP, et al.** Enhancement of bone mass in osteoporotic women with parathyroid hormone followed by alendronate. J Clin Endocrinol Metab. 2000;85:2129-34.

15. **Lane N, Sanchez S, Modin GW, et al.** Parathyroid hormone treatment can reverse corticosteroid-induced osteoporosis: results from a randomized controlled clinical trial. J Clin Invest. 1998;102:1627-33.

16. **Hall GM, Daniels M, Doyle DV, Spector TD.** Effect of hormone replacement therapy on bone mass in rheumatoid arthritis patients treated with or without steroids. Arthritis Rheum. 1994;37:1499-505.

17. **Huddleston JM, Whitford KJ.** Medical care of elderly patients with hip fractures. Mayo Clin Proc. 2001;76:295-8.

18. **Miller PD, Brown JP, Siris ES, et al.** A randomized, double-blind comparison of risedronate and etidronate in the treatment of Paget's disease of bone. Am J Med. 1999;106:513-20.

19. **Cundy T, Wattie D, King AR.** High-dose pamidronate in the management of resistant Paget's disease. Calcif Tissue Int. 1996;58:6-8.

20. **Arden-Cordone M, Siris ES, Lyles KW, et al.** Antiresorptive effect of a single infusion of microgram quantities of zolendronate in Paget's disease of the bone. Calcif Tissue Int. 1997;60:415-18.

SECTION VII

COMMON SYMPTOMS AND COMORBIDITIES

24

■ ■ ■

Fever and Arthritis

Doruk Erkan, MD

Yusuf Yazici, MD

The presence of concurrent fever and arthritis has important diagnostic and therapeutic ramifications. Although the combination of fever and arthritis may be a manifestation of a wide variety of conditions, infectious etiologies are the most important, demanding prompt exclusion or treatment. Furthermore, the presence of an infection in a patient with an underlying systemic inflammatory disorder such as rheumatoid arthritis (RA) or systemic lupus erythematosus (SLE) is not uncommon, and it can be difficult sorting out what findings relate to active disease and which are due to superimposed infection. The practitioner must use all of his acumen to assemble the pertinent facts from the clinical history and physical examination and, with support from laboratory testing, arrive at the correct diagnosis and institute appropriate therapy.

Fever is the pathological elevation of body temperature above the normal circadian range. This is defined as a morning temperature greater than 37.2°C (98.9°F) or an evening temperature greater than 37.7°C (99.9°F). Major fever-producing cytokines in response to infection are interleukin (IL)-1α, IL-1β, tumor necrosis factor (TNF)-α, IL-6, and type I interferons. These cytokines are also widely implicated in the pathogenesis of inflammatory disorders such as RA and SLE and may account for the significant clinical overlap between various infectious and rheumatological conditions.

The differential diagnosis of fever and arthritis is listed in Tables 24-1 and 24-2 and can be classified into five broad categories: infection-related diseases, collagen vascular/inflammatory disorders, crystalline arthropathies, drug-induced illnesses, and other miscellaneous conditions (1,2). Because of the overlapping symptoms and signs of these disorders, a thorough appreciation of their clinical presentations and their nuances facilitates the diagnostic process.

Table 24-1   Infectious Causes of Fever and Arthritis

Bacterial Arthritis	Fungal Arthritis	Viral Arthritis	Reactive Arthritis
Septic arthritis	*Histoplasma capsulatum*	Rubella	Enteric infections
Gonococcal arthritis	*Cryptococcus neoformans*	Human immunodeficiency virus (HIV)	*Chlamdyia* infections
Infective endocarditis	*Coccidioides immitis*	Hepatitis viruses	Acute rheumatic fever
Lyme disease	*Blastomyces dermatitidis*	Parvovirus B19	
Syphilis	*Sporothrix schenckii*	Adenovirus type 7	
Mycobacteria	*Candida* species	Coxsackieviruses	
Whipple's disease		Epstein-Barr virus	
		Mumps	

Table 24-2   Noninfectious Causes of Fever and Arthritis

Connective Tissue Disorders	Crystal-Induced Diseases	Drug-Induced	Miscellaneous
Systemic lupus erythematosus	Gout	Serum sickness disease	Inflammatory bowel disease
Rheumatoid arthritis	Pseudogout	Antibiotics (e.g., minocycline)	Familial Mediterranean fever
Adult-onset juvenile rheumatoid arthritis		Mesalazine	Malignancy
Inflammatory myopathies		Calmette-Guérin bacillus immunotherapy	
Vasculitis		Procainamide	
Sarcoidosis		Hydralazine	
		Isoniazid	
		Methyldopa	
		Chlorpromazine	

Case Presentation

A 28-year-old woman with a history of SLE (photosensitive rash, symmetric polyarthritis, leukopenia, and positive serum test for antinuclear antibodies), who was well controlled with hydroxychloroquine 200 mg twice daily and prednisone 5 mg daily, presents with a new low-grade fever and migratory arthralgias of 1 week duration. During the past 2 days, she developed dis-proportionate pain, warmth, swelling, and erythema of the right knee. Except for a temperature of 38.8°C and the right knee monoarthritis, the physical examination was normal. Initial blood tests revealed only a mild leukocytosis and an elevated erythrocyte sedimentation rate. Twenty-five milli-liters of cloudy synovial fluid were aspirated from the right knee. The white blood cell (WBC) count of the fluid was 20,000/µL with 90% polymorphonu-clear leukocytes, but the Gram stain was negative for organisms. Blood and synovial fluid cultures were negative, but *Neisseria gonorrhoeae* was isolated from pharyngeal cultures. The patient was treated with a third-generation cephalosporin and serial knee joint aspirations, and her symptoms resolved.

Diagnosis

A complete clinical history always offers the most useful information in the evaluation of the patient. Duration of the symptoms, the pattern of the joint involvement, comorbid states, extra-articular manifestations, and environ-mental exposures are particularly important elements. An acute onset of symptoms often suggests a bacterial septic arthritis or crystalline arthropa-thy, whereas a subacute or insidious onset may reflect atypical infection (e.g., mycobacteria, fungi), collagen vascular disease, or other non-infec-tious causes. Septic arthritis most often occurs in a single joint (>90% of cases) and sometimes assumes an oligoarticular pattern (four or fewer joints), but only rarely presents as a polyarthritis (greater than four joints). Crystalline arthropathies may be quite variable in joint distribution; they are commonly monoarticular or asymmetrically oligoarticular, but not uncom-monly polyarticular. Rarely, they masquerade as RA. Patients that are im-munocompromised as the result of underlying illnesses and/or medical treatment are at increased risk for joint infections, as are patients with joint prostheses, known history of active infections, or penetrating joint trauma. A complete review of systems may reveal evidence of systemic illnesses such as SLE or vasculitis. Exposure to new medications, a history of tick bites, sexual history, and exposure to viral illnesses or vaccinations should be explored.

On physical examination, arthritis should be distinguished from soft tissue inflammation surrounding the joint (e.g., in the skin, tendon, or bursa). Although joint mobility is limited on both active and passive range of motion in frank arthritis, patients with tendonitis or bursitis usually have nearly full passive range of motion. After the documentation of fever and arthritis, other clinical features such as rashes, uveitis, oral and genital lesions, tophi, urethritis, and diarrhea will help to further elucidate the diagnosis.

Arthrocentesis is crucial diagnostically and may also be helpful thera-peutically by ridding the joint of pain-inducing and tissue-damaging inflam-matory mediators. Examination of the synovial fluid should include cell count with differential, Gram stain, crystal analysis under polarizing microscopy, and bacterial cultures for aerobic and anaerobic organisms. If clinical suspicion indicates, stains and cultures for fungi and mycobacteria should also be obtained. The characteristics and cellularity of the fluid can often give early indications of probable diagnoses and guide initial management decisions (Table 24-3) (3). Blood cultures should be done to identify a potential hematogenous source of infection. Rarely, when the results of arthrocentesis are not diagnostic, synovial biopsies may be considered. Cultures from synovial biopsies have higher yield and are particularly helpful in cases of mycobacterial or fungal infections. The histopathology may demonstrate significant tissue necrosis and neutrophilic infiltration in infectious arthritis, whereas illnesses like RA or the spondyloarthropathies are characterized by chronic inflammatory changes.

Nongonococcal Septic Arthritis

Acute bacterial arthritis is a rheumatological emergency and should be managed aggressively in order to prevent joint destruction. Septic monoarthritis may be due to direct extension from contiguous infection or to hematogenous spread, but oligoarticular and polyarticular involvement usually reflect concomitant bacteremia. Immunosuppression, direct penetrating trauma, pre-existing joint damage, and chronic illnesses such as rheumatoid arthritis,

Table 24-3   Synovial Fluid Analysis Averaged from Multiple Studies

Diagnosis	Appearance	WBC/mm³	PMN (%)	Microscopy
Normal	Clear yellow	<200	7	
Noninflammatory Osteoarthritis	Clear or slightly turbid	600	13	
Inflammatory Gout	Turbid	21,500	70	Intracellular, negatively birefringent, needle-shaped crystals
Pseudogout	Turbid	14,200	68	Intracellular, positively birefringent, rhomboid and polymorphic crystals
Rheumatoid arthritis	Turbid	19,000	66	
Acute bacterial infections	Very turbid	80,000	90	Positive Gram staining in up to 75%

WBC = white blood cell; PMN = polymorphonuclear leukocyte.
Modified from Krey PR, Lazaro DM. Analysis of Synovial Fluid. Summit, NJ, CIBA-GEIGY; 1992; with permission.

diabetes, cancer, and renal or hepatic disorders are predisposing factors. The presence of constitutional symptoms (fever, chills, rigors), peripheral leukocytosis, a clear source for bacteremia or contiguous infection, and a high synovial fluid leukocyte count (>50,000/mm^3, and certainly >100,000/mm^3) with predominantly polymorphonuclear cells strongly favor the diagnosis. In cases of suspected nongonococcal infectious arthritis, bacteria may be identified by synovial fluid Gram staining in 50% to 75% of cases and by synovial fluid cultures in up to 90%.

Staphylococcus aureus is the most common cause of pyogenic, nongonococcal bacterial arthritis, followed by beta-hemolytic streptococcus and *Streptococcus pneumoniae*. The percentage of gram-negative joint infections is increasing because of the large pool of patients presenting with gram-negative bacteremia (see Table 15-3 in Chapter 15).

Gonococcal Arthritis

Overall, disseminated gonococcemia is the most common cause of infectious arthritis in the young adult population (age 16-50 years). Usually occurring in sexually active patients, 1% to 3% of patients with gonorrhea develop a migratory polyarthritis or monoarthritis. Associated tenosynovitis, especially in the wrist and ankle extensor tendon sheaths, is common. Pain is typically out of proportion to the physical findings. Scattered crops of maculopapular or vesiculopustular skin lesions on an erythematous base on the trunk and extremities are characteristic. Microbiological diagnosis is also commonly made from cultures of other sites such as the oropharynx, urethra, cervix, and rectum.

Infectious Endocarditis

In one series, 44% of patients with infectious endocarditis were found to have musculoskeletal symptoms, typically polyarthralgia and back pain (4). Oligoarthritis or an additive, asymmetrical polyarthritis that precedes fever and the other cardiac and peripheral signs of endocarditis has also been reported (5). Inflammatory arthritis in the setting of infectious endocarditis may be caused by hematogenous infection of the musculoskeletal site or an immunological process triggered by the infection.

Lyme Disease

Lyme disease is caused by the spirochete *Borrelia burgdorferi* transmitted by an *Ixodes scapularis* (*I. dammini*) tick bite. The early phase presents as a nonspecific viral-like syndrome with headache, fever, fatigue, and polyarthralgia without frank arthritis. As many as 70% of patients have the characteristic erythema migrans (EM) rash, an expanding erythematous papule or macule, often with central clearing at the site of the bite. Secondary EM lesions may also be seen at remote locations. A patient who develops EM but is not adequately treated has a 60% chance of developing episodic attacks of asymmetric, waxing, and waning monoarthritis or oligoarthritis of the large joints that are characteristic of late tertiary Lyme disease. The inflammatory arthropathy generally develops several months after the initial infection and commonly affects the knee joint, which tends to be more swollen than painful. Serological testing by enzyme-linked immunosorbent assay (ELISA) supports the diagnosis of Lyme arthritis, but a positive ELISA should always be confirmed by Western blot analysis.

Syphilis

The incidence of syphilis has risen in the United States because of its association with HIV infections. Five to ten percent of patients with secondary syphilis have arthralgias (6). It may also present rarely with symmetrical polyarthritis involving the knees, ankles, and shoulders, and fever. The maculopapular rash on the palms and soles is a distinguishing finding, and serological testing for syphilis can confirm the diagnosis.

Fungal and Mycobacterial Arthritis

A subacute or chronic, progressive destructive monoarthritis or oligoarthritis should raise the suspicion of a fungal or mycobacterial infection. A low-grade fever is typical but may not be prominent. Although acute arthritis may occur with *Candida* or *Blastomyces* infections, the presentation is normally insidious, and the diagnosis is often delayed (7). Conjunctivitis, erythema nodosum, erythema multiforme, or other extraarticular manifestations are commonly associated findings. In tuberculous arthritis, the purified protein derivative (PPD) skin test should be performed but may be falsely negative if the patient is very ill. Diagnosis of mycobacterial and fungal infections often requires arthroscopic synovial biopsy and tissue culture because cultures of the synovial fluid are negative in more than 60% of the patients.

Viral Arthritis

Self-limited oligoarthritis or polyarthritis may be observed with many viral infections and in patients receiving viral vaccines. Among commonly implicated agents are rubella, mumps, hepatitis B, hepatitis C, HIV, adenovirus, Coxsackievirus, Epstein-Barr virus, rubella vaccine, and hepatitis B vaccine (8-12). Parvovirus B19 is a particularly interesting pathogen that characteristically causes a self-limited symmetric polyarthritis resembling RA in adults (13). It is normally acquired from children with erythema infectiosum (fifth disease) and may occur in periodic outbreaks. Serological testing for anti-parvovirus B19 IgM antibodies is the most commonly employed means of evaluating acute infection. The appearance of anti-parvovirus B19 IgG antibodies several weeks after the onset of the acute illness confirms the diagnosis. Although viral arthritides are classically self-limited, there are data that suggest that in some individuals the arthritis may become chronic.

Reactive Arthritis

Reactive arthritis is an inflammatory monoarthritis or oligoarthritis triggered by an infection at a distant mucosal site. Although the joint itself is not directly infected, the microorganism and a component of the joint often share common antigenic epitopes that may lead to an immune-mediated arthritis. Enteric and urogenital infections are the most commonly implicated, and causative organisms include *Salmonella, Shigella, Yersinia, Campylobacter,* and *Chlamydia* among others. The oligoarthritis usually involves large lower extremity joints in an asymmetrical fashion, and patients may rarely develop spine and sacroiliac disease indistinguishable from that of ankylosing spondylitis. Reiter's syndrome is characterized by the classic triad of reactive arthritis, uveitis, and urethritis.

Acute rheumatic fever can occur in adults. An additive polyarthritis postterm may be more common in adults than the classically described migratory polyarthritis of children (14). Pain is frequently more prominent than the objective signs of inflammation. Joint manifestations may occur without skin lesions, carditis, or chorea, but they are invariably accompanied by evidence of a recent group A, beta-hemolytic streptococcal pharyngitis. When positive cultures are not available, elevated titers of anti-streptolysin O antibodies help to make the diagnosis.

Connective Tissue Disorders and Vasculitides

Systemic lupus erythematosus commonly presents with a symmetrical polyarthritis involving the small joints of the hands and feet, as well as many other peripheral joints. Many patients with active SLE have fever, often as high as 40°C, with or without chills. SLE exacerbations are usually associated with other clinical clues such as a typical rash, but fever, especially in those patients already taking corticosteroids or immunosuppressive agents, should alert the physician to strongly consider infection, particularly if a single joint is disproportionately inflamed.

A high spiking fever associated with an evanescent macular rash and polyarthritis are characteristic of adult-onset Still's disease. The presence of lymphadenopathy and hepatosplenomegaly are other clinical hints. Dermatomyositis can early on present with fever and generalized puffiness of the hands in an RA-like picture. Characteristic rashes and proximal muscle weakness should be sought carefully.

Fever and polyarthritis can be the early manifestations of systemic vasculitides like Wegener's granulomatosis, polyarteritis nodosa, Behçet's disease, or relapsing polychondritis (15). Thorough knowledge of the clinical stigmata characteristic of specific conditions is essential in arriving at the appropriate diagnosis and treatment plan.

Crystalline Arthritis

A low-grade fever can be seen in 44% of gout patients, but one should be alert to the possibility of superimposed infection. Moderate peripheral and synovial fluid leukocytosis are common (16), but marked elevations in either or the presence of high fever (>38.5°C) favor infection. It should be noted that in some patients with infectious arthritis, the active inflammation might "strip-mine" uric acid or calcium pyrophosphate crystals off the walls of the joint. Thus, identification of characteristic crystals under polarizing microscopy should not be used to exclude infection, and the synovial fluid should always be examined by Gram staining and culture when fever exists or the white counts are high.

Drug-Induced Fever and Arthritis

Drug reactions always need to be considered as potential causes of fever and joint pains, especially in the setting of a rash (17). Serum sickness is an immune complex disease, which can occur with many drugs, including penicillins, sulfonamides, penicillamine, and propylthiouracil. Fever develops 7 to 12 days after initial exposure and is usually followed by urticaria, arthritis, glomerulonephritis, or myocarditis. A systemic vasculitis may ensue. Other drugs (e.g., minocycline, hydralazine, procainamide, methyldopa, isoniazid, phenytoin) are known to induce a lupus-like syndrome, although severe visceral involvement such as nephritis is rare (18). A combination of fever, vasculitic rash, arthritis, pericarditis, and pericardial effusion has been reported after treatment with mesalazine (19). Symmetric polyarthritis accompanied by fever can be induced by intravesicular Calmette-Guérin bacillus immunotherapy (20).

Miscellaneous

Familial Mediterranean fever is an autosomal recessive disorder, manifested by recurrent episodes of fever, peritonitis, pleuritis, and arthritis. Episodes usually last for 7 to 14 days and then resolve spontaneously. The family history plays an important role in diagnosis.

Hematological disorders such as leukemia, lymphoma, and sickle cell disease can present with joint pain and fever. Often the joint pain is out of proportion to the clinical findings. In children with leukemia, nocturnal pain may be prominent.

Approximately one-third of patients with sarcoidosis present with fever. The Lofgren's syndrome variant of sarcoidosis (erythema nodosum, periarthritis around the ankles, and hilar adenopathy) is often associated with a low-grade fever.

Management

In most cases, an accurate diagnosis will be made promptly and appropriate treatment initiated accordingly. Nonetheless, several management points should be highlighted. If the clinical picture is suspicious for infection (e.g, very high synovial fluid leukocyte count, high fevers with chills or rigors, immunosuppression, concurrent or previous infections), antibiotics should be administered empirically pending the results of cultures even if the Gram stain of synovial fluid is negative (21). Anti-staphylococcus coverage is necessary in patients who are not at risk for gonococcemia, with the addition of antibiotics for gram-negative organisms in immunocompromised patients. The regimen should be adjusted when an organism is identified by culture. The clinician should not be fooled by a synovial leukocyte count that does not appear very elevated in individuals with leukopenia due to SLE, myelosuppression, or a primary bone marrow disease. Patients with underlying joint disorders such as RA or gout present a special challenge. Joints with anatomic derangements are at increased risk for infection, and so the clinician should not reflexively attribute the joint inflammation and fever to a flare of underlying RA or gout. Repeated arthrocenteses are occasionally necessary if there is reaccumulation of synovial fluid and clinical suspicion for infection is still high. With ongoing inflammation, loculations may develop within the joint, potentially resulting in refractoriness to treatment. In such cases, aspiration of the joint from different approaches or surgical debridement may be necessary.

Nonsteroidal anti-inflammatory drugs (NSAIDs) are usually the first-line treatment for most non-infectious causes of fever and arthritis. When NSAIDs are contraindicated or ineffective, systemic or intra-articular corticosteroids are alternatives when infection is reasonably excluded.

Summary

Many patients with rheumatological conditions are prone to infections due to both the disease and potential complications of treatment. Unfortunately, signs and symptoms of infections commonly overlap with those of exacerbations of rheumatological diseases, thereby resulting in diagnostic confusion. Fever needs to be taken very seriously in all patients but particularly in those with underlying rheumatological disorders, and a thorough evaluation should always be performed to exclude infection. At times, concomitant antibiotic therapy for presumptive infection and anti-inflammatory/immunosuppressive medications for control of disease flares may be required for empiric treatment until the definitive cause for fever is identified.

REFERENCES

1. **Pinals RS.** Polyarthritis and fever. N Engl J Med. 1994;330:769-74.

2. **Erkan D, Yazici Y, Paget SA.** Fever and arthritis: narrowing the diagnosis. J Musculoskel Med. 2000;17:676-87.

3. **Krey PR, Lazaro DM.** Analysis of Synovial Fluid. Summit, NJ: CIBA-GEIGY; 1992.

4. **Churchill MA Jr., Geraci JE. Hunder GG.** Musculoskeletal manifestations of bacterial endocarditis. Ann Intern Med. 1977;87:754-9.

5. **Rambaldi M, Ambrosone L, Migliaresi S, Rambaldi A.** Infective endocarditis presenting as polyarthritis. Clin Rheumatol. 1998;17:518-20.

6. **Mindel A, Tovey SJ, Timmins DJ, Williams P.** Primary and secondary syphilis, 20 years' experience. 2. Clinical features. Genitourin Med. 1989;65:1-3.

7. **Katzenstein D.** Isolated *Candida* arthritis: report of a case and definition of a distinct clinical syndrome. Arthritis Rheum. 1985;28:1421-4.

8. **Berman A, Espinoza LR, Diaz JD, et al.** Rheumatic manifestations of human immunodeficiency virus infection. Am J Med. 1988;85:59-64.

9. **Biasi D, De Sandre G, Bambara LM, et al.** A new case of reactive arthritis after hepatitis B vaccination. Clin Exp Rheumatol. 1993;11:215.

10. **Ford DK, Reid GD, Tingle AJ, et al.** Sequential follow up observations of a patient with rubella-associated persistent arthritis. Ann Rheum Dis. 1992;51:407-10.

11. **Frenkel LM, Nielsen K, Garakian A, et al.** A search for persistent rubella virus infection in persons with chronic symptoms after rubella and rubella immunization and in patients with juvenile rheumatoid arthritis. Clin Infect Dis. 1996;22:287-94.

12. **Siegel LB, Cohn L, Nashel D.** Rheumatic manifestations of hepatitis C infection. Semin Arthritis Rheum. 1993;23:149-54.

13. **Stanley JN.** Viral arthritis. In: Klippel JH, Dieppe PA, eds. Rheumatology. London: Mosby; 1998;6:6:1-8.

14. **Gibofsky A, Kerwar S, Zabriskie JB.** Rheumatic fever: the relationships between host, microbe, and genetics. Rheum Dis Clin North Am. 1998;24:237-59.

15. **Hoffman GS, Kerr GS, Leavitt RY, et al.** Wegener granulomatosis: an analysis of 158 patients. Ann Intern Med. 1992;116:488-98.

16. **Raddatz DA, Mahowald ML, Bilka PJ.** Acute polyarticular gout. Ann Rheum Dis. 1983;42:117-22.

17. **Bernstein RM.** Rheumatic complications of drugs and toxins. In: Maddison PJ, Isenberg DA, Woo P, Glass DN, eds. Oxford Textbook of Rheumatology. New York: Oxford University Press; 1998:1689-97.

18. **Elkayam O, Yaron M, Caspi D.** Minocycline-induced arthritis associated with fever, livedo reticularis and pANCA. Ann Rheum Dis. 1996;55:769-71.

19. **Lim AG, Hine KR.** Fever, vasculitic rash, arthritis, pericarditis, and pericardial effusion after mesalazine. BMJ. 1994;308:113.

20. **Clavel G, Grados F, Cayrolle G, et al.** Polyarthritis following intravesical BCG immunotherapy: report of a case and review of 26 cases in the literature. Rev Rhum Engl Ed. 1999;66:115-8.

21. **Dikranian AH, Weisman MH.** Principles of diagnosis and treatment of joint infections. In: Koopman WJ, ed. Arthritis and Allied Conditions, 14th ed. Philadelphia: Lippincott Williams and Wilkins; 2001:2551-69.

25

■ ■ ■

Erythema Nodosum

Arthur M.F. Yee, MD, PhD

E rythema nodosum (EN), first described in the late 18th century by the English dermatologist Robert Willan as a markedly tender subcutaneous nodular lesion with prominent erythema and warmth, is now suspected to be a reflection of underlying systemic inflammatory processes or an adverse drug reaction in most if not all cases. Erythema nodosum affects women four to five times more frequently than men. Its actual incidence is difficult to assess and likely varies from population to population depending on genetic factors and the prevalence of secondary causes such as sarcoidosis or tuberculosis. A fair estimate of the yearly incidence is one to five cases per 100,000 individuals.

The raised nodules occur most commonly on the anterior aspects of the shins and around the ankles, but can also be found less frequently on the thighs and forearms (Figure 25-1). They are usually no more than 2 to 3 cm in diameter but can sometimes be as large as 10 cm. The erythema deepens over time and is followed by local bruising. As the nodule resorbs over several weeks, the pain and discoloration disappear, and the lesion heals without ulceration or scarring.

Although EN is frequently idiopathic, in many case series an underlying illness or etiology can be identified in the majority of cases (Table 25-1). There are well-documented associations with certain infectious diseases, notably tuberculosis and streptococcal infections. It is interesting that in both the northern and southern hemispheres, the incidence of EN is highest in their respective winters and springs, suggesting the importance of infectious agents in many cases. There are also significant associations with other systemic inflammatory diseases such as sarcoidosis, spondyloarthritides, inflammatory bowel diseases, Behçet's disease, and lymphoproliferative disorders. Various medications are also thought to be potential triggers of EN. As demonstrated in three recent studies, the frequency of conditions associated with EN varies from case series to case series (1-3), bringing to

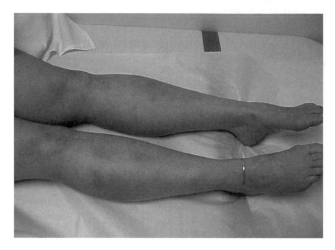

Figure 25-1   Erythema nodosum rash on the pretibial area of the leg in a patient with Löfgren's syndrome. The hyperpigmented nodular lesions eventually develop a deep purple hue and often coalesce to involve the periarticular erythema of the adjacent inflamed ankle.

light the heterogeneity of potential causes and the relative frequency with which they occur in a given population (see Table 25-1).

Histopathologically, EN is a panniculitis, characterized by inflammation around the septal areas of the subcutaneous fat. Lymphocyte and macrophage infiltration occurs early. Later, capillary leakage and prominent local hemorrhaging account for the characteristic cutaneous purpuric discoloration. Venulitis may be present, but arteritis and fat necrosis do not occur. Local deposition of immune complexes containing immunoglobulins and complement components have been documented, which is again consistent with the thought that exogenous triggers may be involved in some cases.

Case Presentation

A 35-year-old woman presented with acute onset of painful and tender erythematous raised skin lesions on both legs. She had been previously healthy and without chronic medical problems. One month before presentation, the patient started taking an estrogen-based oral contraceptive medication. The patient described no other revealing symptoms on a thorough review of systems other than a low-grade fever. The physical examination revealed multiple exquisitely tender, pre-tibial raised nodules that ranged from 2 to 4 cm in diameter. The lesions were warm and erythematous. Erythema nodosum was diagnosed. Laboratory tests revealed an elevated erythrocyte sedimentation rate (ESR) of 55 mm/h but were otherwise unremarkable. A chest X-ray was normal and showed no signs of sarcoidosis, and a tuberculin skin test was non-reactive.

Table 25-1   Conditions Associated with Erythema Nodosum

	Cribier et al.	*Garcia-Porrua et al.*	*Psychos et al.*
Population characteristics			
Number of patients	129	106	132
Female/male	108/21	82/24	110/22
Setting	Strasbourg, France	Lugo, Spain	Ioannina, Greece
Etiologies (% of cases)			
Idiopathic	55	34	35
Streptococcal infection	28	7	6
Sarcoidosis	11	22	28
Tuberculosis	1	5	2
Other infections +/- antibiotics	4	21	14
Enteropathies	1	3	—
Medications alone*	—	3	4
Pregnancy	—	6	—
Malignancy	—	1	—
Other systemic inflammatory illnesses[†]	4	5	—

See References 1 to 3 for data sources.
* Oral contraceptives, NSAIDs, analgesics.
[†] Behçet's disease, Sweet's syndrome, Sjögren's syndrome.

The oral contraceptive was discontinued, and a nonsteroidal anti-inflammatory drug (NSAID) was prescribed. The pain improved significantly, although the rash persisted for several weeks, eventually evolving into a deep purplish bruise. No ulcerations developed, and after several months the skin appeared normal without scarring.

A year later, the patient had another similar episode. This time, however, the patient reported some mild diarrhea and abdominal discomfort for several weeks before the onset of the rash. Laboratory tests again demonstrated an elevated ESR, but now a microcytic anemia was noted on the complete blood count. The patient again responded to NSAID therapy. However, a colonoscopy was performed and revealed ulcerative colitis. Her colitis responded to corticosteroid enemas, and the patient had no further episodes of EN.

Diagnosis

Although EN lesions are quite characteristic and often do not require biopsy, they may occasionally be confused early in the disease for arthropod (e.g, insect or spider) bites or vasculitic diseases such as polyarteritis nodosum or Weber-Christian disease. Key features that distinguish EN from vasculitis are the absence of ulcerations and the absence of scarring.

Although it is appropriate to assure patients that EN lesions are self-limited and nondisfiguring, in the diagnostic evaluation of EN the true challenge to the clinician is the identification of a secondary cause or an associated underlying illness. A thorough history, review of systems, and physical examination are crucial and the most efficient means of attaining this goal. The history may reveal an antecedent upper respiratory tract infection or documented streptococcal infection. Fever is common and occurs in more than half of patients. When accompanied by other constitutional symptoms like anorexia, weight loss, and night sweats, tuberculosis should be considered, especially in endemic areas or in immunosuppressed individuals such as patients infected with the human immunodeficiency virus. A large variety of bacterial, fungal, and viral infections and vaccinations have also been associated with EN.

Erythema nodosum leprosum (ENL) is a multisystem syndrome that affects nearly half of patients with lepromatous leprosy that has as a prominent feature painful cutaneous erythematous nodules generally on the extensor surfaces of the limbs. Prominent systemic features such as peripheral neuritis, uveitis, orchitis, lymphadenitis, and glomerulonephritis can also be present. Although the ENL skin lesion grossly resembles that of classical EN, it differs in that it commonly pustulates and ulcerates, is prone to recur, and more frequently becomes a chronic condition, suggesting that the fundamental pathophysiology does differ. The histopathology also reveals a panniculitis, but concomitant vasculitic features are more common than in classical EN, probably accounting for the propensity to ulcerate.

Erythema nodosum can occur in 8% to 25% of sarcoid patients (4-6). In some series, sarcoidosis accounts for almost one third of cases of EN (3), and so respiratory complaints and physical signs of sarcoidosis such as lupus pernio, lymphadenopathy, and inflammatory arthritis should be sought. The triad of EN, periarticular inflammation around the ankles, and hilar lymphadenopathy is known as Löfgen's syndrome and represents a variant of sarcoidosis that carries a generally favorable overall prognosis (7). Prominent abdominal discomfort, chronic diarrhea, and hematochezia should prompt an investigation for a possible inflammatory bowel disease, in which 2% to 15% of patients may develop EN (8,9). Recurrence of EN can correlate with exacerbations of the bowel disease (10). In Behçet's disease, a rare condition characterized by frequent oral and genital ulcers, thrombophlebitis, and uveitis, EN lesions occur in almost half of all patients (11). Prominent constitutional symptoms should raise the suspicion of a lymphoproliferative malignancy (12).

Many medications have often been thought to be potential causes of EN, but it is usually difficult to establish definitive proof of association and to exclude underlying conditions as less probable causes. For example, antibiotics, especially sulfonamides and penicillins, are commonly implicated as causative agents, but whether the infection being treated or the putative offending drug is the trigger for EN can rarely be definitively established. Among other drugs that have been suspected of causing EN are oral contraceptives, estrogen replacement therapy, NSAIDs, all-*trans* retinoic acid, and filgrastim. However, because EN is a form of cell-mediated hypersensitivity, any medication that can induce this kind of immune response can in theory be a cause of EN.

Investigations

The erythrocyte sedimentation rate and serum concentration of C-reactive protein are usually elevated during an acute EN flare and will normalize with resolution of the rash but are non-specific measures of inflammation.

Plain chest radiography should be obtained on all patients. As many as 25% or more of patients with EN may have an abnormal chest X-ray demonstrating bilateral hilar lymphadenopathy suggestive of sarcoidosis. If the initial chest X-ray is abnormal but not pathognomonic, further investigations such as computed tomography should always be performed to exclude the possibility of indolent malignancies or infections. An intradermal tuberculin test with control antigens (e.g., mumps, *Candida,* and *Trichophyton*) should also be performed.

Throat cultures should be obtained to evaluate for a streptococcal pharyngitis. Serial serum titers of anti-streptolysin O (ASLO) will help to confirm the diagnosis of a streptococcal infection.

If there are prominent abdominal symptoms, occult blood in the stool should be sought, and a gastroenterological consultation and a colonoscopy should be obtained to assess for inflammatory bowel disease.

If the patient is a woman of child-bearing age, a urinary or serological test for β-human chorionic gonadotropin should be examined. In one study, 6% of the cases were associated with pregnancy. Moreover, pregnancy should be excluded before the administration of any medication (e.g., NSAIDs) or exposure to radiological testing that may adversely affect the fetus.

Management

Erythema nodosum is generally a self-limited condition that typically resolves within several weeks. Nonetheless, because the lesions can be exquisitely painful and cosmetically disturbing, it is important to reassure the patient and to institute therapy promptly. Any underlying condition should also be appropriately addressed, and any medication or other exogenous agent suspected as a possible cause should be discontinued.

NSAIDs, given at anti-inflammatory dosages, will normally offer symptomatic relief of the acute EN lesion, although the discoloration may persist even after the tenderness has subsided. The patient should be informed that the most painful period will last about 2 to 3 weeks before gradual waning of symptoms. It should be remembered that anti-inflammatory dosages of NSAIDs are higher than analgesic dosages and are often required for maximal benefit but are also associated with a higher incidence of adverse effects. When EN is non-responsive to NSAIDs, or if there is intolerance or contraindication to these medications, a short course of systemic corticosteroids (starting at prednisone 20-40 mg daily or equivalent with a rapid taper over 1 to 2 weeks) will typically be effective in bringing about relief of the acute inflammation. However, it is crucial that an infectious cause of EN be treated or excluded if corticosteroids are utilized. Potassium iodide (900 mg daily in divided doses) has also been used successfully in many cases of acute EN without significant adverse effects (13).

Rarely, EN may become recurrent or chronic, especially when seen in the setting of an underlying disease. In these cases, maintenance therapy with hydroxychloroquine (200 mg twice daily) has proven effective in controlling the inflammatory process (14). Colchicine (1 to 2 mg daily in divided doses) can also prevent recurrence of EN in certain individuals (15). There are conflicting results as to the effect of thalidomide on EN. One retrospective study reported benefit (16), while a recent prospective study reported exacerbation of EN lesions associated with Behçet's disease (17). In contrast, however, recurrent EN leprosum often has a striking response to thalidomide 100-300 mg nightly (18).

Summary

Erythema nodosum can be quite alarming for the patient because of the associated extreme pain and discoloration. However, EN is generally self-limited, readily treated, and characteristically non-scarring. Nonetheless, EN is very commonly associated with underlying systemic conditions and may often be the initial clue to their presence.

REFERENCES

1. **Cribier B, Caille A, Heid E, Grosshans E.** Erythema nodosum and associated diseases: a study of 129 cases. Int J Dermatol. 1998;37:667-72.

2. **Garcia-Porrua C, Gonzalez-Gay MA, Vazquez-Caruncho M, et al.** Erythema nodosum: etiologic and predictive factors in a defined population. Arthritis Rheum. 2000;43:584-92.

3. **Psychos DN, Voulgari PV, Skopouli FN.** Erythema nodosum: the underlying conditions. Clin Rheumatol. 2000;19:212-6.

4. **Diab SM, Karnik AM, Ouda BA, et al.** Sarcoidosis in Arabs: the clinical profile of 20 patients and review of the literature. Sarcoidosis. 1991;8:56-62.

5. **Baughman RP, Teirstein AS, Judson MA, et al.** Clinical characteristics of patients in a case control study of sarcoidosis. Am J Respir Crit Care Med. 2001;164:1885-9.

6. **Yanardag H, Pamuk ON, Karayel T.** Cutaneous involvement in sarcoidosis: analysis of the features in 170 patients. Respir Med. 2003;97:978-82.

7. **Mana J, Gomez-Vaquero C, Montero A, et al.** Löfgren's syndrome revisited: a study of 186 patients. Am J Med. 1999;107:240-5.

8. **Greenstein AJ, Janowitz HD, Sachar DB.** The extraintestinal complications of Crohn's disease and ulcerative colitis: a study of 700 patients. Medicine. 1976;55-401-12.

9. **Orchard TR, Chua CN, Ahmad T, et al.** Uveitis and erythema nodosum in inflammatory bowel disease: clinical features and the role of HLA genes. Gastroenterology. 2002;123:714-8.

10. **Schorr-Lesnick B, Brandt LJ.** Selected rheumatologic and dermatologic manifestations of inflammatory bowel disease. Am J Gastroenterol. 1988;83:216-23.

11. **Tursen U, Gurler A, Boyvat A.** Evaluation of clinical findings according to sex in 2313 Turkish patients with Behcet's disease. Int J Dermatol. 2003;42:346-51.

12. **Bonci A, Di Lernia V, Merli F, Lo Scocco G.** Erythema nodosum and Hodgkin's disease. Clin Exp Dermatol. 2001;26:408-11.

13. **Schulz EJ, Whiting DA.** Treatment of erythema nodosum and nodular vasculitis with potassium iodide. Br J Dermatol. 1976;94:75-8.

14. **Alloway JA, Franks LK.** Hydroxychloroquine in the treatment of chronic erythema nodosum. Br J Dermatol. 1995;132:661-73.

15. **Yurdakul S, Mat C, Tuzun Y, et al.** A double-blind trial of colchicine in Behçet's syndrome. Arthritis Rheum. 2001;43:2686-92.

16. **Hanza MH.** Treatment of Behçet's disease with thalidomide. Clin Rheumatol. 1986; 5:365-71.

17. **Hamuryudan V, Mat C, Saip S, et al.** Thalidomide in the treatment of the mucocutaneous lesions of Behçet's syndrome. Ann Intern Med. 1998;128:443-50.

18. **Calabrese L, Fleischer AM.** Thalidomide: current and potential clinical applications. Am J Med. 2000;108:487-95.

26

■　■　■

Uveitis

Daniel F. Rosberger, MD, PhD

U veitis, inflammation of the uveal tract (iris, ciliary body, and choroid) (Figure 26-1), is the third leading cause of blindness in the United States, accounting for a tenth of severe vision loss. The hallmarks of this inflammation are the presence of white blood cells and protein transudation (flare) in the aqueous and/or vitreous humors.

Frequently, rather than being an isolated primary ocular condition, uveitis is a secondary manifestation of a systemic disorder, and the differential diagnosis varies greatly depending upon age, genetics, and environment. The most important underlying conditions are the seronegative spondyloarthropathies and sarcoidosis, each accounting for up to 7% of cases seen in uveitis referral centers (1). Attempts have been made to classify uveitis on the basis of etiology, rapidity of onset, chronicity of disease, appearance of the inflammatory precipitates, and whether the cause is endogenous or exogenous in etiology. However, the most clinically useful classification is based upon the location of the inflammation in the eye: anterior versus posterior chamber.

Ocular inflammation damages vascular endothelium, which in turn disrupts the tight junctions of the blood-ocular barrier and causes transudation of plasma proteins (known as a protein flare) and exudation of white blood cells into the eye. Uveitis is often mild and self-limited, but it can also cause severe vision loss due to a variety of mechanisms: damage to the ocular media (e.g., clouding of the aqueous and vitreous, corneal opacification, cataract formation); increased intraocular pressure (glaucoma) from damage to trabecular angle structures responsible for drainage of fluid from the eye; decreased intraocular pressure (hypotony) secondary to damage to the ciliary body structures responsible for aqueous production; irreversible choroidal and retinal scarring; and retinal, choroidal and iris neovascularization. The challenge of treating uveitis involves ameliorating the patients' symptoms and identifying and treating any underlying disease.

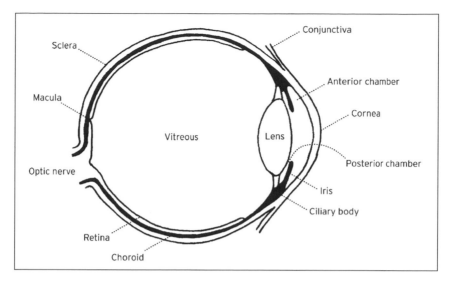

Figure 26-1   Schematic illustration of a sagittal section of the human eye. The uveal tract consists of the iris, the ciliary body, and the choroid. (Illustration by Ms. Lisa Yee.)

Case Presentation

A 43-year-old previously healthy African-American male presented with a 1-month history of mild ocular discomfort in his right eye with moderate injection and tearing that had worsened over the previous 3 days. He reported that his vision was mildly affected but complained of extreme photophobia. Ophthalmological examination was significant for mildly decreased visual acuity in the affected eye with conjunctival and episcleral injection. Moderate anterior chamber cellularity and protein transudation with granulomatous keratic precipitates were noted in the anterior chamber. Intraocular pressure was normal. There were few anterior vitreous cells, but the retina appeared normal. The findings were consistent with acute granulomatous uveitis.

An extensive medical evaluation for a secondary cause of uveitis revealed a mildly elevated serum angiotensin-converting enzyme level and a chest X-ray demonstrating bilateral hilar adenopathy consistent with sarcoidosis. The diagnosis of sarcoid iridocyclitis was made. Because the patient had no systemic or respiratory symptoms, treatment was directed at his ocular problems only. Topical therapy to the right eye with prednisolone acetate 1% (one drop every 30 minutes) and 1% cyclopentolate (one drop three times daily) was initiated. At the same time, a pulmonary consultation was obtained that revealed no pulmonary function abnormalities.

After 1 week, his symptoms were largely improved, but there were still cells in the anterior chamber and anterior vitreous. Treatment was continued, and by 2 weeks there was no longer any active inflammation. The prednisolone acetate and cyclopentolate were successfully tapered off over 2 months. Six months later, however, the patient had an identical recurrence in the same eye that again responded promptly to topical therapy. He was advised that additional recurrences in either eye were certainly possible and that he should report any symptoms immediately. He continues to be followed regularly by his ophthalmologist and pulmonologist.

Anterior Uveitis (Iritis and Iridocyclitis)

Patients with anterior uveitis have inflammation confined to the iris (iritis) and/or ciliary body (iridocyclitis). Acute anterior uveitis presents with symptoms of pain, photophobia, mild to moderate decreased vision, and tearing. Patients with chronic uveitis usually, but not always, have more moderate symptoms.

The defining signs of anterior uveitis are cells and flare in the anterior chamber visualized by slit lamp examination. Often, there are collections of cellular debris and protein on the corneal endothelium called keratic precipitates. These are predominantly composed of polymorphonuclear leukocytes early in the disease process, whereas macrophages and lymphocytes appear later. Keratic precipitates can be either fine and referred to as nongranulomatous, or large ("mutton-fat") and referred to as granulomatous. In granulomatous anterior uveitis, there can also be clusters of cells on the pupillary border and on the iris surface. Some important causes of nongranulomatous and granulomatous anterior uveitis are listed in Table 26-1.

Other signs may include spillover of cells and flare into the anterior vitreous, hypopyon (layering of cells in the anterior chamber), intraocular changes in pressure (either increased or decreased), miosis (constriction of the pupil), engorgement of the perilimbal vasculature, and, with chronicity, adhesions between the iris and anterior lens capsule (posterior synechia).

Diagnosis

A diagnosis of anterior uveitis demands consideration of an underlying etiology, which is present in more than one fourth of cases (Table 26-1). Although no cause is found in a majority of cases, early identification of an associated systemic condition may aid in the treatment of the uveitis and minimizes the sequelae of the underlying condition. Familiarity with these conditions enables the primary care clinician and ophthalmologist to inquire about pertinent symptoms that might otherwise be overlooked in the evaluation of the patient. Rheumatological conditions that are commonly associated with anterior uveitis include the seronegative spondyloarthropathies, sarcoidosis, Behçet's disease, juvenile chronic arthritis, and Lyme disease. Up to 40% of patients with ankylosing spondylitis (AS) present at some point during the course of their illness with anterior uveitis (2). The

Table 26-1 Systemic Causes of Anterior Uveitis and Associated Features

	Frequency*	Systemic Findings	Comments
Acute Non-Granulomatous			
Ankylosing spondylitis	25-40%	Sacroiliitis, spondylitis	Sudden onset, usually unilateral, frequent recurrences, hypopyon
Inflammatory bowel disease	3-11%	Abdominal pain, diarrhea, hematochezia	
Psoriatic arthritis	7-16%	Psoriasis, oligoarthritis	Rarely occurs without arthritis
Reactive arthritis	12-37%	Oligoarthritis, urethritis, precedent GU/GI infection	Hypopyon, usually unilateral
Behçet's disease	30-55%	Mucosal ulcers, vasculitis, thrombophlebitis, pathergy	Hypopyon, usually bilateral
Lyme disease		Erythema migrans, oligoarthritis, serological confirmation	
Herpetic infection (e.g., herpes simplex, varicella zoster)		Vesicular rash	
Acute Granulomatous			
Juvenile chronic arthritis	10-20%	Oligoarticular arthritis, ANA+, RF-	Predominant in girls, frequently bilateral, often painless
Chronic Granulomatous			
Sarcoidosis	15-20%	Hilar adenopathy, erythema nodosum	Often bilateral
Multiple sclerosis	<1%	Oligoclonal bands in CSF, demyelinating disease	Often bilateral
Vogt-Koyanagi-Harada syndrome	65-95%	Fever, CNS symptoms (meningismus, headache), vitiligo	Usually bilateral
Tuberculosis		Abnormal chest X-ray, positive tuberculin test	
Syphilis		Palmar/plantar maculo-papular rash, serological confirmation	

* Percentage of patients with condition with uveitis as a manifestation.
GU = genitourinary; GI = gastrointestinal; ANA = antinuclear antibody; RF = rheumatoid factor; CSF = cerebrospinal fluid; CNS = central nervous system.

prevalence of anterior uveitis across all of the HLA-B27–related seronegative spondyloarthropathies (AS, inflammatory bowel disease, psoriatic arthritis, and reactive arthritis) is between 5% and 10%. Interestingly, the majority of patients with isolated acute anterior uveitis are HLA-B27–positive, suggesting that uveitis and spondylitis represent different points along the same disease spectrum.

A complete ophthalmological examination 1) establishes the presence and quantification of anterior chamber cells, protein flare, and conjunctival and/or perilimbal vascular congestion; 2) characterizes keratic precipitates, intraocular pressure, and lens changes; and 3) determines the presence of cells in the vitreous. Cellularity can also be used as a measure of disease activity and response to therapy.

If the anterior uveitis is a first occurrence, unilateral, and non-granulomatous, careful observation may be considered initially. However, for cases that are recurrent, in which the inflammation is bilateral, or when the inflammation is granulomatous, the evaluation should include complete blood count (CBC), erythrocyte sedimentation rate (ESR), tuberculin skin testing, and chest X-ray. When clinically appropriate, serological testing for syphilis and *Borrelia burgdorferi* should also be obtained.

Additional testing can be further guided by features of the presenting history and extraocular signs and symptoms that may suggest a specific etiology (for example, colonoscopy to assess for inflammatory bowel disease).

Management

Therapy is directed toward treating the underlying condition if one is identified. If an ophthalmologist is not already involved, immediate consultation should be sought for evaluation and assistance with management of the local inflammation. Delayed or ineffective management of ocular inflammation may rapidly result in permanent vision loss. Suppression of inflammation is usually accomplished with topical corticosteroids (e.g.. prednisolone acetate 1% ocular drops). Initial dosing is one drop every 30 minutes, which is then titrated down to the interval sufficient to suppress the presence of aqueous cells. This may take several weeks. After the presence of aqueous cells have completely resolved, an attempt to slowly taper the drops may be made, typically with gradual dose reductions on a weekly basis. However, if the taper is too rapid, there may be a recurrence necessitating an increase in the dosage. In conjunction with the topical corticosteroids, cycloplegic agents (cyclopentolate, homatropine, scopolamine, or atropine) are also used in the initial phase of therapy to prevent ciliary spasm and to prevent or disrupt synechia formation.

In cases where there has been an inadequate response to topical therapy, a depot injection of corticosteroids (methylprednisolone 40-80 mg) can be given into the subtenon space located beneath the posterior episcleral fascia. There are substantial risks to subtenon injections, including inadvertent perforation of the globe that can result in hemorrhage, retinal detachment, or blindness. In addition, injections are contraindicated in patients with a history of corticosteroid-induced increases in intraocular pressure or glaucoma. Moreover, subtenon injections often need to be repeated periodically.

When both topical and subtenon corticosteroids have been ineffective and especially when vision has been affected by the development of cystoid macular edema (Figure 26-2), systemic corticosteroids should be considered. Initial systemic corticosteroid therapy should be aggressive (e.g., 1.5 mg/kg/d of prednisone or equivalent), and dosages should be tapered slowly only after the desired affect has been achieved, typically after 2 to 3 weeks. Systemic nonsteroidal anti-inflammatory drugs (NSAIDs) also have a role in the maintenance therapy of uveitis patients. For example, approximately 70% of patients with HLA-B27–associated uveitis may remain relapse-free while on a daily dose of NSAIDs.

In cases where corticosteroids are contraindicated, where the uveitis has not been responsive to maximal systemic corticosteroids, or where it has been impossible to reduce the daily dose of prednisone below 15 mg, various immunomodulating agents have been utilized to control the active inflammatory process. Included among some of the more commonly employed agents are azathioprine, methotrexate, mycophenolate mofetil, cyclosporine, tacrolimus, cyclophosphamide, and chlorambucil. As reviewed recently by an expert panel of clinicians, most of the evidence for the use of these drugs is from uncontrolled case series (3). However, reasonably large controlled studies supporting the use of azathioprine (2.5 mg/kg/d) and cyclosporine (10-15 mg/kg/d) have been published (4,5). At present, the effectiveness of inhibitors of tumor necrosis factor such as infliximab and etanercept is not clearly established but may not be as impressive as for inflammatory arthritic diseases (6).

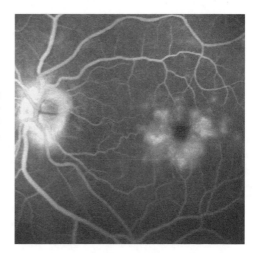

Figure 26-2 Late frames of a left fundus fluorescein angiogram demonstrating the typical optic nerve and macular hyperfluorescence due to dye leakage in a uveitis patient with cystoid macular edema.

Frequently, patients with anterior uveitis develop secondary glaucoma. This can result from blockage of the open angle trabecular meshwork with cellular debris from severe anterior chamber inflammation, neovascularization of the iris and angle, formation of inflammatory synechiae causing angle closure, or as an idiosyncratic response to corticosteroid therapy. Treatment consists of controlling the underlying inflammation, managing the increased intraocular pressure with topical glaucoma medications, and, when necessary, surgical interventions that create an alternative route for the outflow of aqueous fluid (e.g. trabeculectomy). If the increase in intraocular pressure is believed to be an adverse effect of corticosteroids, an attempt should be made to taper the dose or to add a corticosteroid-sparing agent. Alternatively, corticosteroids with lower pressure-elevating properties (e.g., fluorometholone or loteprednol) can be used, but unfortunately in clinical practice these agents generally demonstrate less potent anti-inflammatory effects than conventional corticosteroid agents.

Posterior Uveitis

Patients with posterior uveitis may present with symptoms of blurred vision, photophobia, and pain. The majority of cases are idiopathic, but important secondary causes are described in Table 26-2, of which sarcoidosis, Wegener's granulomatosis, and Behçet's syndrome are of particular interest to the rheumatologist.

The defining signs of posterior uveitis are white blood cells in the vitreous. There may also be retinal infiltrates, choroidal infiltrates, retinal (often macular) edema, and vascular sheathing. Optic nerve edema as well as retinal hemorrhages and exudates may also be present. Patients with posterior uveitis may also have all of the signs of anterior uveitis, including conjunctival injection, white blood cells and protein flare in the aqueous, and posterior synechiae. In addition, secondary retinal detachment, glaucoma, cataract formation, and choroidal neovascularization can occur.

Diagnosis

The diagnostic evaluation of posterior uveitis begins with a complete history and physical examination to try to elucidate an underlying systemic cause. A complete ophthalmological examination, including careful binocular indirect ophthalmoscopy with careful attention to the inferior ora serrata, slit lamp biomicroscopy of the vitreous, macula, optic disc and vessels, and intraocular pressure measurement, is required. The diagnostic evaluation is guided by the clinical presentation but should always include a CBC, chest X-ray, tuberculin skin testing, and serological testing for syphilis to assess for common treatable causes. Additional testing where appropriate may include *Toxoplasma* serologies, angiotensin-converting enzyme, ESR,

Table 26-2   Systemic Causes of Posterior Uveitis and Associated Features

	*Frequency**	*Systemic Findings*
Sarcoidosis	10-15%	Hilar adenopathy, erythema nodosum
Behçet's disease	20-55%	Mucosal ulcers, vasculitis, thrombophlebitis, pathergy
Vogt-Koyanagi-Harada syndrome	40-95%	Fever, CNS symptoms (menigismus, headache), vitiligo, alopecia
Wegener's granulomatosis	2-3%	Upper and lower respiratory tract inflammation, renal disease
Multiple sclerosis	1-2%	Oligoclonal bands in CSF, demyelinating disease
Tuberculosis		Abnormal chest X-ray, positive tuberculin test
Lyme disease		Erythema migrans, oligoarthritis, serological confirmation
Whipple's disease		Gastrointestinal symptoms, PAS+ macrophages in jejunal lamina propria, PCR
Toxoplasmosis		Congenital infection in 95%, serological confirmation
Syphilis		Palmar/plantar maculopapular rash, serological confirmation
Endophthalmitis		Immunosuppression, bacteremia

* Percentage of patients with conditioin with uveitis as a manifestation.
CNS = central nervous system; CSF = cerebrospinal fluid; PAS = periodic acid-Schiff; PCR = polymerase chain reaction.

lumbar puncture, or serological testing for *B. burgdorferi* and human immunodeficiency virus.

In cases where a bacterial or fungal infectious etiology is suspected (e.g. endophthalmitis) or a "masquerade syndrome" (reticulum cell sarcoma) is entertained, a diagnostic vitrectomy can be performed to obtain specimens for analysis, stain, and culture. More recently, polymerase chain reaction analysis of vitreous specimens has led to the diagnosis of viral and parasitic infections in selected cases.

Management

As with anterior uveitis, non-infectious posterior uveitis is managed by beginning with aggressive local and systemic corticosteroid therapy, systemic NSAIDs, and when necessary immunomodulatory agents. Moreover, management is also dictated by identification and treatment of underlying causes. An ophthalmologist should always be part of the management team.

Sarcoidosis, Behçet's disease, and Vogt-Koyanagi-Harada syndrome are three non-infectious systemic inflammatory conditions that are distinctive in that either or both anterior and posterior uveitis can be prominent ocular manifestations (1,7). As described in Chapter 11, sarcoidosis is characterized by non-caseating granulomatous infiltration of virtually any organ system. In some series, uveitis eventually affects up to 24% of sarcoid patients and is usually an early manifestation, often preceding the initial diagnosis of sarcoidosis (8). Sarcoid-associated posterior uveitis is treated similarly to anterior uveitis with the exception that posterior disease more frequently requires subtenon and systemic corticosteroids, especially in the presence of cystoid macular edema. If retinal neovascularization occurs due to retinal capillary non-perfusion, pan-retinal photocoagulation is indicated. Anterior uveitis may be more common among black patients with sarcoidosis, whereas posterior involvement may be more common in white patients (8).

Vogt-Koyanagi-Harada syndrome is a rare inflammatory disease that can involve the eyes (uveitis), skin (alopecia and vitiligo) and central nervous system (encephalopathy, meningitis, cranial neuropathy) (9). Behçet's disease is characterized by recurrent oral and genital ulcers, but uveitis, various cutaneous manifestations, and vascular disease are also part of the clinical picture. Uveitis in both of these conditions often requires systemic corticosteroids and immunomodulating drugs (10,11).

Uveitis can occur at any time in 2% to 3% of patients with Wegener's granulomatosis and is an important cause of vision loss when left untreated (12). Chronic inflammation of the upper or lower respiratory tract (e.g., otitis, sinusitis, or pulmonary infiltrates) or renal disease should raise suspicion for this disorder. Aggressive immunosuppressive therapy with oral cyclophosphamide (0.5-3.0 mg/kg daily) in conjunction with systemic corticosteroids is usually required to preserve vision in Wegener's granulomatosis (13).

Uveitis in Lyme disease has been treated with oral systemic antibiotics in early mild disease, but the threshold to use intravenous therapy is low (14).

In one series, toxoplasmosis accounted for 10% of all cases of uveitis seen in a referral center. Initial management of toxoplasmosis can be vigilant observation if the inflammation is mild and if the retinochoroidal lesions are small and do not threaten the optic nerve or macula. If an anterior chamber reaction is present, topical corticosteroids and cylcoplegics are instituted. In cases where the lesions are large or close to the optic nerve or fovea or if the vitritis is severe, systemic antibiotics (e.g., sulfadiazine, pyrimethamine, or clindamycin) are used, and systemic corticosteroids are added once antimicrobial therapy is instituted. Patients taking pyrimethamine need folinic acid supplementation.

In the presence of posterior uveitis secondary to suspected syphilis and positive serologies, a lumbar puncture for cellular determination and/or serology is indicated. If the lumbar puncture results are positive, the patient should be treated for neurosyphilis with intravenous antibiotics.

Endophthalmitis is an ocular emergency and needs to be treated as quickly as possible with intravitreal antibiotics and corticosteroids. The cause may be an antecedent intraocular surgery or trauma or bacteremic spread from a distal site (often in immunocompromised patients or in intravenous drug abusers). The Endophthalmitis Vitrectomy Study demonstrated a benefit from vitrectomy in patients with visual acuity of light perception or worse, while patients with hand motions vision or better are treated with a vitreous paracentesis. All patients should receive broad-spectrum intravitreal antibiotics. Specimens are sent to the laboratory for identification and sensitivities to confirm and, if necessary, adjust antibiotic selections. The timing of intravitreal corticosteroid therapy is controversial but is usually administered in acute cases concurrently with antibiotics. Intravenous antibiotics are indicated only in endogenously derived endophthalmitis and are directed toward the systemic infectious source.

Summary

Uveitis is an important cause of blindness, and early diagnosis and intervention is necessary for minimizing morbidity. Although most commonly idiopathic in nature, uveitis is often seen as part of systemic inflammatory illnesses, both infectious and non-infectious in etiology. Identification of underlying conditions is essential not only for the appropriate management of the ophthalmological problem but also for reducing complications associated with the systemic disease. Close collaboration between the internist, rheumatologist, and ophthalmologist is crucial for optimal care of the patient.

REFERENCES

1. **Rothova A, Buitenhuis HJ, Meenken C, et al.** Uveitis and systemic disease. Br J Ophthalmol. 1992;76:137-41.
2. **Banares A, Hernandez-Garcia C, Fernadez-Gutierrez B, Jover JA.** Eye involvement in the spondyloarthropathies. Rheum Dis Clin North Am. 1998;24:771-84.
3. **Jabs DA, Rosenbaum JT, Foster S, et al.** Guidelines for the use of immunosuppressive drugs in patients with ocular inflammatory disorders: recommendations of an expert panel. Am J Ophthalmol. 2000;130:492-513.
4. **Yazici H, Pazarli H, Barnes CG, et al.** A controlled trial of azathioprine in Behçet's syndrome. N Engl J Med. 1990;322:281-5.
5. **Nussenblatt RB, Palestine AG, Chan CC, et al.** Randomized, double-masked study of cyclosporine compared to prednisolone in the treatment of endogenous uveitis. Am J Ophthalmol. 1991;112:138-46.
6. **Smith JR, Levinson RD, Holland GN, et al.** Differential efficacy of tumor necrosis factor inhibition in the management of inflammatory eye disease and associated rheumatic disease. Arthritis Rheum. 2001;45:252-7.
7. **Smith JR, Rosenbaum JT.** Management of uveitis: a rheumatologic perspective. Arthritis Rheum. 2001;46:309-18.
8. **Rothava A, Alberts C, Glasius E, et al.** Risk factors for ocular sarcoidosis. Doc Ophthalmol. 1989;72:287-96.

9. **Snyder DA, Tessler HH.** Vogt-Koyanagi-Harada syndrome. Am J Ophthalmol. 1980;90:69-75.

10. **Rubsamen PE, Gass JD.** Vogt-Koyanagi-Harada syndrome: clinical course, therapy, and long-term visual outcome. Arch Ophthalmol. 1991;109:682-7.

11. **Hamuryudan V, Ozyazgan Y, Hizli N, et al.** Azathioprine in Behçet's syndrome: effects on long-term prognosis. Arthritis Rheum. 1997;40:769-74.

12. **Hoffman GS, Kerr GS, Leavitt RY, et al.** Wegener granulomatosis: an analysis of 158 patients. Ann Intern Med. 1992;116:488-98.

13. **Guillevin L, Cordier J-F, Lhote F, Cohen P, et al.** A prospective, multicenter, randomized trial comparing steroids and pulse cyclophosphamide versus steroids and oral cyclophosphamide in the treatment of generalized Wegener's granulomatosis. Arthritis Rheum. 1997;40:2187-98.

14. **Winward KE, Smith JL, Culberson WW, Paris-Hamelin.** Ocular Lyme borreliosis. Am J Ophthalmol. 1989;108:651-7.

27

Low Back Pain

Charis F. Meng, MD

L ow back pain (LBP) is a common problem affecting up to 80% of the general population, with the highest prevalence in the fifth to seventh decades of life (1,2). Most cases of acute LBP resolve spontaneously, but up to 10% of cases become chronic. Acute pain is defined as that which lasts less than 6 weeks. Subacute pain lasts up to 12 weeks, and when it persists after 12 weeks, the pain is defined as chronic. The subsequent disability from chronic LBP and its attendant costs in billions of dollars annually are well established. Although a discussion of low back pain can comprise volumes, a systematic approach to evaluation will efficiently lead to an appropriate therapeutic plan in the vast majority of cases.

Although the causes of LBP are many and not always well understood, review of the skeletal anatomy of the lumbosacral spine is helpful in teasing out many different pain syndromes (Figure 27-1). The most common causes are mechanical and include disc herniation, spinal stenosis, spondylosis, spondylolisthesis, or lumbar strain (3). In the primary care setting, such mechanical etiologies for LBP represent more than 97% of cases.

The facet joints, periosteum, meninges, blood vessels, muscle, and ligaments are all innervated with pain fibers and thus are all pain-sensitive structures. Various chemical mediators have been implicated in the transmission of spinal pain, including substance P, somatostatin, cholecystokinin, vasoactive intestinal peptide, and bradykinin (4). A herniated intervertebral disc causes pain by impingement of adjacent structures, but whether degeneration of the disc itself can generate pain is a matter of debate in view of the absence of pain fibers in the disc (3). One area of active interest is how herniated discs spontaneously resorb. Recent work suggests, for example, that macrophage infiltration and production of matrix metalloproteinases may participate in the resorption of herniated discs. Further elucidation of such mechanisms may eventually offer novel therapeutic options in expediting recovery in patients with LBP from disc herniation.

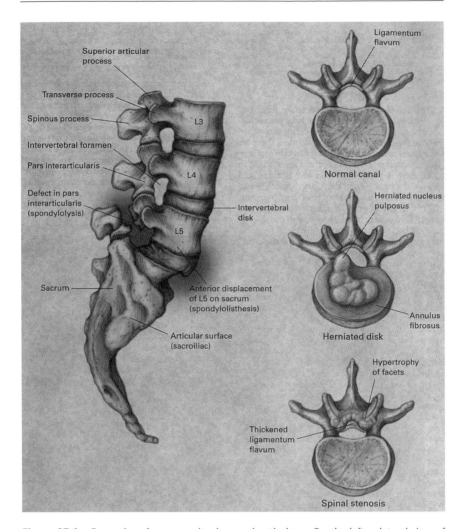

Superior articular process

Transverse process

Spinous process

Intervertebral foramen

Pars interarticularis

Defect in pars interarticularis (spondylolysis)

Sacrum

L3

L4

L5

Intervertebral disk

Anterior displacement of L5 on sacrum (spondylolisthesis)

Articular surface (sacroiliac)

Ligamentum flavum

Normal canal

Herniated nucleus pulposus

Annulus fibrosus

Herniated disk

Hypertrophy of facets

Thickened ligamentum flavum

Spinal stenosis

Figure 27-1   Examples of common lumbosacral pathology. On the left, a lateral view of the lumbosacral spine shows the bony and soft tissue components of the spine and illustrates spondylolisthesis and spondylolysis. On the right, a superior view shows the normal canal (*top*) compared with the narrowed canal space due to a herniated disc (*middle*) and spinal stenosis (*bottom*). (From Deyo R, Weinstein J. Low back pain. N Engl J Med. 2001; 344:363-70; with permission.)

Various factors contribute to the development of chronic low back pain. Acute low back pain, regardless of specific cause, is thought to induce paraspinal muscle spasms, which then become an independent source of painful stimuli. Progressive immobility, deconditioning, and increased body weight may then potentiate this vicious cycle (5). It is clear that while an exceedingly common problem, LBP and its pathogenesis are far from being fully understood.

Case Presentation 1

A 37-year-old active and athletic man with a 1-month history of intermittent right-sided low back pain developed an acute exacerbation of his symptoms while lifting a heavy object. He also complained of new radiating pain and paresthesias down his right buttock and lateral aspect of his leg to the dorsum of his foot. On physical examination, there was mildly restricted motion of his back in all planes with palpable tenderness along the paraspinal musculature. Straight-leg raise testing was positive on the right leg at 45 degrees, but there were no focal neurological deficits. Nonsteroidal anti-inflammatory drugs (NSAIDs) were prescribed. Physical therapy was recommended, but the patient declined citing a lack of time. His symptoms waxed and waned for 3 months, at which time he had another acute exacerbation that interfered significantly with his desk job. A seated position was particularly uncomfortable, and he frequently needed to lie flat for pain relief.

Magnetic resonance imaging (MRI) demonstrated a herniated disc at the L4/L5 intervertebral space with impingement on the L5 nerve root. An epidural corticosteroid injection provided temporary relief for 3 months, during which time he consented to physical rehabilitation and "back school" for back protection exercises and techniques. His radicular symptoms resolved, and although he continued to have intermittent low back pain, it was greatly improved. He has incorporated back exercises into his usual athletic activities.

Case Presentation 2

A 75-year-old generally active woman presents with the complaint of low back pain. She reports intermittent low back pain for many years that in general has not hampered her activities and has been symptomatic only with prolonged activities. X-rays of the lumbosacral spine 4 years ago revealed scoliosis and multilevel degenerative changes, and the patient was prescribed physical therapy that reduced her discomfort. However, although she conscientiously performs her back exercises daily, her back pains have become more frequent and severe over the past year. She also reports that when she walks upright, the pain radiates down to her left foot, causing her to walk stooped forward or to sit in order to relieve the discomfort. Acetaminophen and NSAIDs helped originally but as of late have been ineffective in controlling her pain, and she is unable to maintain her usual exercise routine. She denies muscle weakness and urinary and bowel incontinence. X-rays show progression of the osteoarthritis.

The patient attempted another course of supervised physical therapy but was unable to continue because of pain. Acupuncture also did not help. MRI revealed mild central canal stenosis at several levels and marked foraminal compromise at the L3/L4 interspace with bilateral nerve root impingement. A series of epidural corticosteroid injections did not offer sustained relief.

A surgical consultation was obtained, and the patient subsequently underwent a laminectomy to decompress the nerve root impingement. Postoperatively, the patient progressed steadily with a closely monitored rehabilitation program. She continued to do well after discharge, regularly performing her prescribed exercises and returning to her usual activities, with only occasional and minimal back discomfort.

Diagnosis

Clinical History

A complete medical history is crucial in the evaluation of LBP. Although the vast majority of back pain cases are of musculoskeletal origin and self-limited, a minority of patients who initially present with LBP may have referred symptoms due to a malignancy, infection, visceral organ disease, or abdominal aneurysms and may require immediate intervention (Table 27-1). A history of night pain, fevers, chills, night sweats, weight loss, or change in bowel habits should alert the clinician to these possible etiologies. Updated age-appropriate screening tests for malignancy are important. Risk factors for osteoporosis need to be sought in women with acute back pain attributable to vertebral compression fractures.

The quality of pain is frequently an important clue in determining the cause of LBP. Colicky pain raises the possibility of referred pain from abdominal or pelvic organs. Malignancy should be suspected when pain is nocturnal, not linked to specific movements, associated with constitutional

---

Table 27-1   "Red Flags" in the Evaluation of Low Back Pain

Suspect cancer or infection if:
- History of cancer
- Unexplained weight loss
- Immunosuppression
- Intravenous drug use
- History of urinary infection
- Pain increased by rest or nocturnal pain
- Fever
- Age >50

Suspect spinal fracture if:
- History of significant trauma
- Risk factors for osteoporosis
- Age >70

Suspect cauda equina syndrome if:
- Bladder dysfunction
- Urinary retention
- Overflow incontinence
- Bowel dysfunction
- Loss of anal sphincter tone
- Fecal incontinence
- Saddle anesthesia
- Progressive motor weakness

Suspect abdominal aortic aneurysm if:
- Risk factors for atherosclerosis
- Palpable pulsatile mass in abdomen or abdominal bruit
- Pain in back, chest or scrotum
- Calcified aorta on plain radiograph

Modified from Datta D, Mirza SK, White AA III. Low back pain. Textbook Rheumatol Updates. 2001;1:1-15; with permission.

symptoms, or refractory to treatment. Spinal infections can cause acute severe pain associated with systemic symptoms such as fever, chills, and sweats. They are usually hematogenous in origin (particularly in intravenous drug users) but can be due to contiguous infections introduced during local injections. Pain that improves with activity or is associated with morning stiffness or peripheral joint synovitis may reflect a seronegative spondyloarthropathy such as ankylosing spondylitis. An abdominal aortic aneurysm can cause back pain that does not change appreciably with rest or activity and can be palpated as a pulsatile mass in the abdomen. Fibromyalgia is suspected when there appears to be disproportionate tenderness over the gluteal area and other stereotypic points in the presence of a generally normal examination and vague complaints of fatigue, depression, or irritable bowel symptoms. Table 27-2 summarizes common clinical features of different causes of low back pain.

Back pain that radiates down below the knee suggests a radiculopathy (pathology of a single spinal nerve root) and may be associated with lower extremity paresthesias and weakness. Radiculopathic pain may be exacerbated by coughing, sneezing, or Valsalva maneuvers. Sciatica is pain or paresthesias in the distribution of the sciatic nerve that receives contributions from the L4-S1 nerve roots. Symptoms of sciatica may result from disease processes anywhere from the level of these individual nerve roots to the egress of the sciatic nerve itself from the pelvis (e.g., entrapment by the piriformis muscle).

Table 27-2   Clinical Presentations of Different Causes of Low Back Pain

Diagnosis	Clinical Presentation
Disc disease	Back pain that improves with rest, worsens with lifting and bending over, nerve root impingement signs
Spinal stenosis	Back pain that improves with flexion and rest, worsens with standing and extension, leg heaviness, neurogenic claudication, nerve root impingement signs
Spondyloarthropathy	Sacroiliac pain, morning stiffness, back pain that improves with exercise, presenting in a young man
Spinal tumor	History of malignancy, weight loss, night sweats, back pain on recumbency or at night, elevated sedimentation rate
Spinal infection	History of intravenous drug use, instrumentation or systemic infection, fever, chills, severe back pain, leukocytosis, elevated sedimentation rate
Fibromyalgia	Tenderness at multiple stereotypic points, normal general examination and laboratory tests
Fracture	History of trauma or osteoporosis risk factors, sudden onset of back pain, kyphosis, presenting in postmenopausal women

Spinal stenosis pain classically improves with back flexion and worsens with extension, causing the patient to stoop forward or sit for pain relief (Table 27-3). In contrast, nerve impingement by a herniated disc is often exacerbated by prolonged sitting and relieved with back extension. Patients with spinal stenosis may be more comfortable walking uphill or while bent forward rather than downhill or upright, as is characteristic of a patient with a herniated disc. The presence of leg weakness or heaviness, paresthesias, or incontinence should be assessed as indications of more advanced neurological compromise. Bowel or bladder incontinence, in particular, requires immediate attention as a possible sign of cauda equina syndrome (see Table 27-1).

It is important to ask the patient how the LBP affects the activities of daily living. Does the pain interfere with walking, working, household chores, sports activities, or sleep? The impact of LBP on function is clinically relevant and allows the physician to assess the severity of the pain in a semi-quantitative manner. Functional outcomes are as important as pain measures in assessing treatment effectiveness.

Physical Examination

A complete medical examination should be performed to determine whether LBP is a local musculoskeletal problem or a part of a systemic or non-musculoskeletal process. Particular attention should be directed to the examination of the abdomen, pelvis, vasculature, axial and peripheral skeleton, and nervous system.

The examination of the lumbosacral spine begins with inspection of the alignment and curvature of the spine, which may reveal deformities such as kyphosis or scoliosis. Straightening of the normal lumbar lordosis suggests ligamentous strain. Severe pain on percussion raises the possibility of a spinal infection. The palpation of tender and trigger points (e.g., muscle spasm, myofascial pain, fibromyalgia), the costovertebral angles (e.g.,

Table 27-3   Differentiating Between Pain from Disc Disease and Pain from Spinal Stenosis

	Discogenic Low Back Pain	*Spinal Stenosis Pain*
Standing/walking	Decreased	Increased
Sitting	Increased	Decreased
Valsalva maneuver	Increased	No change
Bending	Increased	Increased with extension, decreased with flexion
Lifting	Increased	No change
Bed rest	Decreased	Decreased

Modified from Lipson SJ. Low back pain. In: Kelley EN, Ruddy S, Harris ED Jr, Sledge CB, eds. Textbook of Rheumatology, 5th ed. Philadelphia: WB Saunders; 1997: 439-56; with permission.

pyelonephritis), the sciatic notch (e.g., piriformis syndrome), and the sacroiliac joints (e.g., sacroiliitis) is helpful. With range-of-motion testing of the lumbosacral spine, spinal stenosis is suggested if the pain is caused by or worsened by back extension, a position that further narrows the spinal canal. In contrast, nerve impingement caused by a herniated disc may be relieved by back extension and exacerbated with back flexion. The straight leg-raising test of Lasègue places the L4, L5, and S1 nerve roots under tension; a positive test occurs when the typical radiating pain is reproduced. The level at which the raised leg elicits pain is recorded. The test has high sensitivity but low specificity. Alternatively, in a positive crossed straight-leg raising test, radicular pain occurs in the contralateral leg; this is less sensitive but more specific (6). The presence of confirmatory dural tension signs, gait disturbances, inability to heel and toe walk, and evidence of vascular insufficiency should be sought. Neurogenic pseudoclaudication is a characteristic manifestation of spinal stenosis. The clinical presentations of different nerve root impingement syndromes are summarized in Table 27-4.

Laboratory Testing

Unless the medical history or physical examination suggests a systemic disorder or visceral abnormality, laboratory testing for the initial evaluation of LBP

Table 27-4 Differentiating Levels of Nerve Root Impingement

Nerve Root	Intervertebral Space	Pain Radiation from Back	Sensory Dysfunction	Straight Leg Raise	Knee Jerk	Ankle Jerk	Motor Weakness*
L3	L2-L3	To buttocks and anterior knee	Knee region	Usually negative	Normal	Normal	Quadriceps
L4	L3-L4	To buttocks, posterior thigh, and inner calf	Medial part of lower leg	Occasionally positive	Abnormal	Normal	Quadriceps, anticus
L5	L4-L5	To buttocks and dorsum of foot and great toe	Dorsum of foot and great toe	Positive	Normal	Normal	Anterior tibialis, great toe extensor, gluteus medius
S1	L5-S1	To buttocks, sole of foot and heel	Heel or lateral foot	Strongly positive	Normal	Abnormal	Gastrocnemius, hamstring, gluteus maximus

*Only the more obvious and functional muscles are listed.
Modified from Cailliet R. Low Back Pain Syndrome, 5th ed. Philadelphia: FA Davis; 1995; with permission.

is rarely necessary. The decision to obtain tests (such as complete blood count, erythrocyte sedimentation rate, serum chemistries, blood cultures, or serum and urine protein electrophoreses) should be guided by the level of clinical suspicion for infection, malignancy, or systemic inflammatory disorders.

Imaging Studies

Likewise, imaging studies for acute back pain in the absence of systemic symptoms are generally not needed. The clinical picture guides most initial diagnostic and therapeutic decisions (7). Because degenerative changes in the intervertebral discs, facet joints, and vertebral bodies are all common findings, controlled studies show that there is actually poor correlation between clinical symptoms and plain radiographic signs of degeneration per se (8). Reasons to consider imaging of the spine include associated neurological symptoms or signs, refractory pain, or the anticipation of an invasive procedure such as an epidural steroid injection or surgery.

When indicated, plain radiographs with anteroposterior and lateral views are commonly ordered first. They often show degenerative changes such as intervertebral disc space narrowing, osteophyte formation, and facet joint arthritis, and are helpful in visualizing misalignments such as scoliosis or kyphosis. Spondylolysis, a defect in the pars interarticularis secondary to neural arch weakness, is a risk factor for spondylolisthesis, the displacement of one vertebral body on another (see Figure 27-1), most commonly an anterior slipping of L4 on L5. Resulting spinal instability can be seen on lateral flexion and extension views. Plain radiography may also demonstrate evidence for malignant disease (e.g., osteolytic lesions) or metabolic bone diseases (e.g., compression fractures).

Although detailed visualization of bony structures may be further obtained with computed tomography (CT), MRI is generally better for the evaluation of soft tissues such as intervertebral discs and associated encroachment on neural structures. Gadolinium contrast adds additional resolution and, for example, may help distinguish disc herniation from post-surgical scarring.

Imaging tests are useful for confirmation of diagnoses but should not supercede the clinical impression. The presence or extent of common structural abnormalities such as degenerative disc disease and spinal stenosis often do not correlate with the clinical picture. In addition, early disc disruptions, facet degeneration, arachnoiditis, and soft tissue lesions may be missed on CT and MRI. CT-discography may be more sensitive than MRI in identifying early disc disease and may be helpful when MRI is negative. However, because it is an invasive procedure, it is used judiciously.

Electrophysiological Studies

Electromyography (EMG) and nerve conduction velocity (NCV) studies may demonstrate nerve root compression, demyelination, or inflammation.

EMG/NCV studies are often helpful in supporting the clinical impression and imaging studies when the diagnosis of radiculopathy is still unclear. Electrophysiological studies may better define the extent of neurological involvement. They can also discriminate between acute and chronic lesions, but, like imaging studies, they must be placed in the context of clinical findings. However, it should be noted that spinal stenosis can be quite severe and symptomatic even in the face of normal electrophysiological studies.

Management

Complete resolution of acute LBP due to mechanical causes typically occurs within 2 months. For this reason, a trial of conservative therapy, typically consisting of short-term bedrest, NSAIDs, muscle relaxants, and analgesics, is recommended for most cases. Massage, traction, short-term bracing, hot packs, and other physical therapeutic modalities are also used.

Although bedrest has been historically prescribed for acute LBP, well-designed studies have shown that patients randomized to shorter periods of bedrest (i.e., less than 2 days) had better outcomes than those who were prescribed longer periods of bedrest (8). Prolonged bed rest is not an effective treatment for acute LBP and may, in fact, delay recovery because of muscle disuse and resultant weakness. Remaining active and gradual, progressive return to ordinary activities result in less chronic disability and a more rapid return to work (9).

NSAIDs are widely prescribed for LBP. A systematic review of 51 trials suggested that NSAIDs are effective for short-term symptomatic relief in patients with acute LBP (10). However, NSAID use in chronic LBP is less well established and may be complicated by increased risks due to associated adverse effects, particularly in the elderly. Non-narcotic analgesic agents such as acetaminophen or tramadol may be more appropriate in patients with contraindications to NSAIDs. Muscle relaxants can also be helpful on a short-term basis when there is a concomitant element of muscle spasm.

Opioid analgesic therapy is often useful in severe acute LBP but is more controversial in the management of chronic LBP. One review of several uncontrolled case series of chronic LBP patients suggested that chronic opioid analgesic therapy was safe and effective for refractory cases (11). Substance abuse disorders, psychiatric disorders, and certain occupational factors are relative contraindications to chronic opioid analgesia. Methods for monitoring for drug dependence include contracts, family interviews, and periodic drug testing. Prevention of constipation is mandatory, particularly in the elderly.

Physical Treatment Modalities

Formal back exercises may be initiated after the acute pain phase has passed for at least 2 weeks. Exercises are aimed at strengthening the lower abdominal and back muscles and improving lumbopelvic flexibility. It should be emphasized to the patient that the primary goal is not to treat the acute pain but to help prevent recurrences. Therefore, it must be made clear that exercises as part of a home program should be continued indefinitely to maintain good back health. However, although physical exercise is widely recommended for LBP, data supporting this approach are actually limited. Some investigators report improved pain, function, and return to work, whereas others suggest that no definitive conclusions about the benefits of exercise therapy or which specific types of exercise are the most effective can be made (12,13). However, in view of the general safety of exercise, it should always be considered as part of an overall treatment plan.

Lifestyle modifications aimed at learning appropriate lifting and back protection techniques, increasing aerobic fitness with low-impact activities, and weight reduction in obese patients should also be emphasized (14). These measures are reinforced in "back schools" that educate and train LBP patients about ergonomics, posture, body mechanics, exercise, psychology, and self-management techniques.

At times, therapeutic injections for LBP can be administered into the painful soft tissues, trigger points, sacroiliac joints, facet joints, discs, nerve roots, and epidural space. The injections may contain local anesthetics and corticosteroids and are generally well tolerated and safe. Advocates cite their use as a short-term measure for relief of acute pain or exacerbations of chronic pain, thereby decreasing the need for analgesics and deferring potential surgery. However, definitive and convincing evidence for the long-term benefit of such injections is lacking (15).

Although traction has historically enjoyed popularity, the role of traction in the treatment of LBP has been controversial. Ostensibly, traction has been thought by some to distract and unload the spine and to enforce bedrest. However, traction has been found to be no more effective than sham traction in alleviating pain, improving functional status, restoring range of motion, or reducing work absenteeism (16).

Complementary Modalities

Acupuncture has become a popular complementary treatment for LBP. Derived from traditional Chinese medicine, acupuncture is a method of stimulating specific points on the body with fine, metallic needles to relieve pain and treat other medical problems. These so-called "acupoints" are often located near nerves and neuromuscular junctions, and there is an approximately 70% correlation with trigger points. Acupuncture has been shown to stimulate the release of endorphins. Several systematic reviews of controlled trials of acupuncture for LBP have suggested benefit but have been unable to conclude whether there was unequivocal superiority to placebo (17). Thus, the role of acupuncture for chronic LBP currently remains unclear. Nonetheless, due to its superior safety profile, acupuncture may be appropriate for patients who are unable to tolerate or who are unresponsive to conventional therapy.

Spinal manipulation is another widely utilized complementary treatment for LBP. However, a systematic review of 36 randomized methodologically sound clinical trials comparing spinal manipulation with other treatments, including placebo therapy, did not find spinal manipulation efficacious for patients with LBP (18).

Surgical Approaches

Surgery is indicated only in the setting of fixed or progressive neurological deficits or refractory back pain (Table 27-5). It should only be considered when there is an identifiable anatomic defect that clearly corresponds to symptoms and signs. Spinal procedures in which defined surgical indications are less clear are associated with poorer outcomes. The physician should work with the surgeon to judge the optimal timing of surgery. Nonemergency spinal surgery should occur after at least 4-6 weeks of conservative treatment but before the development of worsening neurological deficits. Common procedures include laminotomy, laminectomy, open discectomy, microdiscectomy, and spinal fusion.

A small portion of the lamina is excised in a laminotomy, whereas in a laminectomy, the lamina is removed completely. Discectomy removes the nucleus pulposus from the intervertebral space. These decompression procedures are performed in cases of spinal stenosis (laminotomy/laminectomy) and herniated disc (discectomy). A spinal fusion may also be performed when spinal instability is present or a likely anticipated post-operative complication. However, spinal fusion as first-line surgical treatment may be

Table 27-5   Indications for Surgical Referral Among Low Back Pain Disorders

Diagnosis	Indications for Surgical Referral
Herniated disc	Bowel or bladder dysfunction; numbness in saddle distribution; bilateral leg pain, weakness, or numbness; severe or progressive neurological signs or symptoms or persistent motor weakness or radiculopathy after 4-6 weeks of conservative therapy
Spinal stenosis	Neurological signs and symptoms as for herniated discs; disabling back and leg pain with confirmatory imaging tests of spinal stenosis
Spondylolisthesis	Neurological signs and symptoms as for herniated discs; disabling back and leg pain with confirmatory imaging tests of spinal stenosis; severe back pain or radiculopathy with severe functional impairment lasting a year or longer

Modified from Deyo R, Weinstein J. Low back pain. N Engl J Med. 2001;344:363-70; with permission.

appropriate in young patients with symptoms directly related to lumbar instability, when decompression requires removal of facet joints and the disc, or when post-surgical pain due to worsening vertebral slippage occurs after simple decompression (19).

Potential post-operative morbidities must be reviewed with the patient before proceeding with surgery. Post-surgical scar formation after lumbar spine surgery is frequently symptomatic. Moreover, the donor site for autologous bone graft used for spinal fusion is another site for possible post-surgical pain and dysesthesia. Arachnoiditis is another potential complication, causing post-operative back and/or leg pain. Microdiscectomies are associated with relatively little morbidity and are thus preferred if appropriate to the clinical picture.

Summary

Acute low back pain is a highly prevalent condition that is usually mechanical in nature and is generally self-limited. However, when LBP becomes chronic, disability to the individual and costs to society can be significant. The initial evaluation of LBP is aimed at excluding systemic and visceral causes, which can generally be achieved by obtaining a thorough medical history and physical examination. Extensive laboratory and radiological testing is usually unnecessary during the acute phase. Imaging is appropriate for patients with neurological deficits, refractory symptoms, or clinical evidence of systemic, visceral, or vascular disease. Conservative treatment is usually effective, with injections and surgery reserved for the minority of patients with refractory or neurological symptoms.

REFERENCES

1. **Kelsey, JL, White AA.** Epidemiology of low back pain. Spine. 1980;6:133-42.
2. **Borenstein, DG.** Epidemiology, etiology, diagnostic evaluation, and treatment of low back pain. Curr Opin Rheumatol. 1999;11:151-7.
3. **Borenstein, DG.** Epidemiology, etiology, diagnostic evaluation and treatment of low back pain. Curr Opin Rheumatol. 1996;8:124-9.
4. **Weinstein J.** Neurogenic and nonneurogenic pain and inflammatory mediators. Orthop Clin North Am. 1991;22:235-46.
5. **Roland MO.** A critical review of the evidence for a pain-spasm-pain cycle in spinal disorders. Clin Biomech. 1986;1:102-9.
6. **Deyo RA, Rainville J, Kent DL.** What can the history and physical examination tell us about low back pain? JAMA. 1992;268:760-5.
7. **Jarvik JG, Deyo RA.** Diagnostic evaluation of low back pain with emphasis on imaging. Ann Intern Med. 2002;137:586-97.
8. **Atlas SJ, Volinn E.** Classics from the spine literature revisited: a randomized trial of 2 versus 7 days of recommended bed rest for acute low back pain. Spine. 1997;22:2331-7.

9. **Waddell G, Feder G, Lewis M.** Systematic reviews of bed rest and advice to stay active for acute low back pain. Br J Gen Pract. 1997;47:647-52.

10. **van Tulder M, Scholten RJ, Koes BW, Deyo R.** Nonsteroidal anti-inflammatory drugs for low back pain: a systematic review within the framework of the Cochrane Collaboration Back Review Group. Spine. 2000;25:2501-13.

11. **Brown RL, Fleming MF, Patterson JJ.** Chronic opioid analgesic therapy for chronic low back pain. J Am Board Fam Pract. 1996;9:191-204.

12. **Hazard R, Fenwick J, Kalisch S, et al.** Functional restoration with behavioral support: a one-year prospective study of chronic low back pain. Spine. 1989;14: 157-61.

13. **Koes BW, Bouter LM, Beckerman H, et al.** Physiotherapy exercises and back pain: a blinded review. Br Med J. 1991;302:1572-6.

14. **Leboeuf-Yde C.** Body weight and low back pain: a systematic literature review of 56 journals reporting on 65 epidemiologic studies. Spine. 2000;25:226-37.

15. **Koes BW, Scholten RJ, Mens JM, Bouter LM.** Efficacy of epidural steroid injections for low back pain and sciatica: a systematic review of randomized clinical trials. Pain. 1995;63:279-88.

16. **Beurskens AJ, de Vet HC, Koke AJ, et al.** Efficacy of traction for nonspecific low back pain: 12-week and 6-month results of a randomized clinical trial. Spine. 1997;22:2756-62.

17. **van Tulder M, Cherkin D, Berman B, et al.** The effectiveness of acupuncture in the management of acute and chronic low back pain. Spine. 1999;24:1113-23.

18. **Koes BW, Assendelft WJ, van der Heijden GJ, Bouter LM.** Spinal manipulation for low back pain: an updated systematic review of randomized clinical trials. Spine. 1995;21:2860-71.

19. **Brunon J, Chazal J, Chirossel JP, et al.** When is spinal fusion warranted in degenerative lumbar spinal stenosis? Rev Rhum Engl Ed. 1996;63:44-50.

28

■ ■ ■

Raynaud's Phenomenon

Arthur M.F. Yee, MD, PhD

Raynaud's phenomenon is typically described as episodic vasospasm of the fingers and toes, usually in response to cold or stress. Other acral sites, including the tip of the nose, the ears, and the nipples, may also be involved. Raynaud's phenomenon is caused by an exaggerated constriction of the affected small arteries resulting in the classical color changes from pallor (loss of perfusion) to cyanosis (deoxygenation) to erythema (hyperemic reperfusion), although this triphasic progression is not always present and is not required for diagnosis. In mild cases, patients may complain only of cold-induced color changes but, with more pronounced ischemia, paresthesias and pain may be present; in the worst cases, digital ulcers, infections, and loss of tissue may ensue. Rarely, vasospasm can involve visceral organs, including the heart, lung, and gastrointestinal tract.

Raynaud's phenomenon is a common ailment, occurring in 5% to 15% of the general population, with a greater prevalence in colder climates. Women are more frequently affected than men. When there is no underlying causative illness, the condition is known as *primary Raynaud's phenomenon,* which is generally mild and normally presents in younger patients (less than 30 years old). However, in approximately 10% to 15% of cases, Raynaud's phenomenon evolves into or is seen in the context of another medical condition (usually a collagen vascular disorder) or after exposure to an environmental factor (usually drugs or trauma); this is termed *secondary Raynaud's phenomenon* (Table 28-1) (1). Secondary Raynaud's phenomenon in the setting of a rheumatic disease is most commonly associated with systemic scleroderma, mixed connective tissue disorder (MCTD), and systemic lupus erythematosus (SLE) and may present at the time of diagnosis or may precede diagnosis by many years.

Regulation of vasomotor activity involves the interaction of the endothelium, arterial smooth muscles, compliance of the vascular wall, and

Table 28-1   Some Conditions Associated with Secondary Raynaud's Phenomenon

Rheumatologic Disorders*
- Limited systemic sclerosis (95%)
- Diffuse systemic sclerosis (85%)
- Mixed connective tissue disease (85%)
- Systemic lupus erythematosus (55%)
- Rheumatoid arthritis (20%)
- Sjögren's syndrome (20%)

Vascular Disorders
- Thromboangiitis obliterans (Buerger's disease)
- Brachiocephalic atherosclerosis
- Atheroembolic disease
- Prinzmetal angina
- Arteriovenous fistula

Hematologic Disorders
- Cryoglobulinemia
- Polycythemia
- Cold-agglutinins
- Paraproteinemia

Endocrine Disorders
- Hypothyroidism

Endocrine Disorders (*cont'd*)
- Pheochromocytoma
- Carcinoid syndrome

Medications, Drugs, and Toxins
- Beta-blockers
- Ergots (e.g., ergotamine, methysergide)
- Sympathomimetics (e.g., ephedrine, pseudoephedrine, cocaine, amphetamines)
- Tobacco products
- Vinblastine, vincristine, bleomycin
- Polyvinyl chloride
- Type 1 interferons (i.e., alpha and beta)

Traumatic and Occupational Causes
- Hand-arm vibration syndrome (e.g., jackhammer operation)
- Frostbite
- Large vessel trauma (e.g., thoracic outlet syndrome, crutch pressure)

* Numbers in parentheses indicate the percentage of patients with the condition that have Raynaud's phenomenon.

the autonomic and sensory innervation of the vessel (2). In Raynaud's phenomenon, vasoconstriction appears to be highly dependent on the activity of sympathetic nerves (particularly the α_2-adrenergic fibers) that course through the adventitial layer of the arteries and innervate vascular smooth muscle. Specific inhibition of α_2-adrenergic receptors but not α_1-adrenergic improves symptoms of primary Raynaud's phenomenon (3). In addition, β-adrenergic blockers are well known precipitants or aggravators of Raynaud's phenomenon, perhaps due to unopposed α-adrenergic activity (4).

Because of comorbid factors that contribute to ischemia, patients with secondary Raynaud's phenomenon tend to have poorer outcomes than patients with primary disease. These factors include hypercoagulability, atherosclerosis, vasculitis and other inflammatory changes, infection, and fixed structural changes of the vascular wall; aberrations in any one factor often exacerbates others. Exogenous factors such as certain drugs (e.g., sympathomimetics, nicotine) and trauma can further promote or worsen the ischemic process.

Case Presentation

A 23-year-old woman presents with twelve months of discomfort and color changes in her fingers and toes when exposed to the cold. She had no significant medical problems and was taking no prescribed medications, and there was no family history of rheumatic diseases. She was a light smoker and reported moderate caffeine intake. At first, her symptoms were mild, characterized by blanching and numbness of the tips of all of her fingers when she handled frozen objects. Later, however, when she walked out into mildly cold weather without gloves or mittens, her fingers quickly turned blue and became painful. She also noticed pain in her toes with cold exposure. She began avoiding winter sports and other activities that would subject her to cold environments. In the summer, air conditioning was uncomfortable for her. The review of symptoms revealed only that she would occasionally wake up in the morning with hand and wrist stiffness that improved over the course of an hour. She described these symptoms as being qualitatively different from the sharper pains induced by the cold. On rare occasions, she would take over-the-counter ibuprofen that improved her morning joint stiffness.

The patient's fingers and toes were dusky on examination, but there were no active digital ulcers or evidence of past ulcerations. The Allen test was normal. The rest of her physical examination was normal without any mucocutaneous or musculoskeletal abnormalities. Routine laboratory testing (complete blood count, blood chemistries, and urinalysis) was normal, although she had a positive antinuclear antibody (ANA) test at a titer of 1:80 in a diffuse pattern.

The patient was diagnosed with Raynaud's phenomenon, possibly in the context of an undifferentiated collagen vascular disorder. Behavioral modifications (e.g., avoidance of unwarranted exposure to cold and discontinuation of smoking) and amlodipine 5 mg daily during periods of cold reduced the frequency and severity of attacks. After five years, she continues to be evaluated every three to four months, with good control of her Raynaud's phenomenon and without evidence of further evolution to a systemic illness.

Diagnosis

Although various formal techniques such as digital blood pressure monitoring, skin temperature testing, and dynamic videomicroscopy under cold provocation have been developed for the assessment of Raynaud's phenomenon, these tests are generally employed for clinical studies only. In clinical practice, the diagnosis of Raynaud's phenomenon can almost always be made based on clinical history. Emphasis should be placed on the identification of any underlying conditions, and a complete medical history should be ascertained. Skin thickening, telangiectasias, cutaneous calcinosis, sclerodactyly (thickening of the skin of the digits), or symptoms of upper or lower gastro-intestinal dysmotility should raise suspicion for systemic scleroderma. SLE should be considered if there is inflammatory arthritis, typical mucocutaneous manifestations (malar rash, discoid rash, photosensitivity, and/or mucosal ulcers), or pleurisy. Past and present exposures to drugs, chemicals, trauma, and other potentially injurious exogenous factors should be ascertained.

In mild cases of primary Raynaud's phenomenon, the physical examination is often normal unless vasoconstriction is provoked by cold. Cyanosis, active digital ulcerations, and infections can be seen in more severe cases (Fig. 28-1). With chronic disease, evidence of past ulcerations and infection such as digital pitting and scarring can be present. Loss of tissue at the tuft of the digits reflects long-standing ischemia and can be demonstrated by acral osteolysis on plain radiography (Fig. 28-2). Raynaud's phenomenon characteristically affects multiple digits; thus, when there is a single ischemic digit present, other vascular conditions such as thrombosis, embolism, or obstruction should be considered.

A thorough physical examination is essential to evaluate for an underlying systemic condition. Again, typical mucocutaneous or musculoskeletal signs can point to scleroderma, SLE, MCTD, or overlapping collagen vascular diseases. Two simple techniques can also be helpful in identifying patients with early scleroderma: nailfold capillaroscopy and palpation for tendon friction rubs (5,6). Nailfold capillaroscopy can be performed with a standard ophthalmoscope set at a high diopter (>20) after mineral oil application on the nailfolds to enhance visualization. Normal capillary loops are not easily

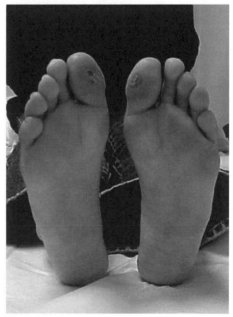

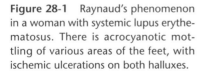

Figure 28-1   Raynaud's phenomenon in a woman with systemic lupus erythematosus. There is acrocyanotic mottling of various areas of the feet, with ischemic ulcerations on both halluxes.

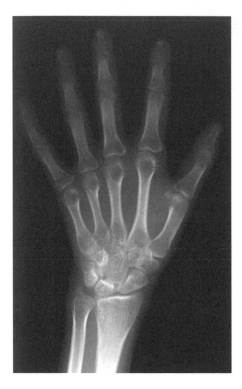

Figure 28-2 Osteolysis of the distal phalanges in severe Raynaud's phenomenon secondary to scleroderma. Plain radiographs of the hands show loss of soft tissue in the tufts of the fingers and resorption of bone in the distal phalanges due to long-standing severe ischemia.

seen but, even in early scleroderma, enlarged and tortuous capillary loops can be observed. In order to detect tendon friction rubs due to diffuse scleroderma, the palmar surface of the examiner's fingers is placed over the tendon being examined while the patient actively moves the underlying joint through maximal range of motion. A friction rub may feel like a "squeaking" rubbing sensation. The most reliable places to elicit a friction rub are the extensor and flexor tendons of the wrists and fingers, the triceps tendons, the patellar tendons, and the tendons of the ankles (anterior and posterior tibial, peroneal, and Achilles' tendons). Any suspicion of an underlying collagen vascular disorder should prompt a formal rheumatologic consultation.

Laboratory Testing

Laboratory testing is important mostly for seeking out secondary causes of Raynaud's phenomenon. An anemia of chronic disease, thrombocytosis, or an elevated sedimentation rate is suggestive of a systemic inflammatory illness. SLE may be characterized by leukopenia or thrombocytopenia. Occult renal disease (e.g., elevated serum creatinine, active urinary sediment or proteinuria) may point to the possibility of early SLE or scleroderma.

Serologic testing for antinuclear antibodies (ANA) can sometimes be helpful for prognostic purposes. Whereas the vast majority of patients with

Raynaud's phenomenon do not develop a secondary condition (7), over one half of patients with clearly high serum levels of ANA at the time of presentation will eventually be diagnosed with a systemic rheumatologic disease (8). However, the clinician must be cautious about the use of ANA testing. There is great variability in technique and sensitivity, and often results are reported as simply "positive" or "negative". The significance of low circulating levels of ANA is questionable. A positive test for ANA should always be taken in the context of the complete clinical picture and, in the absence of other clinical manifestations, warrants only regular clinical monitoring to assess for the development of a systemic disease.

Autoantibodies against other antigens offer specificity for certain diseases: anti-dsDNA antibodies for SLE, anti-ribonucleoprotein (RNP) antibodies for MCTD, anti-centromere antibodies for limited scleroderma (or the CREST syndrome), and anti-Scl-70 antibodies for diffuse scleroderma. Although these antibodies, particularly anti-RNP antibodies, are associated with poorer prognoses (9), routine testing is not recommended unless demanded by the clinical picture for confirmation of a diagnosis.

Radiological Testing

Radiological tests are generally not necessary for the diagnosis of Raynaud's phenomenon but can be helpful in evaluating other potential causes of digital ischemia. When required for objective measurements, noninvasive vascular laboratory testing such as Doppler studies of the superficial palmar arch and proximal arteries or finger photoplethysmography and blood pressure monitoring can be obtained. Echocardiography is indicated to assess for the presence of cardiac sources of thromboembolic disease or an atrial myxoma. Conventional arteriography or magnetic resonance angiography is only necessary if a fixed proximal occlusion is suspected or if microsurgical revascularization is contemplated. Sympathetic nerve blockade should be performed during angiography to prevent vasospasm.

Management

Appropriate treatment of Raynaud's phenomenon depends on the severity of the disease and the presence of comorbid conditions and may require any combination of behavioral modifications, pharmacologic agents, and surgical interventions (Table 28-2). Treatment of underlying diseases in secondary Raynaud's phenomenon is also essential.

Nonpharmacological Therapies

Elimination of factors that may precipitate attacks of Raynaud's phenomenon is central to treatment. Avoidance of cold temperatures and the use of warm

Table 28-2   Therapeutic Options for the Management of Raynaud's Phenomenon*

Behavioral and Non-Pharmacologic Approaches
- Avoidance of cold temperatures
- Lined hand and footwear
- Discontinuation of tobacco products
- Discontinuation of offending medications, drugs, or toxins
- Avoidance of trauma
- Stress management and relaxation techniques
- Biofeedback
- Conditioning exercises

Vasodilator Therapies
- Calcium channel blockers (e.g., nifedipine, nicardipine, amlodipine, diltiazem)
- Prazosin
- Hydralazine
- Topical nitrate ointments
- Newer and investigational pharmacologic approaches (serotonin antagonists, selective serotonin reuptake inhibitors, phosphodiesterase inhibitors, angiotensin-converting enzyme inhibitors, angiotensin II type 1 receptor antagonists, prostaglandin analogues)
- Sympathetic nerve blockade

Anti-Infective Prevention and Therapy
- Local ulcer care
- Systemic antibiotics
- Debridement

Anticoagulation
- Aspirin
- Folic acid
- Warfarin
- Low molecular weight heparins

Surgical Interventions
- Digital sympathectomy/adventitial stripping
- Investigational approaches (microsurgical revascularization, skin grafting)

* These modalities are generally implemented concomitantly in order to address different mechanisms of ischemia. Anticoagulation with warfarin or heparins is usually indicated for severe cases. Surgical intervention is typically reserved for the most severe or refractory cases or in circumstances in which a digit is at imminent risk for permanent damage or loss.

clothing, coverings for the hands and feet, and electrical or chemical warming devices that can be inserted into handwear or footwear are simple and effective measures. Medications or substances like beta-blockers or cocaine that can exacerbate Raynaud's phenomenon should be discontinued. Cessation of tobacco use is mandatory. Activities that may lead to traumatic injury (e.g., piano playing, typing, the use of vibratory tools) should be minimized.

It is notable that in clinical trials a favorable placebo effect can be seen in over 40% of patients with Raynaud's phenomenon, suggesting that psychological approaches can also be helpful in reducing symptoms. Emotional stress increases vasoconstriction, and so relaxation techniques and stress modification using meditation or psychotherapeutic means can be helpful. Some patients respond to biofeedback techniques by which they are trained to increase finger temperature in response to reinforcing signals. Another approach is through the use of conditioning exercises in which the hands are repeatedly exposed to warm water while the rest of the body is exposed to cold temperatures. Over time, cold stimulus may elicit a warm-hand response, reflecting conditioned relaxation of the affected arteries. Biofeedback and conditioning can often help patients with primary Raynaud's phenomenon but are less effective for individuals with secondary disease, probably because of concomitant nonvasospastic causes of ischemia.

Vasodilators

A variety of pharmacologic agents have been employed to minimize vasospasm and to dilate ischemic arteries. The use of vasodilators is clearly more effective in primary Raynaud's phenomenon than in secondary Raynaud's phenomenon (especially that associated with scleroderma) in which structural fibrotic changes of the vascular wall render the vessels less responsive to these medications. Use of vasodilators may also cause unanticipated hypoperfusion of ischemic vessels by lowering systemic blood pressure. Similarly, vessels that are less affected by Raynaud's phenomenon may have a better response to vasodilator therapy and may "steal" blood flow from more ischemic nearby arteries. Thus, worsening of symptoms can sometimes result from the administration of these agents, warranting reduction of dosages.

Calcium channel blockers (e.g., nifedipine, nicardipine, amlodipine, diltiazem), which act by relaxing vascular smooth muscle, are the most widely studied class of agents, and ample studies have shown modest but clear benefit (10,11). Longer-acting preparations appear to be more effective and better tolerated. Dosages should be titrated to minimal amounts required for efficacy without adverse effects such as hypotension, headache, lightheadedness, and flushing. Calcium channel blockers may also aggravate upper and lower gastrointestinal dysmotility problems in patients with scleroderma.

The α_1-adrenergic receptor inhibitor prazosin (1 to 2 mg three times daily) is also effective for controlling vasospasm (3). Hydralazine (10-50 mg four times daily) is another commonly used potent vasodilator. Small bedtime test doses of prazosin and hydralazine are recommended at the onset of therapy to minimize adverse effects such as hypotension, lightheadedness, and syncope before increasing dosages to therapeutic ranges. Some clinicians feel that tachyphylaxis can be a problem with prazosin and hydralazine.

Topical nitroglycerin ointments applied to the base of ischemic digits are convenient and have modest effectiveness in primary Raynaud's phenomenon. The mechanism of action is thought to be due to increased nitric oxide (NO) vasodilatory activity. However, systemic absorption is significant and associated with adverse effects, most notably headaches (12). Recently, an investigational NO-generating system (sodium nitrite and ascorbic acid in a water soluble gel) designed to stimulate local NO production and activity has been shown to increase digital blood flow in patients with primary Raynaud's phenomenon without significant systemic hemodynamic effects (13).

Iloprost, a prostacyclin analogue with vasodilatory and platelet-inhibitory properties, has been evaluated as both an intravenous and oral medication for the treatment of Raynaud's phenomenon secondary to scleroderma. Intravenous iloprost, administered daily through a central vein catheter in a monitored setting for five days, appears to be effective for short-term alleviation of Raynaud's phenomenon but is expensive and not currently available in the United States. Oral iloprost has not shown clear effectiveness. Other agents currently being considered as possible therapies for Raynaud's phenomenon include serotonin antagonists, selective serotonin reuptake inhibitors, phosphodiesterase inhibitors (e.g., sildenafil), angiotensin-converting enzyme inhibitors, and angiotensin II type 1 receptor antagonists.

Sympathetic Nerve Blockade

Temporary sympathetic nerve blockade can be performed proximally or distally in the acute management of a severe exacerbation of Raynaud's phenomenon. This technique can serve several purposes. It is very effective for pure analgesia. It can be used as a "bridge" until more definitive management plans are determined. Finally, in a minority of cases, it may even abort an attack of Raynaud's phenomenon.

Infection Control

Prevention and prompt treatment of ischemic digital infections are crucial for preservation of tissue. Simple cuts and abrasions can progress quickly in an ischemic zone to aggressive infections and should not be taken lightly. When indicated, systemic antibiotics should be prescribed; these must include coverage for *Staphylococcus aureus*. Occasionally, surgical incision and debridement are necessary, but this can be associated with wound-healing difficulties because of poor digital perfusion.

Anticoagulation

Chronic vasoconstriction and hypoperfusion can result in local vascular stasis and hypercoagulability and ultimately in the development of microthrombi. Accordingly, although large controlled studies are lacking, anti-platelet agents such as aspirin or anticoagulants such as warfarin or heparins are often used as adjuvants to vasodilators in maximizing perfusion.

There has been recent interest in the observation that patients with primary Raynaud's phenomenon and Raynaud's phenomenon secondary to scleroderma have elevated circulating levels of homocysteine (14). Because this metabolite is thought to be procoagulant and vasculotoxic, some investigators have advocated the use of folic acid (e.g., 1 mg daily) supplementation to lower blood homocysteine levels.

Surgical Options

Sympathectomy, the microscopic surgical disruption of sympathetic innervation to the digital arteries, has become a more widely used treatment for refractory Raynaud's phenomenon and a "finger-at-risk" for severe ischemic damage. Digital sympathectomy involves the dissection of the adventitial layer of the digital arteries resulting in 1) the elimination of the sympathetic fibers that traverse this tissue, 2) the removal of encasing fibrotic tissue that causes a fixed obstruction of the vessel, and 3) possibly increased postoperative responsiveness to vasodilators (15). This procedure can acutely restore perfusion and when performed by an experienced surgeon is associated with few complications. Because the affected arteries in the fingers are physically decompressed, digital sympathectomy is more effective than more proximal cervicothoracic sympathectomies.

Microsurgical revascularization and skin grafting are other investigational surgical procedures aimed at preserving viable tissue, but their long-term outcomes and benefits are less clear.

REFERENCES

1. **Spencer-Green, G.** Outcomes in primary Raynaud phenomenon. Arch Int Med. 1998;158:595-600.
2. **Block JA, Sequeira W.** Raynaud's phenomenon. Lancet. 2001; 357:2042-8.
3. **Freedman RR, Baer RP, Mayes MD.** Blockade of vasospastic attacks by α_2-adrenergic but not α_1-adrenergic antagonists in idiopathic Raynaud's's disease. Circulation. 1995;92:1448-51.
4. **Brand FN, Larson MG, Kannel WB, McGuirk JM.** The occurrence of Raynaud's phenomenon in a general population: the Framingham Study. Vasc Med. 1997;2: 296-301.
5. **Steen VD, Medsger TA Jr.** The palpable tendon friction rub: an important physical examination finding in patients with systemic sclerosis. Arthritis Rheum. 1997;40: 1146-51.
6. **Cutolo M, Grassi W, Cerinic MM.** Raynaud's phenomenon and the role capillaroscopy. Arthritis Rheum. 2003;48:3023-30.
7. **Gerbracht DD, Steen VD, Ziegler GL, et al.** Evolution of primary Raynaud's phenonmenon (Raynaud's disease) to connective tissue disease. Arthritis Rheum. 1985; 28:87-92.

8. **Landry GJ, Edwards JM, McLafferty RB, et al.** Long-term outcome of Raynaud's syndrome in a prospectively analyzed patient cohort. J Vasc Surg. 1996;23:76-8.

9. **Ihata A, Shirai A, Okubo T, et al.** Severity of seropositive isolated Raynaud's phenomenon is associated with serological profile. J Rheumatol. 2000;27:1686-92.

10. **White CJ, Phillips WA, Abrahams WA, et al.** Objective benefit of nifedipine in the treatment of Raynaud's phenomenon: a double-blind controlled study. Am J Med. 1986;80:623-5.

11. **Wise RA, Malamet R, Wigley FM.** Acute effects of nifedipine on digital blood flow in human subjects with Raynaud's phenomenon: a double-blind placebo controlled trial. J Rheumatol. 1987;14:278-83.

12. **Teh LS, Manning J, Moore T, et al.** Sustained-release transdermal glyceral trinitrate patches as a treatment for primary and secondary Raynaud's phenomenon. Br J Rheumatol. 1995;34:636-41.

13. **Tucker AT, Pearson RM, Cooke ED, Benjamin N.** Effect of nitric-oxide-generating system on microcirculatory blood flow in skin of patients with severe Raynaud's syndrome: a randomised trial. Lancet. 1999;354:1670-5.

14. **Levy Y, George J, Langevitz P, et al.** Elevated homocysteine levels in patients with Raynaud's syndrome. J Rheumatol. 1999;26:2383-5.

15. **Yee AMF, Hotchkiss RN, Paget SA.** Adventitial stripping: a digit-saving procedure in refractory Raynaud's phenomenon. J Rheumatol. 1998;25:269-76.

SECTION VIII

PHARMACOLOGICAL AGENTS

29

■ ■ ■

Non-Steroidal Anti-Inflammatory Drugs

David J. Chang, MD

Non-steroidal anti-inflammatory drugs (NSAIDs) possess anti-inflammatory, analgesic, and anti-pyretic properties and are commonly prescribed agents for rheumatic conditions. Currently there are over 20 NSAIDs available in the United States (Table 29-1), including newer agents which selectively inhibit cyclooxygenase-2 (COX-2), resulting in a safer gastrointestinal profile than older NSAIDs. Some NSAIDs are available in delayed-release formulations that allow for less frequent dosing; others are designed as rapid-release formulations that provide a faster onset of action than the parent compound. Systemic NSAIDs can also be delivered in parenteral forms, rectal suppositories, and oral suspensions. Topical NSAIDs such as ophthalmic drops or ointments are also available for local indications and carry fewer systemic adverse effects.

Mechanism of Action

The primary mechanism of action of NSAIDs is mediated through the inhibition of the enzyme cyclooxygenase (COX) resulting in the decreased metabolism of arachadonic acid into pro-inflammatory prostaglandins, especially prostaglandins of the E series. Acetylsalicylic acid (aspirin) acetylates and *irreversibly* inhibits COX activity, while the non-aspirin NSAIDs cause *reversible* COX inhibition. NSAIDs are also known to inhibit the production of thromboxane and prostacyclin. Thromboxane is involved in platelet-mediated hemostasis, whereas prostacyclin inhibits platelet aggregation and also acts as a vasodilator.

Two distinct isoforms of COX have been identified. Cyclooxygenase-1 (COX-1) is found constitutively in most tissues and cell types and is involved

Table 29-1   Dosing and Indicated Uses of Non-Steroidal Anti-Inflammatory Drugs (NSAIDs) Available in the United States

Drug (Trade Name)	Dosing Interval	Usual Dose Range (mg/d)	Some Approved Indications and Selected Uses
Salicylates			
Acetylsalicylic acid (aspirin)*,**	4-6×/d	1000-6000	Pain, OA, RA, spondylo-arthropathies, JRA, arthritis and pleurisy associated with SLE
Nonacetylated Salicylates			
Choline magnesium trisalicylate (Trilisate)†	BID-TID	1500-4000	OA, RA, acute painful shoulder
Salsalate (Disalcid)	BID-TID	1500-5000	OA, RA
Non-Salicylates			
Diflunisal (Dolobid)	BID	500-1500	Pain, OA, RA
Etodolac (Lodine)*	BID-TID	600-1200	Pain, OA, RA
Fenoprofen (Nalfon)	TID-QID	900-3200	Pain, OA, RA
Flurbiprofen (Ansaid)	BID-QID	100-300	OA, RA
Ibuprofen (many brands)†	TID-QID	1200-3200	Pain, OA, RA, JRA
Indomethacin (Indocin)*,†,**	TID-QID	50-200	OA, RA, AS, acute painful shoulder, gout
Diclofenac (Voltaren)*,+	BID-QID	100-200	OA, RA, AS
Ketoprofen (Orudis)*	TID-QID	100-300	Pain, OA, RA
Ketorolac (Toradol)#	QID	40	Pain
Meclofenamate (Meclomen)	TID-QID	200-400	OA
Mefenamic acid (Ponstel)	QID	500-1000	Pain
Meloxicam (Mobic)	QD	7.5-15	OA
Nabumetone (Relafen)	QD-BID	1000-2000	OA, RA
Naproxen (Naprosyn, Aleve)*,+,†	BID	500-1500	Pain, OA, RA, JRA, AS, tendinitis, bursitis, gout
Oxaprozin (Daypro)	QD-BID	600-1800	OA, RA
Piroxicam (Feldene)	QD	10-20	OA, RA
Sulindac (Clinoril)	BID	300-400	OA, RA, AS, acute painful shoulder, gout
Tolmetin (Tolectin)	TID-QID	1200-1600	OA, RA, JRA
COX-2 Selective Inhibitors			
Celecoxib (Celebrex)	QD-BID	200-400	Pain, OA, RA
Valdecoxib (Bextra)	QD-BID	10-40	Dysmenorrhea++, OA, RA

OA = osteoarthritis; RA = rheumatoid arthritis; JRA = juvenile rheumatoid arthritis; AS = ankylosing spondylitis; SLE = systemic lupus erythematosus.

 * Available in delayed-release formulations.
 + Available in rapid-release formulations.
 † Available in oral suspension.
 # Available in parenteral formulation.
 ** Available as rectal suppositories.
 ++ Approved for dysmenorrhea but not pain.

in homeostatic housekeeping functions such as the protection of the stomach from injury and the maintenance of the normal functioning of platelets.

The other isoform, COX-2, is usually absent in most normal tissues and cells but can be induced by factors such as pro-inflammatory cytokines. Inducible COX-2 is expressed in tissues and cells (e.g., monocytes, macrophages, endothelial cells, chondrocytes, synovial cells) that participate in inflammatory processes. It is believed that inhibition of COX-2 is the mechanism by which NSAIDs provide clinical efficacy, whereas the inhibition of COX-1 contributes to many of the adverse effects. Different NSAIDs vary greatly in their relative inhibitory effects on COX-1 and COX-2. The drugs with the highest COX-2/COX-1 selectivity ratios (rofecoxib, celecoxib, valdecoxib) are considered to be "selective" COX-2 inhibitors, because the inhibition of COX-1 at therapeutic levels of the drugs is minimal. Although diclofenac, etodolac, and meloxicam also preferentially inhibit COX-2, these agents lose this advantage at higher therapeutic doses where clinically significant COX-1 inhibition occurs.

Clinical Uses

All NSAIDs have anti-inflammatory, analgesic, and anti-pyretic properties. Typically, higher doses of NSAIDs are required to achieve anti-inflammatory effects than those needed for analgesia. In clinical trials, all non-salicylate NSAIDs have generally shown similar clinical efficacy in the treatment of osteoarthritis and rheumatoid arthritis. Non-acetylated salicylates (e.g., salsalate, trisalicylate) are probably less effective but potentially safer than standard non-salicylate NSAIDs, because they are not potent inhibitors of prostaglandin synthesis. Although NSAIDs may alleviate the symptoms associated with rheumatic diseases, they do *not* alter the natural history of the inflammatory or destructive processes associated with some of the disorders such as rheumatoid arthritis.

Most NSAIDs are approved for the treatment of osteoarthritis and rheumatoid arthritis. Historically, indomethacin has been considered one of the more effective NSAIDs in the treatment of gout and ankylosing spondylitis. However, there are now other NSAIDs formally approved for the treatment of these disorders as well as for the management of juvenile rheumatoid arthritis, tendinitis, bursitis, acute shoulder pain, and acute pain (including dysmenorrhea) (see Table 29-1).

Short courses as needed of NSAIDs with rapid onset of action are particularly useful in the treatment of acute or intermittent pain, such as in the setting of surgery. NSAIDs with longer duration of action reduce the frequency of dosing and improve patient compliance, which is particularly important in patients with chronic conditions who require continuous therapy. Concurrent use of more than one NSAID does not increase efficacy, although adverse effects are additive. Consequently, combination NSAID therapy is *not* recommended.

Toxicities

NSAIDs are associated with many adverse effects, but gastrointestinal (GI), anti-platelet, and renal effects are the most common and clinically relevant (Table 29-2). Most toxicities are related to the inhibition of COX-1 and the resultant loss of protective prostaglandins, although idiosyncratic reactions are also encountered. Prescribing the lowest effective dose is clinically prudent because side effects related to the GI tract and kidneys are largely dose-dependent. Complete blood counts, serum electrolytes, blood urea nitrogen, serum creatinine, and hepatic transaminases should be performed within 4 to 8 weeks of initiating NSAID therapy and every 2 to 3 months thereafter to minimize and monitor for potential toxicities. Regular testing (e.g., three times yearly) for occult blood in the stool is also important to screen for NSAID-induced gastrointestinal bleeding. In the elderly, patients with comorbidities, and individuals that are anticipated to be on chronic NSAID therapy, baseline blood testing should be performed before initiating treatment.

Gastrointestinal Effects

COX-1 is expressed in the gastric mucosa and is responsible for the production of gastroprotective prostaglandins. Inhibition of COX-1 predisposes

---

Table 29-2   Toxicities of Non-Steroidal Anti-Inflammatory Drugs

- Gastrointestinal Effects
  - —Gastroduodenal ulcers, bleeding, perforation, and obstructions
  - —Dyspepsia, abdominal pain, nausea, vomiting, and diarrhea
  - —Liver transaminase elevation
  - —Esophagitis and esophageal strictures
  - —Intestinal ulcers, strictures, and obstructions
  - —Cholestasis
- Anti-Platelet Effects
- Renal Effects
  - —Sodium retention, fluid retention, and edema
  - —Elevation in blood pressure
  - —Hyperkalemia
  - —Acute renal failure
  - —Nephrotic syndrome with interstitial nephritis
  - —Acute papillary necrosis
- Hypersensitivity Reactions
- Neurologic Effects
  - —Tinnitus and hearing loss
  - —Aseptic meningitis, headaches, and confusion
- Hematologic Effects
  - —Aplastic anemia, hemolytic anemia, neutropenia, agranulocytosis, and thrombocytopenia

---

the gastric mucosa to injury (1). The Food and Drug Administration estimates that upper GI ulcers, gross bleeding, or perforations occur in approximately 1% of patients treated with NSAIDs for 3 to 6 months, then increases to 2% to 4% among patients treated for one year. In the setting of NSAID use, gastric ulcers are three times more common than duodenal ulcers. These estimates are based primarily on experience with traditional non-selective NSAIDs, irrespective of any concurrent medications including gastroprotective agents. It is very likely that these numbers are significantly lower among patients treated with COX-2 inhibitors and among patients receiving gastroprotective agents. Factors associated with increased risks of developing significant GI complications are advanced age, history of prior ulcers, concomitant use of corticosteroids, higher doses of NSAIDs, simultaneous use of more than one NSAID, concomitant administration of anticoagulants, and the presence of serious systemic disorders such as cardiovascular disease or severe rheumatoid arthritis.

A decreased incidence of serious GI side effects has been demonstrated with the selective COX-2 inhibitors rofecoxib and celecoxib even when administered at higher than recommended chronic dosages. Data from the VIGOR trial, in which over 8000 patients with rheumatoid arthritis were treated for a median of 9 months, showed a 54% risk reduction of GI perforations, obstructions, symptomatic ulcers, and upper GI bleeding for rofecoxib-treated patients compared with patients treated with standard therapeutic dosages of naproxen (2). In the CLASS study of over 8000 osteoarthritis and rheumatoid arthritis patients, in which the median duration of treatment was at least 6 months, patients taking celecoxib had a 41% risk reduction of significant upper GI events compared to patients treated with standard therapeutic dosages of ibuprofen or diclofenac as an aggregate (3). It is likely that valdecoxib provides similar reductions in GI side effects as rofecoxib and celecoxib, but results of comparably large outcomes studies are not currently available.

With concomitant use of aspirin, patients taking either traditional NSAIDs or COX-2 inhibitors will have an increased incidence of serious GI adverse events, but further studies are warranted to determine whether there is a significant difference between the two groups. A subanalysis at 6 months from the CLASS study of patients taking up to 325 mg of aspirin per day demonstrated no difference in significant GI complications when the celecoxib group was compared with the group treated with either ibuprofen or diclofenac (3). However, this lack of difference could be related to the high dose of aspirin allowed in the study, and it is possible that an aspirin dose of 81 mg per day or lower may yield a clinically important difference.

Non-acetylated salicylates, etodolac, and meloxicam at lower doses may also have lower risks of significant GI events than other non-COX-2 selective NSAIDs because of their relative COX-2 selectivity. Large GI outcomes trials similar to those conducted with rofecoxib and celecoxib, however, have not been performed with the non-acetylated salicylates or etodolac to substantiate the possible improved GI safety. Two short-term GI tolerability studies comparing the lowest dose of meloxicam to diclofenac and piroxicam over a 28-day treatment period demonstrated numerically, but not statistically significant, lower rates of perforations, ulcers, or bleeds among meloxicam-treated patients.

Individuals who are at an increased risk of developing NSAID-induced gastric or duodenal ulcers may benefit from gastroprotective prophylactic therapy. The prostaglandin analogue misoprostol, proton pump inhibitors, and high doses of histamine-2 receptor blockers have all been shown to reduce the incidence of NSAID-induced gastric and duodenal ulcers (4). However, only misoprostol has been demonstrated to clearly prevent the more severe complications of perforations, obstruction, and bleeding associated with NSAID-induced gastric ulcers. Sucralfate and antacids have not been shown beneficial in preventing gastroduodenal ulcerations.

NSAIDs administered as rectal suppositories or as parenteral injections do not offer a safer GI profile than those administered orally, because inhibition of gastroprotective prostaglandin production occurs after systemic absorption of the drug.

In addition to serious gastrointestinal events, dyspepsia, abdominal pain, nausea, vomiting, and diarrhea are well-known common side effects of NSAIDs. Dyspepsia will probably develop in at least 10% to 20% of patients. Liver transaminase elevation of two to three times the upper limits is frequently seen early in therapy but generally is clinically unimportant and reversible upon discontinuation of the NSAID.

Less common but increasingly appreciated gastrointestinal side effects are esophagitis, esophageal strictures, and small and large intestine ulcers, strictures, and obstructions. Cholestasis has also been reported among NSAID users.

Anti-Platelet Effects

Through the inhibition of COX-1, traditional NSAIDs (except for non-acetylated salicylates such as salsalate and trilisate) reduce the production of thromboxane, which is involved in platelet activation. The end result is the decreased ability of platelets to aggregate and provide effective hemostasis. Coupled with the potential for gastric injury, this diminished platelet-mediated hemostasis may further augment the risk and severity of gastrointestinal bleeding induced by non-selective NSAIDs.

Because aspirin irreversibly affects platelet function, discontinuing aspirin approximately one to two weeks (i.e., the average circulatory life of platelets) before major surgery is reasonable to reduce the risk of perioperative bleeding. However, the effect of other non-selective NSAIDs on platelets is reversible, and the duration of reduced platelet function correlates with the serum half-life of the drug. For these NSAIDs, discontinuation of the drug for approximately four to five half-lives before surgery is adequate.

This is usually less than two to three days for NSAIDs dosed more than twice daily and typically three to five days for most NSAIDs dosed once or twice daily. Piroxicam, whose half-life is greater than 24 hours, is an exception and may require discontinuation at least one week before invasive procedures.

COX-2 inhibitors do not appear to significantly affect platelet thromboxane production or aggregation. Consequently, these agents need not be discontinued before surgery. Patients with osteoarthritis taking COX-2 inhibitors have continued their medication up to the day of surgery for total knee replacement without an increase in intraoperative or postoperative bleeding (5). The lack of platelet effects has also allowed for the safe pre-emptive administration of selective COX-2 inhibitors before surgery, resulting in reduced pain and postoperative opioid use and potentially offering a novel paradigm in the approach to acute pain management. COX-2 inhibitors may be used concomitantly with warfarin, but careful monitoring of the international normalized ratio should still be maintained.

There is ongoing concern regarding the cardiovascular safety of COX-2 inhibitors. It has been conjectured that selective inhibition of COX-2 may enhance pro-thrombotic effects of COX-1-generated thromboxanes (6). Retrospective reviews of randomized clinical trials of rofecoxib and celecoxib have failed to reveal differences between either agents with comparator traditional NSAIDs and placebo in regard to increased cardiovascular thrombotic events (7,8). However, a large retrospective post-marketing study of elderly patients (65 years or older) suggested that there was a dose-dependent increased risk of acute myocardial infarction with rofecoxib therapy when compared with celecoxib and no-NSAID use (9). Based on these data and the results of subsequent supporting epidemiological studies, rofecoxib was voluntarily withdrawn from the market by its manufacturer in September 2004.

An additional concern is the ability of some NSAIDs to antagonize the cardioprotective effect of aspirin. In a recent study, the inhibitory effects of aspirin on thromboxane formation and platelet aggregation were shown to be blocked by a single 400 mg dose of ibuprofen given within 2 hours of the aspirin dose (10). These effects were not observed with rofecoxib, diclofenac, or acetaminophen. It remains uncertain whether these in vitro observations translate into a clinical loss of the cardioprotective effect of aspirin and whether other NSAIDs also share these properties.

Renal Effects

Both COX-1 and COX-2 are constitutively expressed in the kidneys. COX-1 is ubiquitous in the kidneys and found mostly in the vasculature, thin loop of Henle, and collecting ducts. COX-2 is localized to the vasculature, cortical macula densa, and medullary interstitial cells; the expression of COX-2 in these areas increases with age. Both enzymes are probably involved in homeostatic function of producing vasodilatory prostaglandins.

Prostaglandin E2 and prostacyclin are renal vasodilators critical in preserving adequate renal blood flow in the state of volume depletion. NSAIDs as well as COX-2 inhibitors inhibit the synthesis of both prostanoids, and up to 5% of patients treated with these agents develop clinically relevant nephrotoxicities including edema and worsening hypertension (11). Fortunately, most of the effects are fully reversible when the drug is discontinued. Renal side effects result from inhibition of prostaglandin synthesis and, accordingly, patients whose renal function is largely prostaglandin-dependent are more likely to develop toxicities than are healthy individuals. The patients at increased risk are those who are volume-depleted, such as those with severe congestive heart failure, hepatic cirrhosis, diuretic use, restricted sodium intake, hemodynamically significant bleeding, and septic shock (12). Elderly persons, patients receiving angiotensin-converting enzyme inhibitors, and individuals with chronic renal disease of any etiology are also at increased risk for worsening renal function. Every attempt should be made to avoid the use of NSAIDs, including COX-2 inhibitors, in individuals with even modest renal insufficiency. Most NSAIDs are extensively eliminated through renal excretion. Accordingly, although these drugs may be used in the setting of end-stage renal disease, patients on dialysis may have prolonged drug exposure, potentially subjecting them to increased toxicities.

Sodium retention with associated fluid retention and edema is a common side effect of NSAIDs, occurring in approximately 3% of patients. Typically, this occurs within the first week of therapy and is usually mild and reversible upon discontinuation of the offending agent. Inhibition of prostaglandin E2 is believed to cause increased sodium and water reabsorption in the distal tubules. Both non-selective NSAIDs and COX-2 inhibitors have been associated with peripheral edema, suggesting that homeostatic sodium excretion is at least in part a COX-2–mediated event (12).

Elevation in blood pressure is another common toxicity of NSAIDs and COX-2 inhibitors. Two large meta-analyses have demonstrated that blood pressure measurements increase approximately 3 to 5 mm with the administration of NSAIDs (13,14). The elevations are greatest among patients with pre-existing hypertension and in those being treated with diuretics, beta-blockers, and angiotensin-converting enzyme inhibitors.

Hyperkalemia is an uncommon NSAID-induced electrolyte abnormality. A possible mechanism is decreased prostaglandin-mediated renin release, leading to diminished aldosterone secretion. The end result is decreased renal potassium excretion. Stopping the NSAID reverses the hyperkalemia. COX-2 inhibitors probably cause hyperkalemia to the same extent as standard NSAIDs.

Acute renal failure is a rare complication caused by diminished renal perfusion after inhibition of prostacyclin production. The onset is usually within days of starting therapy and occurs more rapidly with NSAIDs with short half-lives. It is likely that acute renal failure in the high-risk population can also be seen with COX-2 inhibitors.

Rare adverse renal events include nephrotic syndrome with interstitial nephritis and acute papillary necrosis. Nephrotic syndrome usually develops several days to months after starting therapy. The mechanism for this event is hypothesized to be a shunting of the arachidonic acid pathway away from prostaglandins towards increased production of leukotrienes, which may be involved in affecting vascular permeability in the glomerular and peritubular capillaries. The proteinuria may ultimately resolve but that may take up to a year after discontinuation of the offending NSAID. Acute papillary necrosis, unlike the other renal toxicities, is a permanent, albeit rare, form of kidney damage that is caused by a massive overdose of NSAIDs in the setting of volume depletion.

No NSAID is without renal toxicities. Because COX-2 is constitutively expressed in the kidney, COX-2 inhibitors also have renal toxicities comparable to standard NSAIDs. Future studies may be helpful in determining if the lack of COX-1 inhibition in the kidneys by these agents may mitigate the severity or frequency of the toxicities.

Other Adverse Effects

Hypersensitivity reactions such as rashes, urticaria, photosensitivity, and Stevens-Johnson syndrome have been reported among NSAID users. An interesting side effect is the cross-reactivity between aspirin and NSAIDs in triggering asthma, especially among patients with vasomotor rhinitis and nasal polyposis. Recent studies with these patients, however, have demonstrated a lack of cross-reactivity between aspirin and the COX-2 inhibitor rofecoxib, suggesting that COX-1 inhibition is a potential initiating event of aspirin-sensitive asthma (15).

Of the neurological adverse events, tinnitus and hearing loss are commonly associated with high doses of aspirin and non-acetylated salicylates but may also occur less frequently with other NSAIDs. Both of these side effects are reversible upon discontinuation. Aseptic meningitis, headaches, and confusion are potential toxicities but rarely encountered. The cause is unknown but may be more common in individuals with histories of migraine headaches or systemic lupus erythematosus.

Aplastic anemia, hemolytic anemia, neutropenia, agranulocytosis, and thrombocytopenia are rare hematologic complications of NSAIDs.

Contraindications and Precautions

Although NSAIDs are widely used, their ubiquity should not be interpreted as a reflection of absolute safety. These are potent medications with important and potentially serious adverse effects, particularly when used in the elderly or in individuals with chronic and multiple medical problems.

Aspirin and traditional NSAIDs should be used with extreme caution, if at all, in the setting of underlying gastritis, peptic ulcer disease, or gastrointestinal bleeding, because these drugs may cause or exacerbate hemorrhaging. Concurrent use of systemic corticosteroids magnifies this risk. Even the use of COX-2 selective inhibitors is not completely without hazard, because partial inhibition of COX-1 can still occur at therapeutic concentrations (16). Complete blood counts should be regularly followed to identify new anemia due to gastrointestinal blood loss.

Patients with bleeding diatheses or taking anticoagulants should be assessed thoroughly before the start of aspirin or traditional NSAID treatment to determine whether the risks of therapy warrant the potential benefits. COX-2 selective agents may be better options for these individuals, because they do not significantly affect platelet function.

Both traditional NSAIDs and COX-2 inhibitors can worsen pre-existing renal insufficiency and should be used with extreme caution, if at all, in patients with impaired renal function. Other patients at risk for nephrotoxicity include individuals with low effective blood volume and reduced renal perfusion. Alternative means of treatment that do not affect kidney function are strongly encouraged, such as acetaminophen for osteoarthritis or corticosteroids for acute gout. However, if the decision is made to use these medications in these patients, close monitoring of renal function is mandatory.

As for all medications, NSAIDs should be used during pregnancy only if the potential benefits justify the potential risks to mother and fetus. No definitive information is available as to whether NSAIDs are teratogenic. Hemorrhagic complications to both mother and fetus have been reported with high dosages of aspirin (>10 g/d). However, low dosages of aspirin (<325 mg/d), such as those used for the prevention/treatment of complications of pregnancy such as preeclampsia and anti-phospholipid syndrome, are quite safe and justified. Similarly, while the use of NSAIDs should generally be avoided in the third trimester of pregnancy because they may increase the risk of premature closure of the ductus arteriosus and fetal pulmonary hypertension, aspirin therapy is appropriate in those special cases.

Low concentrations of aspirin and NSAIDs can be distributed to breast milk and can rarely cause complications in the nursing infant such as bleeding. This is much more likely with chronic high-dose NSAID therapy and highly unlikely with sporadic occasional use.

Conclusion

Traditional NSAIDs and selective COX-2 inhibitors are extremely useful and widely prescribed medications. While generally safe, they can have potentially serious adverse effects, and it is crucial that clinicians remain vigilant for these complications, particularly in the elderly, in patients being treated chronically, and in those with comorbid or confounding conditions that may put them at increased risk. Like all medications, use of these drugs should be tailored to the individual patient. The drugs should be utilized at the lowest possible effective dose in order to minimize adverse events and only after other, safer options have been employed.

REFERENCES

1. **Wolfe MM, Lichtenstein DR, Singh G.** Gastrointestinal toxicity of nonsteroidal antiinflammatory drugs. N Engl J Med. 1999;340:1888-99.

2. **Bombardier C, Laine L, Reicin A, et al.** Comparison of upper gastrointestinal toxicity of rofecoxib and naproxen in patients with rheumatoid arthritis. VIGOR Study Group. N Engl J Med. 2000;343:1520-8.

3. **Silverstein FE, Faich G, Goldstein JL, et al.** Gastrointestinal toxicity with celecoxib versus nonsteroidal anti-inflammatory drugs for osteoarthritis and rheumatoid arthritis. The CLASS study: a randomized controlled trial. JAMA. 2000;284:1247-55.

4. **Lanza FL.** A guideline for the treatment and prevention of NSAID-induced ulcers. Members of the Ad Hoc Committee on Practice Parameters of the American College of Gastroenterology. Am J Gastroenterol. 1998;93:2037-46.

5. **Reuben SS, Fingeroth R, Krushell R, Maciolek H.** Evaluation of the safety and efficacy of the perioperative administration of rofecoxib for total knee arthroplasty. J Arthroplasty. 2002;17:26-31.

6. **Belton O, Byrne D, Kearney D, et al.** Cyclooxygenase-1 and -2 dependent prostacyclin formation in patients with atherosclerosis. Circulation. 2000;102:840-5.

7. **Reicin AS, Shapiro D, Sperling RS, et al.** Comparison of cardiovascular thrombotic events in patients with osteoarthritis treated with rofecoxib versus nonselective nonsteroidal anti-inflammatory drugs (ibuprofen, diclofenac, and nabumetone). Am J Cardiol. 2002;89:204-9.

8. **White WB, Faich G, Whelton A, et al.** Comparison of thromboembolic events in patients treated with celecoxib, a cyclooxygenase-2 specific inhibitor, versus ibuprofen or diclofenac. Am J Cardiol. 2002;89:425-30.

9. **Solomon DH, Schneeweiss S, Glynn RJ, et al.** Relationship between selective cyclooxygenase-2 inhibitors and acute myocardial infarction in older adults. Circulation. 2004;109:2068-73.

10. **Catella-Lawson F, Reilly MP, Kapoor SC, et al.** Cyclooxygenase inhibitors and the antiplatelet effects of aspirin. N Engl J Med. 2001;345:1809-17.

11. **Frishman WH.** Effects of nonsteroidal anti-inflammatory drug therapy on blood pressure and peripheral edema. Am J Cardiol. 2002;89:18D-25D.

12. **Whelton A.** Renal and related cardiovascular effects of conventional and COX-2-specific NSAIDs and non-NSAID analgesics. Am J Ther. 2000;7:63-74.

13. **Pope JE, Anderson JJ, Felson DT.** A meta-analysis of the effects of nosteroidal anti-inflammatory drugs on blood pressure. Arch Intern Med. 1993;153:477-84.

14. **Johnson AG, Nguyet TV, Day RO.** Do non-steroidal anti-inflammatory drugs affect blood pressure? A meta-analysis. Ann Intern Med. 1994;121:289-300.

15. **Szczeklik A, Nizankowska E, Bochenek G, et al.** Safety of a specific COX-2 inhibitor in aspirin-induced asthma. Clin Exp Allergy. 2001;31:219-25.

16. **Cryer B, Feldman M.** Cyclooxygenase-1 and cyclooxygenase-2 selectivity of widely used nonsteroidal anti-inflammatory drugs. Am J Med. 1998;104:413-21.

30

■　■　■

Corticosteroids

Stephen A. Paget, MD

S oon after the initial clinical use of corticosteroids (CS) in 1948, these extraordinary anti-inflammatory agents were thought to be "miracle cures" and, as such, were employed in the treatment of many systemic, disabling and refractory disorders. The number of diseases in which CS have been found useful has increased far beyond the three originally reported by Hench and his associates: rheumatoid arthritis (RA), systemic lupus erythematosus (SLE), and rheumatic fever (1,2). While some of the initial enthusiasm continued because CS lived up to expectations in extricating patients from previously "non-treatable" disorders, the list and severity of side effects began to grow. Recently, Balow aptly described these complications as ranging from minor to severe, early to late, flagrant to insidious, expected to rare, and tolerable to intolerable. Because CS combine "the good, the bad and the ugly," they exemplify the prototypic "double-edged sword" with which patients and their physicians need to strike an extremely fine balance between the beneficial and detrimental effects of these agents.

Now, over 50 years after the Nobel Prize was awarded for the use of CS in the treatment of RA, an appropriately healthy respect for their many effects has evolved. Through the vast accumulation of basic research data and clinical experience with CS, there is now greater appreciation of their therapeutic effects, safer steroid preparations and dosing regimens, and the need to develop and employ steroid-sparing medications. However, as the molecular mechanisms of pathogenesis of inflammatory diseases become more fully elucidated, it is hoped that more targeted medications will become available and that there will be fewer situations that necessitate aggressive or prolonged CS therapy.

Mechanisms of Action

Molecular and Cellular Effects

Corticosteroids broadly and profoundly inhibit many immune and inflammatory processes, rendering them potent and versatile agents in the treatment of rheumatologic disorders. After binding of CS to specific cytosolic receptors, the resulting complex translocates to the nucleus and modulates the expression of various genes. One well-characterized system is nuclear factor-κB (NF-κB), a ubiquitous and central transcription factor involved in the promotion of immune and inflammatory responses (3). Free NF-κB binds to specific sites in the promoter regions regulating the expression of genes coding for various proteins such as cytokines like tumor necrosis factor (TNF)-α, proteolytic enzymes, and adhesion molecules. Consequently, the inhibition of NF-κB activity by CS results in the disruption of a cascade of various inflammatory events. At the cellular level, these effects translate broadly into processes such as the inhibition of neutrophil migration to sites of inflammation; interference of leukocyte, endothelial cell, and fibroblast functions; and suppression of the production and the effects of pro-inflammatory humoral factors.

Although the cause and pathogenesis of many inflammatory and immunologically mediated disorders are not fully elucidated, the unregulated localization of leukocytes at sites of inflammation, their subsequent activation, and the generation of secretory products are processes that are common to these conditions and contribute to tissue damage. Pharmacologic doses of CS dramatically inhibit the accumulation and action of leukocytes at these sites of inflammation. CS antagonize macrophage differentiation and many of its functions, inhibit neutrophil adhesion to endothelial cells, block molecular events associated with endothelial cell activation, and suppress fibroblast proliferation (4). Many factors influence the magnitude of these effects, including the dosage and route of administration of CS and the type and differentiation state of the target cell population. Host factors, such as the rate of CS metabolism or target tissue sensitivity, also modify the physiologic responses to CS.

The immunosuppressive effects of CS are also directed towards the trafficking and function of lymphocytes. The generation and proliferation of helper, suppressor, and cytotoxic T lymphocytes are inhibited by CS. T-cell functions, like the expression of cytokines such as interleukin (IL)-2, interferon-γ, and IL-6, are also inhibited by CS. In contrast to T cells, B cells are relatively resistant to the immunosuppressive effects of CS. However, high doses of CS can lead to reduced immunoglobulin synthesis.

This impressive profile of immune- and inflammation-altering effects of CS account for their extraordinary ability to control diverse disorders that are dominated by immune and inflammatory dysfunction, such as systemic lupus erythematosus, asthma, pemphigus, polymyositis, multiple sclerosis, and ulcerative colitis. Moreover, when used in conjunction with appropriate antimicrobial agents, the anti-inflammatory effects of CS have also been exploited successfully and safely in limiting tissue damage caused by inflammation in various infectious diseases such as meningitis, tuberculosis, and *Pneumocystis carinii* pneumonia.

Clinical Pharmacology

Corticosteroids are 17-hydroxy, 21-carbon steroid molecules whose principal, naturally occurring form is cortisol (hydrocortisone). Many synthetic CS derivatives have been developed via the modification of various sites on the cortisol molecule. Their therapeutic and adverse effects are strongly determined by dosage and dose schedules, routes of administration, biologic half-lives, and anti-inflammatory and mineralocorticoid effects (Table 30-1).

Several important clinical considerations can be gleaned from structure-function analysis and knowledge of different metabolic and biologic properties of various CS (Tables 30-1 and 30-2):

1. Synthetic agents were developed by modifying various sites on the cortisol molecule in order to enhance the anti-inflammatory and reduce the mineralocorticoid (Na^+-retaining) activity. In general, for clinical purposes, agents with lower mineralocorticoid effects are associated with fewer problems with fluid retention and hypertension. Nonetheless, although dexamethasone has the lowest mineralocorticoid effect, it is rarely employed in the treatment of systemic inflammatory disorders because its very long half-life carries greater potential for other CS-related adverse effects.

Table 30-1   Pharmacological Properties of Corticosteroids

Drug	Duration of Action (hr)	Plasma $T^{1/2}$ (min)	Approximate Relative Potency		
			Gluco-corticoid	Mineralo-corticoid	Dose Equivalence
Short-Acting					
Cortisone	8-12	90	0.8	0.8	25
Cortisol (hydrocortisone)	8-12	80-110	1	1	20
Intermediate-Acting					
Prednisone	12-36	180	4-5	0-0.8	5
Prednisolone	12-36	115-200	4-5	0-0.8	5
Methylprednisolone	12-36	150-180	5-6	0-0.5	4
Triamcinolone	12-36	200	4-5	0	4
Long-Acting					
Dexamethasone	36-72	240	30	0	0.5-0.7

2. Minor differences in plasma half-life contrast with the marked differences in potency and duration of biologic activity. Thus the chronic use of dexamethasone will yield many more CS-related side effects than an equivalent dose of prednisone.

3. The 11-keto CS, cortisone and prednisone, must be activated in the liver by conversion to their respective 11-hydroxyl metabolites, cortisol (hydrocortisone), and prednisolone. Thus severe hepatic dysfunction may alter the metabolism of cortisone and prednisone and attenuate their clinical efficacy. Also, only cortisol and prednisolone can be used for parenteral therapy, which is often necessary when the patient cannot take oral medications. They are often used in the setting of a severe, systemic inflammatory disorder in which an immediate clinical response is required or when intestinal absorption is compromised by gastrointestinal dysfunction or edema.

4. Differences in the structure of various CS derivatives result in useful differences in potency, mineralocorticoid effect and pharmacokinetic profiles (see Tables 30-1 and 30-2) that can be utilized in specific clinical settings. For example:

   • For the routine control of a clinically stable inflammatory disorder, an intermediate-acting CS such as prednisone given in a single daily, morning dose is usually adequate.

   • In the setting of an active, systemic inflammatory disorder, especially one that is organ- or life-threatening, "around-the-clock" disease suppression is mandatory; thus an intermediate-acting CS would be used in a two-, three- or four-times daily dosing schedule. Once disease control is achieved, a once daily suppression regimen can be introduced.

   • Short-acting preparations are employed in the peri-operative period in order to avoid adrenal insufficiency in patients who have received oral CS for more than 3 weeks within the past year. They are also used for maintenance adrenal replacement therapy in patients with chronic adrenal insufficiency.

Clinical Uses

Treatment Options

With broader knowledge about the clinical effectiveness of CS and greater appreciation of their negative effects, alternative treatment regimens have been sought in order to optimize the outcomes and minimize the risks of CS therapies. While specific CS preparations for systemic use have remained the same for many years, distinct treatment approaches as to which preparations may be more appropriate in which clinical situations have evolved

Table 30-2   Clinical Uses of Corticosteroids

Drug	Brand Name	Preparation/Dose	Clinical Use	Comments
Oral				
Prednisone	Generic drug with many trade names (e.g., Orasone)	Tablets; 1 mg, 5 mg, 10 mg, 20 mg	Most commonly used oral steroid for treatment of inflammatory disorders	Least expensive oral steroid
Prednisolone	Generic drug with many trade names	Tablets; 1 mg, 2.5 mg, 5 mg	Commonly used oral steroid for inflammatory disorders; useful in patients with hepatic dysfunction	May be more effective in patients with liver disease or malabsorption
Methylprednisolone	Medrol	Tablets; 2 mg, 4 mg, 8 mg, 16 mg, 32 mg	Commonly used oral steroid; useful in patients with hepatic dysfunction	More expensive than prednisone; may be more effective in patients with liver disease
Dexamethasone	Decadron	Tablets; 0.25 mg, 0.50 mg, 0.75 mg, 1.5 mg, 4.0 mg	Rarely used for long-term treatment of inflammatory disorders	Long biologic half-life increases risk of steroid side effects
Hydrocortisone	Hydrocortone	Tablets; 10 mg	Used primarily for primary or secondary adrenal insufficiency	Used because of its mineralocorticoid and glucocorticoid activity
Parenteral				
Hydrocortisone phosphate	Hydrocortone	IV, IM 50 mg vials	In patients on long-term oral steroid, used in the peri-operative period or in periods of stress; rarely used for the control of inflammation	Short half-life; fluid and salt retention

Parenteral (*cont'd*)

Methylprednisolone sodium succinate	Solu-Medrol	IV, IM	Commonly used in the setting of severe systemic inflammatory disorders or in patients who cannot absorb oral steroids	Less fluid and salt retention than cortisol
Dexamethasone phosphate	Decadron	IV, IM, IA	Rarely used for the long-term treatment of inflammatory disorders	Long biologic half-life can lead to greater side effects
Adrenocortico-tropin (ACTH)	Co-syntropin	IM , IV, SQ	Used primarily for testing of adrenal function; rarely used for acute gout	Not for patients on chronic steroids
Locally Deposited				
Methylprednisolone acetate	Depo-Medrol	For IA, IL, IM	Commonly used for IA injections	Post-injection inflammation rarely
Triamcinolone hexacetonide	Aristospan	For IA use	Commonly used for IA injections	Post-injection inflammation rarely

IV = intravenous; IM = intramuscular; IA = intra-articular; SQ = subcutaneous; IL = intralesional.

in response to cumulative clinical experience. Also, appropriate aggressiveness of dosing tailored to the clinical scenario helps minimize toxicities.

Some typical CS regimens that have been employed in the treatment of inflammatory disorders are given below. Table 30-3 summarizes the dose ranges for prednisone and methylprednisolone.

High-Dose Therapy

Daily oral prednisone 40-80 mg or an equivalent (in a single or divided dose schedule) is commonly used for the treatment of active and severe inflammatory disorders such as SLE with visceral manifestations, severe asthma, or inflammatory bowel disease. The main objective of this regimen is to rapidly control inflammation and prevent tissue damage and irreversible organ dysfunction. Once the acute inflammation is brought under control, the dosage can be tapered by 5 to 10 mg every several days to weeks and consolidated to a more physiological and safer single daily dose. Higher initial or cumulative dosages and prolonged treatment courses increase the likelihood of major side effects.

Alternate-Day Therapy

Alternate-day regimens were initially used in children as an attempt to minimize growth-retardation secondary to CS and then later adapted more generally as a means of maintaining disease control while limiting toxicities (5). Initial disease control is mandatory *before* switching to an every-other-day schedule. Once control of active disease is achieved with daily CS therapy, the dosage can be doubled on the "on" day while gradually tapered to zero on the "off" day. Alternatively, one can taper the dose on the "off" day, eventually reaching an every-other-day regimen. Afterwards, the "on" day dose is then tapered slowly, with close observation of the disease activity. The effectiveness of the every-other-day regimen is unclear. Some rheumatologists believe it inadequate for controlling the constant inflammatory processes in systemic illnesses such as RA or SLE. Every-other-day dosing, in fact, has been associated with an increased risk of vision loss in giant cell arteritis and is not recommended for this condition (6).

Rapid Tapers

Short pulses of oral low-to-moderate dose CS are commonly employed in the treatment of non-organ- or life-threatening manifestations of diseases

Table 30-3   Daily Dose Ranges of Prednisone and Methylprednisolone

Low	Prednisone <20 mg; methylprednisolone <16 mg
Moderate	Prednisone 20-40 mg; methylprednisolone 16-32 mg
High	Prednisone 40-80 mg; methylprednisolone 32-64 mg
Intravenous "pulse"	Methylprednisolone 250-1000 mg IV × 1-3 days

such as RA and SLE. This approach attempts to rapidly reset the inflammatory thermostat, allowing other medications such as non-steroidal anti-inflammatory drugs to more effectively maintain disease control. A typical course may be prednisone 10 mg PO bid tapering by 5 mg per day over a total of four days, with the evening dose reduced first. Higher or lower initial dosages may be chosen depending upon the activity of the disease or the patient's prior experience.

Extended Tapers

In certain conditions such as polymyalgia rheumatica (PMR) and giant cell arteritis, systemic CS therapy may be maintained for months to years and tapered very slowly. While many different taper schedules have been used for these disorders, it is clear that overly rapid reduction of dosages often results in relapses and ultimately in a greater cumulative exposure to CS (6). For PMR, a typical daily starting dose may be prednisone 20 mg that can then be tapered by 2.5 mg weekly down to 10 mg within a month. Subsequently, the daily dose can often be reduced by 1 mg weekly down to 5 mg, after which the taper can be continued by 1 mg monthly until prednisone is discontinued or symptoms recur. There is great variability in patient response in PMR, and so the CS taper schedule will need to be adjusted accordingly. Compared with PMR, an overly rapid CS taper in GCA has a narrower margin for error and may have serious consequences such as vision loss. For GCA, a typical daily starting dose may be prednisone 40-60 mg. Once disease activity is completely suppressed, the daily dose can be tapered by 5-10 mg monthly until 20 mg, after which the taper should be slowed to 2.5 mg monthly. Below 10 mg, an even slower taper may be required (e.g., 1 mg increments every 1-2 months).

"Bridge" Therapy

Certain disease-modifying anti-rheumatic drugs (DMARDs) such as methotrexate for RA or hydroxychloroquine for SLE generally take weeks to bring about adequate disease control. During this "window" of disease activity, low-dose daily prednisone (e.g., 5-7.5 mg) maintains disease control and improves function until the therapeutic effects of the DMARD are realized. However, once CS are started, it is often difficult to taper the dose quickly without inciting a disease flare. This must be considered carefully, especially when "bridge therapy" is employed for more than two weeks. "Bridge therapy" can easily become chronic therapy with all of its attendant side effects.

Intravenous "Pulse" Therapy

High-dose, long-term courses of prednisone (e.g., 60-80 mg/d for more than 4-6 weeks), while effective in controlling most inflammatory states, also predictably lead to major side effects. Alternative, safer disease-controlling CS regimens have been sought. "Pulse" therapy, most commonly intravenous methylprednisolone 1 g daily for three days, has been used in the treatment of active SLE with severe visceral involvement and renal transplant rejection since the 1970s. This ultra-high, but limited, treatment approach seems to be quite effective in controlling severe inflammatory conditions such as lupus glomerulonephritis while reducing the incidence of many undesired effects associated with daily oral CS therapy (7). "Mini-pulses" have also been used with regimens varying from methylpred-nisolone 1 g/d for 1-2 days to 250 mg/d for 1-3 days (8). The exact dosing is guided by the severity of the inflammation, presence of or potential for organ damage, and past therapeutic responses by the patient.

In many circumstances, a single intravenous CS "pulse" is prescribed to maximally suppress systemic inflammation at the outset of CS therapy without anticipating the need for further intravenous boluses and given just before the start of daily oral CS dosing. For example, systemic vasculitis that threatens an end-organ like a peripheral nerve may be treated with a single intravenous methylprednisolone "pulse" followed by a gradual oral prednisone taper and cytotoxic therapy. In other conditions, extensive clinical experience has led to more formal scheduled approaches. In lupus nephritis, for example, intravenous CS boluses are often administered on a monthly basis for several months, frequently in conjunction with immuno-suppressive/cytotoxic therapy, until the disease is deemed controlled (9).

Intralesional or Locally Administered Steroids

In order to avoid the use of systemic steroids, various local CS therapies have been devised. Specific CS preparations have been developed to more easily, more safely, and more effectively control inflammation in different body sites. However, although these therapeutic approaches tend to be safer than systemic steroids, they are not totally free of side effects, especially if used chronically.

Topical CS are used for the treatment of various types of dermatitis and injectable CS for joint or soft tissue inflammation (Table 30-4). Other examples include injected epidural CS for lumbar disc disease or spinal stenosis, ocular CS drops for inflammatory eye disorders, and inhaled CS for asthma or

---

Table 30-4   Sample Methylprednisolone Dosages for Intra-Articular and Soft Tissue Corticosteroid Injections

- Large joint (shoulder, hip, knee): 60-80 mg

- Medium joint (wrist, ankle, elbow): 20-40 mg

- Small joint (interphalangeal, metacarpophalangeal): 10 mg

- Bursa (e.g., subacromial, subdeltoid, anserine): 20-40 mg

- Tenosynovium (e.g., trigger finger, bicipital): 10-20 mg

- Carpal tunnel or tarsal tunnel: 20-40 mg

chronic sinusitis. Cortisone enemas may be helpful for inflammatory bowel disease localized to the rectum and CS suppositories for the inflammation caused by hemorrhoids.

Adrenocorticotropic Hormone (ACTH)

Because a great variety of adrenocorticosteroids are secreted in response to ACTH and the exact levels of steroid secretion are unpredictable, ACTH has not been employed for general clinical use. The one area in which ACTH has been used with some regularity, albeit uncommonly, is in the treatment of acute crystalline arthritis. Intramuscular injection of 40 U of ACTH can be quite effective in the treatment of acute exacerbations of gout or pseudo-gout. However, similar clinical responses can be obtained with the use of oral systemic CS preparations such as prednisone, without the need for par-enteral administration. Today, the use of ACTH is generally limited to the ACTH stimulation test for the evaluation of adrenal insufficiency.

Replacement/Supplementation Therapy for Known or Suspected Adrenal Insufficiency

Patients treated with chronic steroids or those receiving cortisol replacement therapy because of hypothalamic-pituitary-adrenal (H-P-A) hypofunction should be considered at risk for CS-withdrawal syndrome or cardiovascular collapse in the setting of severe physiologic stress or surgery. The duration of CS therapy, the highest dose, and the total cumulative dose have long been considered important predictors of the suppression of the H-P-A axis (10). In general, for practical purposes, patients treated with more than prednisone 5 mg daily (or equivalent) for more than 2 to 4 weeks within the past year should be considered to have some degree of H-P-A dysfunc-tion (11). Recent studies indicate that the rate of cortisol production in normal subjects is two to three times lower than previously believed. In healthy adults, the adrenal glands produce about 50 mg of cortisol per 24 hours during minor surgery and 75-150 mg per 24 hours during major surgery. A 1994 consensus paper makes reasonable and clear recommen-dations for the dose and duration of CS supplementation perioperatively: a total of 25 mg of hydrocortisone (or equivalent) for minor stress; hydrocor-tisone 50-75 mg (or equivalent) for moderate stress; and hydrocortisone 100-150 mg (or equivalent) or more daily given parenterally for one to three days for surgeries involving major stress (e.g., coronary artery by-passes, bowel resections, arthroplasties) (12). A commonly employed regi-men for major surgery is 100 mg of intravenous hydrocortisone one hour before surgery and then 100 mg every 8 hours for the first day (300 mg total dose on day one). The hydrocortisone dose is then halved for each of the subsequent two days. The patient is then usually able to reinstitute the oral preparation that existed pre-operatively. In patients who receive CS topically (i.e., inhalation, intranasally, transdermally, or by enema), H-P-A suppression is rarely clinically significant. Thus additional CS is generally unnecessary during minor or moderate surgical procedures or illnesses, as long as their clinical course is uncomplicated and closely observed for signs of adrenal insufficiency.

General Principles of Corticosteroid Use

To optimize the outcome of CS therapy and to "win the (short-term) battle *and* the (long-term) war" against disease and complications of therapy, the physician should

- Be reasonably assured of the diagnosis and that infection and cancer have been excluded.
- Initially consider other treatment approaches besides CS for the disease-specific clinical problem.
- Use CS only if other, less toxic options have been exhausted; if the disease is life-, tissue- or organ-threatening; or if clinical experience supports their use.
- Fully educate the patient and family on the potential positive and negative effects of CS treatment and how they might impact specifically upon the treated individual.
- Understand the natural history and pathogenesis of the disease being treated and the anticipated response of the disease process to CS.
- Carefully match the aggressiveness of the disease with the CS regimen. Define disease outcomes measures and use them as therapeutic milestones.
- Appreciate the unique pharmacologic characteristics of the various CS preparations.
- Understand the clinical effects of differing CS dose schedules and routes of administration.
- Choose a dose and dosing schedule that will optimally control the disorder, then taper the medication as fast as possible, preferably to zero, recognizing that the shortest course of CS with the lowest initial and cumulative dose is the safest.
- Obtain in-depth knowledge of alternative disease-modifying and steroid-sparing therapeutic modalities and recognize when their use may more optimally control disease activity while simultaneously reducing CS requirements.
- Recognize that CS-related side effects may mimic the signs of the active disease itself (e.g., steroid myopathy in the setting of myositis).
- Treat the patient, not a laboratory test (e.g., never simply "chase the sedimentation rate").

Adverse Effects

No CS regimen is completely free of potential short- or long-term adverse effects, which can vary from the mild and self-limited (e.g., memory lapses, acne) to major or life-threatening (e.g., osteonecrosis of a hip, overwhelming infection and sepsis). In general, side effects are dose-related; higher initial and cumulative doses and longer treatment courses increase the likelihood of treatment complications. Table 30-5 lists some of the many potential CS side effects. Patients vary tremendously with regard to the side effect profile that may develop acutely or over time. Although most patients on chronic CS will develop weight gain, facial swelling, easy bruising, emotional lability, and a mild leukocytosis, fewer will develop major infections, diabetes mellitus, proximal muscle weakness, and osteonecrosis.

It is important for the clinician to institute preventive measures for all patients started on chronic CS. These include 1) effective monitoring for and protection against osteoporosis, 2) immunization against influenza, pneumococcus, and other organisms, and 3) close observation and prompt treatment for hypertension, hyperglycemia, and hyperlipidemia. Elderly patients, patients with diabetes, hypertension, heart disease, or osteoporosis, and patients who are receiving immunosuppressive therapy have an increased propensity for some of the more severe CS-related side effects.

For the rheumatologist, osteoporosis stands out from the myriad adverse effects associated with CS use. Within several weeks of chronic CS therapy, loss of bone mass can be appreciated (13). Accordingly, the American College of Rheumatology (2001) has recommended that measures to prevent osteoporosis be taken if a patient is on at least 5 mg daily of prednisone for

Table 30-5 Adverse Effects of Chronic Corticosteroid Therapy

	Common	Uncommon
Skin		
Easy bruisability (ecchymoses, petechiae)	✓	
Thin, fragile skin	✓	
Striae	✓	
Facial erythema	✓	
Acne	✓	
Hirsuitism (facial)	✓	
Atrophy (post-injection)		✓
Impaired wound healing	✓	
Ophthalmologic		
Posterior subcapsular cataracts	✓	
Glaucoma, increased intraocular pressure		✓
Exophthalmos		✓

(Cont'd)

Table 30-5   Adverse Effects of Chronic Corticosteroid Therapy *(Cont'd)*

	Common	Uncommon
Cardiovascular		
Hypertension	✓	
Hyperlipoproteinemia, premature atherosclerosis	✓	
Congestive heart failure (in patients with cardiac dysfunction)		✓
Metabolic		
Diabetes, hyperglycemia	✓	
Diabetic ketoacidosis		✓
Negative nitrogen balance	✓	
Truncal obesity	✓	
Sodium retention, edema	✓	
Secondary adrenal insufficiency (>5 mg prednisone, >3 weeks)	✓	
Suppression of growth in children	✓	
Gastrointestinal		
Peptic ulcer, primarily gastric, hemorrhage	✓	
Diverticulitis, cholecystitis		✓
Fatty liver with hepatomegaly		✓
Pancreatitis		✓
"Silent" intestinal perforation		✓
Neurologic/Psychiatric		
Benign intracranial hypertension or pseudotumor cerebri		✓
Alterations in mood, depression, insomnia, euphoria, appetite increase	✓	
Psychosis		✓
Bone and Musculoskeletal		
Myopathy	✓	
Osteoporosis, fragility fractures	✓	
Osteonecrosis	✓	
Joint pains associated with steroid taper (pseudorheumatism)		✓
Hematologic/Immunologic		
Neutrophilia, monocytopenia, lymphopenia	✓	
Suppressed delayed-type hypersensitivity	✓	
Infection		
Increased risk for all bacterial, viral, mycobacterial, fungal, and protozoal infections, particularly at high CS doses for long periods of time or when used in conjunction with other immunosuppressants	✓	

more than 3 months (14). However, some clinicians advocate intervention even if patients are anticipated to be on CS therapy for as little as 2 weeks. Intervention should include adequate calcium and vitamin D supplementation and possibly anti-resorptive medications such as alendronate or risedronate (15,16). Teriparatide, an analogue of human parathyroid hormone, has also proven to be beneficial (17). The management of CS-induced osteoporosis is discussed more fully in Chapter 23.

Precautions

Corticosteroid therapy should be kept at the minimum required to control disease activity in order to reduce the risks of developing or exacerbating adverse effects. Close vigilance should be given particularly to patients with pre-existing conditions such as hypertension, dyslipidemias, diabetes mellitus, glaucoma, or osteoporosis that could be worsened with prolonged CS use. Corticosteroids increase the risk of gastrointestinal bleeding and attendant complications in patients receiving non-steroidal anti-inflammatory drugs, and their use should be monitored especially carefully in this population.

Although in certain infection syndromes such as *Pneumocystis carinii* pneumonia and severe tuberculosis the anti-inflammatory effects of CS therapy when given with appropriate anti-microbial agents limit permanent organ damage, CS must be prescribed with care in patients with infections because of their immunosuppressive properties. Also, while early observations had suggested the contrary, high doses of CS have not been shown to improve prognosis in patients with sepsis and may in fact be associated with increased mortality in some circumstances (18,19).

At typical dosages, non-fluorinated CS such as prednisone and methylprednisolone do not cross the placenta and can be used safely during pregnancy. Fluorinated CS like dexamethasone *do* cross the placenta and *should not* be used during pregnancy if fetal exposure is not desired. Corticosteroids are minimally distributed in milk but should nevertheless be prescribed with caution in nursing mothers.

Future Directions

Despite major advances in understanding the pathogenesis of inflammatory disorders over the past 50 years, we still rely on corticosteroids for the treatment of innumerable illnesses (20). As illustrated by the experience with deflazacort, recent attempts at altering the chemistry of the cortisol molecule in order to optimize therapeutic benefits and minimize adverse effects have failed. Although early studies suggested that deflazacort could adequately control inflammation without causing concomitant steroid-induced osteoporosis, it was later demonstrated that when equipotent doses of deflazacort to prednisone were compared, the putative bone-sparing capacity was lost. Nonetheless, ongoing attempts at chemical manipulations may still lead to the eventual development of the "perfect" steroid preparation for clinical use.

The development of new targeted biologic modifiers and increased use of non-steroidal immunosuppressive medications will, no doubt, markedly improve the treatment of inflammatory disorders and reduce reliance on CS for disease control. For example, the effective use of anti-TNF-α medications such as adalimumab, etanercept, and infliximab in rheumatoid arthritis has, thus far, been accompanied by marked reductions in CS requirements. However, whether such medications will, in the long run, enable the physician to avoid CS therapy entirely or use significantly lower and safer CS regimens remains to be seen.

REFERENCES

1. **Hench PS, Kendall EC, Slocumb CH, Polley HF.** The effect of a hormone of the adrenal cortex (17-hydroxy-11-dehydrocorticosterone: compound E) and of pituitary adrenocorticotropic hormone on rheumatoid arthritis. Proc Staff Meet Mayo Clin. 1949;24:181-97.

2. **Hench PS, Kendall EC, Slocumb CH, Polley HF.** Effects of cortisone acetate and pituitary ACTH on rheumatoid arthritis, rheumatic fever and other conditions. Arch Intern Med. 1950;85:545-666.

3. **Barnes PJ, Karin M.** Nuclear factor-κB: a pivotal transcription factor in chronic inflammatory diseases. N Engl J Med. 1997;336:1006-71.

4. **Boumpas DT, Chrousos GP, Wilder RL, et al.** Glucocorticoid therapy for immune-mediated diseases: basic and clinical correlates. Ann Intern Med. 1993; 119:1198-1208.

5. **Hunder GG, Sheps SG, Allen GL, Joyce JW.** Daily and alternate-day corticosteroid regimens in treatment of giant cell arteritis: comparison in a prospective study. Ann Intern Med. 1975;82:613-8.

6. **Fauci AS.** Alternate-day corticosteroid therapy. Am J Med. 1978;64:729-35.

7. **Kimberly RP.** Glucocorticoid therapy for rheumatic diseases. Curr Opin Rheumatol. 1992;4:325-31.

8. **Smith MD, Bertouch JV, Smith AM, et al.** The clinical and immunological effects of pulse methylprednisolone therapy in rheumatoid arthritis. I: Clinical effects. J Rheumatol. 1988;15:229-35.

9. **Illei GG, Austin HA 3rd, Crane M, et al.** Combination therapy with pulse cyclophosphamide plus pulse methylprednisolone improves long-term renal outcome without adding toxicity in patients with lupus nephritis. Ann Intern Med. 2001;135:248-57.

10. **Chrousos GP.** The hypothalamic-pituitary-adrenal axis and immune-mediated inflammation. N Engl J Med. 1995;332:1351-62.

11. **LaRochelle GE, LaRochelle AG, Ratner RE, Borenstein DG.** Recovery of the hypothalamic-pituitary-adrenal (HPA) axis in patients with rheumatic diseases receiving low-dose prednisone. Am J Med. 1993;95:258-64.

12. **Salem M, Tainsh RE Jr, Bromberg J, et al.** Perioperative glucocorticoid coverage: a reassessment 42 years after emergence of a problem. Ann Surg. 1994;219:416-25.

13. **Laan RFJM, van Riel PLCM, van de Putte LBA, et al.** Low-dose prednisone induces rapid reversible axial bone loss in patients with rheumatoid arthritis: a randomized, controlled study. Ann Intern Med. 1993;119:963-8.

14. Recommendations for the prevention and treatment of glucocorticoid-induced osteoporosis; 2001 update. American College of Rheumatology Ad Hoc Committee on Glucocorticoid-Induced Osteoporosis. Arthritis Rheum. 2001;44:1496-1503.

15. **Sambrook PN, Kotowitz M, Nash P, et al.** Prevention and treatment of glucocorticoid-induced osteoporosis: a comparison of calcitriol, vitamin D plus calcium, and alendronate plus calcium. J Bone Miner Res. 2003;18:919-24.

16. **Wallach S, Cohen S, Reid DM, et al.** Effects of risedronate treatment on bone density and vertebral fractures in patients on corticosteroid therapy. Calcif Tissue Int. 2000;67:277-85.

17. **Lane N, Sanchez S, Modin GW, et al.** Parathyroid hormone treatment can reverse corticosteroid-induced osteoporosis: results of a randomized controlled clinical trial. J Clin Invest. 1998;102:1627-33.

18. **Bone RC, Fisher CJ, Clemmer TP, et al.** Early methylprednisolone treatment for septic syndrome and the adult respiratory distress syndrome. Chest. 1987;92:1032-6.

19. **Luce JM, Montgomery AB, Marks JD, et al.** Ineffectiveness of high-dose methylprednisolone in preventing parenchymal lung injury and improving mortality in patients with septic shock. Am Rev Respir Dis. 1988;138:62-8.

20. **Lamberts SWJ, Bruining HA, deJong FH.** Drug therapy: corticosteroid therapy in severe illness. N Engl J Med. 1997;337:1285-92.

31

■ ■ ■

Disease-Modifying
Anti-Rheumatic Drugs

Joseph A. Markenson, MD

Arthur M.F. Yee, MD, PhD

Disease-modifying anti-rheumatic drugs (DMARDs), a heterogeneous group of agents frequently used for the control of many chronic systemic inflammatory disorders, represent the state-of-the-art in the practice of rheumatology (Table 31-1). Whereas DMARDs were still largely reserved for the most severely affected patients as recently as two decades ago, the current therapeutic paradigm usually involves early use of DMARDs to prevent irreversible damage to tissues and organs. Ostensibly, DMARDs are thought to act at various points in the immune system, thereby modulating inflammatory processes, and many (although not all) are truly immunosuppressive. However, the mechanisms of action of most DMARDs (e.g., methotrexate) have not been fully defined (1). The exceptions are the newer biological DMARDs such as etanercept, infliximab, anakinra, and adalimumab, which are targeted against very specific proinflammatory cytokine components of the immune system (2).

The definition of DMARDs is elusive. In the strictest sense, DMARDs are defined in the context of rheumatoid arthritis (RA) as agents with the capacity to alter the natural history of the disease. According to the American College of Rheumatology Ad Hoc Committee on Clinical Guidelines (1996), DMARDs are described as having "the potential to reduce or prevent joint damage, preserve joint integrity and function, and, ultimately, to reduce the total costs of health care and maintain economic productivity of the patient with RA." However, this characterization carries flaws. For example, a recent study has suggested that corticosteroids may retard progression of joint erosions in RA (3), yet most rheumatologists would not consider them to be DMARDs. In fact, many clinicians would categorically exclude corticosteroids

Table 31-1   Characteristics of Commonly Used Disease-Modifying Anti-Rheumatic Drugs

Medication	Dose Range/ Route of Administration	Capacity to Affect Joint Erosions in RA*	Major Side Effects	Monitoring Protocols
Adalimumab	40 mg every 1-2 wks; SQ	+	Injection-site reaction, infection, TB, cyto- penias, autoimmunity	CBC, PPD, CXR
Anakinra	100 mg/d; SQ	+	Injection-site reaction, infection, cytopenias	CBC
Auranofin	3-9 mg qd; oral	0	Rash, diarrhea	CBC, urinalysis
Azathioprine	2-3 mg/kg; oral	+	Liver, fever, bone marrow, neoplasm, infection	CBC, LFT
Cyclophos- phamide	2 mg/kg/d; oral 0.5-1 g/m²/ month; IV	+	Infection, cytopenias, infertility, neoplasm, marrow, bladder	CBC, electrolytes, urinalysis
Cyclosporine	2-5 mg/kg/d; oral	+	Hypertension, renal, marrow, infection, neoplasm	CBC, Cr, BP
Etanercept	25 mg twice weekly or 50 mg weekly; SQ	+	Injection-site reaction, infection, TB, cyto- penias, autoimmunity	CBC, PPD, CXR
Gold sodium thiomalate	50 mg/wk; IM	+	Rash, renal, marrow	CBC, urine
Hydroxy- chloroquine	200 mg bid; oral	0	Maculopathy, rash, diarrhea	Ophthalmologi- cal examina- tions, G6PD
Infliximab	3-10 mg/kg wk 0, 2, 6, then q 8 wks; IV	+	Infusion reaction, infection, TB, cyto- penias, autoimmunity	CBC, PPD, CXR
Intravenous immuno- globulin	1-2 g/kg usually in divided doses; IV	N/A	Infusion reactions, constitutional symp- toms, CHF, serum sickness	IgA levels, vital signs, cardio pulmonary
Leflunomide	100 mg/d × 3d, then 10-20 mg/d; oral	+	Diarrhea, liver, GI, marrow, infection	CBC, LFT, hepa- titis screen
Methotrexate	7.5-25 mg/wk; oral, SQ, or IM	+	Liver, marrow, lung, infection, lymphoma	CBC, LFT, Cr, CXR, hepa- titis screen
Mycophenolate mofetil	250-1000 mg bid; oral	N/A	Marrow, infection, GI	CBC, LFT
Sulfasalazine	1-1.5 g bid; oral	+	Rash, GI, leukopenia, oligospermia	CBC, LFT, G6PD

* "+" denotes agents that have shown the capacity to affect the progression of erosions in rheumatoid arthritis. "0" denotes agents for which consistent evidence of the ability to affect erosions is lacking.
RA = rheumatoid arthritis; CBC = complete blood count; GI = gastrointestinal intolerance; LFT = liver function tests; Cr = serum creatinine; BP = blood pressure monitoring; TB = tuberculosis; PPD = purified protein derivative; CXR = chest X-ray; G6PD = glucose-6-phosphate dehydrogenase; N/A = not available; CHF = congestive heart failure.

from this class of drugs, and, indeed, others would accept steroid-sparing properties as a defining criterion. Accordingly, although agents such as anti-malarial drugs have not been proven to limit the development of erosions, they are nonetheless considered by a significant number of practitioners to be DMARDs. Further confounding the issue is the increasing use of many of these drugs in inflammatory diseases other than RA, thereby rendering outcome measures specific to RA such as joint erosions inapplicable.

DMARDs are neither corticosteroids nor nonsteroidal anti-inflammatory drugs (NSAIDs). They are all suspected or known to modulate processes involved in immune functions, and the intent of their use is not to suppress acute inflammation but rather to induce or maintain chronic control of disease activity. Clinical rationales for the use of DMARD therapy are diverse and often include addressing inadequate response to other agents like NSAIDs or cortico-steroids; minimizing corticosteroid-induced adverse effects; inducing or main-taining disease remission; and preventing irreversible end-organ damage. Weeks to months of use may be required before a fair assessment of the clinical effec-tiveness of a DMARD can be realized, although the newer biological agents like etanercept or infliximab may show benefit even after several days. Moreover, months or years may be needed to demonstrate retardation of erosions in RA.

DMARDs vary widely with regard to clinical indications, expected effec-tiveness, potential toxicities, costs, and routes of administration. The choice of a DMARD depends on the nature and severity of disease, the presence and type of comorbid conditions, the use of concomitant medications, and responses to previous therapies. Other factors specific to individual patients such as family planning (Table 31-2) and medical insurance issues must also commonly be factored into the final decision. Moreover, because it is anticipated that patients will require long-term DMARD treatment, regular and vigilant monitoring for adverse effects is mandatory.

Before initiating DMARD therapy, a thorough discussion with the pa-tient regarding the goals of therapy, the anticipated benefits and the ex-pected time required to achieve them, and the potential risks should be conducted. Baseline laboratory tests (e.g., complete blood counts [CBC] or biochemical profile) are recommended generally, but other, more specific tests (e.g., urinalysis, tuberculin skin testing, chest X-ray, hepatitis serolo-gies) may be necessary depending on the medication being considered.

The DMARDs discussed in this chapter are those of greatest clinical in-terest and use in the modern practice of rheumatology. Appendix A pro-vides DMARD generic and trade names.

Methotrexate

Clinical Uses

Methotrexate, the most commonly prescribed and best studied DMARD for the treatment of RA, has generally been considered the "gold standard" against which all other agents are measured. Methotrexate may be used as monotherapy or as the cornerstone in a DMARD combination approach and has been shown to retard the development of joint erosions. In addition, methotrexate is commonly used in the treatment of seronegative spondyloarthropathies, particularly in psoriatic arthritis, and has been found to be effective in treating joint involvement in systemic lupus erythematosus (SLE), inflammatory myositis, limited forms of Wegener's granulomatosis and other vasculitides, sarcoidosis and other interstitial lung diseases, and psoriasis.

Mechanism of Action

Methotrexate inhibits dihydrofolate reductase, which converts folate to its active metabolite, which in turn is required for the biosynthesis of purines and of the amino acids serine and methionine. Thus, methotrexate affects both polynucleotide and protein synthesis. Therapeutic concentrations of methotrexate may also result in the inhibition of 5-aminoimidazole-4-carboxamide ribonucleoside (AICAR) transformylase, resulting in the increase of intracellular AICAR concentrations and ultimately in the release of adenosine, a potent endogenous anti-inflammatory agent.

The eventual effects of methotrexate on immunity and inflammation are multiple, but those that appear to be pertinent to the treatment of inflammatory diseases include inhibition of B cell, monocyte/macrophage, and neutrophil functions and reduction of pro-inflammatory cytokine production such as tumor necrosis factor (TNF)-α and interleukin (IL)-1, IL-6, and IL-8.

Dosing and Administration

Methotrexate can be administered orally, subcutaneously, or intramuscularly. Bioavailability after an oral dose is greater than 70%. Parenteral routes are usually used in patients who cannot tolerate or respond inadequately to oral dosing or who are suspected of having malabsorption syndromes. Dosing usually begins at 7.5-10 mg weekly and is increased by 2.5 mg increments every 1 to 2 weeks until clinical improvement is seen, usually after several weeks. The typical effective dose range is 15-25 mg weekly. The maximal weekly dose is generally held to be 25 mg, although higher doses may occasionally be required.

Because methotrexate is cleared through urinary excretion, dose reduction or increased dosing interval is necessary in patients with renal insufficiency. Methotrexate should not be used in patients whose creatinine clearance is less than 60% of normal and in those with end-stage renal disease. In addition, because NSAIDs decrease glomerular filtration and inhibit renal tubular secretion of methotrexate, concomitant use warrants vigilant monitoring.

Table 31-2   Disease-Modifying Anti-Rheumatic Drugs and Fertility, Pregnancy, and Lactation

Medication	FDA Category*	Female Fertility	Male Fertility	Miscarriages	Teratogenicity	Neonate	Breastfeeding
Adalimumab	B	No long-term data	No long-term data	No long-term data	No long-term data	No long-term data	Use with caution
Anakinra	B	No long-term data	No long-term data	No long-term data	No long-term data	No long-term data	Use with caution
Auranofin	C	Probably no effect	Probably no effect	No clear increased risk	No consistent pattern	No known toxicity	Use with caution
Azathioprine	D	Probably no effect	Probably no effect	No clear increased risk	No consistent pattern	No known toxicity	Use with caution
Cyclophos-phamide	D	Ovarian failure, especially over age 30	Oligospermia; azoospermia	Abortifacient	Especially in first trimester	Immuno-suppression	Contra-indicated
Cyclosporine	C	No long-term data	No long-term data	Possible increased risk	No consistent pattern	Possible pre-maturity and low birth rate	Contra-indicated
Etanercept	B	No long-term data	No long-term data	No long-term data	No long-term data	No long-term data	Use with caution
Gold sodium thiomalate	C	Probably no effect	Probably no effect	No clear increased risk	No consistent pattern	No clear toxicity	Use with caution

Hydroxy-chloroquine	C	Probably no effect	Probably no effect	No clear increased risk	No consistent pattern	No clear toxicity	Use with caution
Infliximab	C	No long-term data	No long-term data	No long-term data	No long-term data	No long-term data	Use with caution
Intravenous immunoglobulin	C	Probably no effect	Probably no effect	No clear increased risk	No consistent pattern	No clear toxicity	Use with caution
Leflunomide	X	No long-term data	No long-term data	No long-term data	No long-term data	No long-term data	Contra-indicated
Methotrexate	X	Rare long-term effects	Temporary oligospermia	Abortifacient	Especially in first trimester	Immunosuppression	Contra-indicated
Mycophenolate mofetil	C	No long-term data	No long-term data	No long-term data	No long-term data	No long-term data	Contra-indicated
Sulfasalazine	B; consider D in third trimester	Probably no effect	Temporary oligospermia; abnormal sperm and dysmotility	No clear increased risk	No consistent pattern	Hyperbilirubinemia in preterm neonate	Use with caution

FDA categories for medication use during pregnancy: A = no known risks based on controlled studies; B = no evidence of risk in humans; C = risk cannot be excluded; D = positive evidence of risk, but benefit may outweigh risk; X = contraindicated; benefit does not outweigh risk.

Safety Issues and Adverse Effects

Anorexia, nausea, vomiting, diarrhea, alopecia, and oral sores are the most common adverse effects. Most of these are nuisances and generally resolve with dose reduction or divided dosing. Folic acid 1-5 mg daily or folinic acid 2.5-10 mg weekly (given at least 8 hours after the methotrexate dose) should be routinely administered to prevent many of these minor side effects (4). Rheumatoid nodules, particularly small, painful ones on the digits, may paradoxically appear or increase in number or size after the start of methotrexate therapy, even as the patient shows clinical improvement otherwise.

Hepatotoxicity is an important consideration with methotrexate, and abnormalities in serum liver function and enzyme tests are fairly common (5). However, although irreversible damage such as hepatic fibrosis or cirrhosis can occur, this is a rare complication of methotrexate use in RA, occurring in less than 0.1% of patients. Before considering methotrexate therapy, concomitant risk factors for liver disease, such as significant alcohol use, diabetes mellitus, chronic hepatitis, or morbid obesity, should be sought.

Although rare, bone marrow suppression presenting as leukopenia, anemia, thrombocytopenia, or pancytopenia may occur (6). Significant immunosupresssion leading to infections may occur in certain patients, particularly in those concomitantly treated with corticosteroids. The development of B cell non-Hodgkin's lymphoma has been reported in the setting of methotrexate therapy. Intriguingly, a reversible lymphoma-like lymphoproliferative disorder that resolves with discontinuation of methotrexate has also been described.

Methotrexate may also cause interstitial pulmonary disease, which can occur at any time (7). In some patients, this may occur as an unexplained dry cough. In others, it may be quite fulminant with fever, hypoxia, eosinophilia, and interstitial infiltrates and nodules. Although the incidence of pulmonary toxicity is rare, there is no specific therapy except for the discontinuation of methotrexate, supportive respiratory care, and possibly a short course of corticosteroids. Outcome is variable, but one study has reported a mortality rate as high as 17%.

Although methotrexate has not been associated with permanent ovarian dysfunction, it is an abortifacient and a teratogen, and, accordingly, counseling on contraceptives should be performed before the start of therapy. Methotrexate should be discontinued in women for at least three ovulatory cycles and in men for at least 3 months before attempting conception. Both men and women previously treated for hematological malignancies with high-dose methotrexate have had normal offspring.

Monitoring

Complete blood count, liver function and enzyme tests, renal function, hepatitis B and C serologies, and chest X-ray should be evaluated before methotrexate is initiated.

Serial clinical and laboratory evaluations should be performed at least every 6 weeks and more frequently while the dosage of methotrexate is being increased. Laboratory examination should include CBC and serum biochemistries to assess kidney and liver function (particularly hepatic transaminases and albumin).

Routine baseline and serial liver biopsies are not advocated by the American College of Rheumatology in RA patients considering or taking methotrexate who do not have underlying clinical or biochemical evidence of liver disease (8). Current recommendations are to obtain a liver biopsy if there are serum hepatic transaminase elevations or persistent hypoalbuminemia unrelated to active disease on any three consecutive serial observations or five out of nine evaluations. Evidence of high-grade liver disease requires discontinuation of methotrexate. It must be noted that these recommendations were specifically developed for patients with RA and may not be extended to patients with other illnesses such as psoriatic arthritis or sarcoidosis.

Leflunomide

Clinical Uses

Leflunomide is an oral DMARD approved for treatment of RA. In multiple clinical trials it has been shown effective in reducing signs and symptoms of RA and in retarding radiographic progression of the disease, both as a single agent and in combination with methotrexate. Because leflunomide is a relatively new medication, its experience in other diseases is limited.

Mechanism of Action

Leflunomide is converted into its active metabolite M1, which is thought to inhibit dihydroorotate dehydrogenase, a key enzyme in the de novo synthesis of the pyrimidine ribonucleotide uridine monophosphate (rUMP). In lymphocytes, low intracellular rUMP activates the tumor suppressor P53 protein, which then arrests cell division in the G1 stage of the cell cycle. By stopping lymphocyte cell division, leflunomide inhibits clonal expansion of memory T cells. In theory, reducing memory T cells in the joint may limit the conversion of synoviocytes into more destructive phenotypes and thereby slow joint damage.

Dosing and Administration

Therapy with leflunomide is initiated with a loading dose of 100 mg daily administered orally for 3 days followed by a maintenance dose of 20 mg daily. The maintenance dose can be decreased to 10 mg daily in patients who are intolerant of the higher dose or in patients who develop adverse effects. Dose adjustments should be made in the setting of significant renal insufficiency.

Safety Issues and Adverse Effects

In the phase III clinical trials, the most frequently reported side effects with leflunomide therapy were alopecia, rashes, hypertension, fluid retention, and gastrointestinal complaints (especially diarrhea, which can be quite pronounced) (9). Liver transaminase elevations are also common but generally return to normal upon dose reduction or discontinuation of the drug. However, postmarking surveillance has identified several deaths resulting from liver disease in the context of leflunomide use. Concomitant methotrexate therapy has been implicated as a potential risk factor for increased hepatotoxicity, but a causative association has yet to be firmly established.

Leflunomide is extremely toxic to a developing fetus and has been classified as a class X drug by the Food and Drug Administration. Because of its long half-life, leflunomide should be discontinued for at least 4 months before attempting conception. If complete elimination of leflunomide and M1 from the body is desired because of pregnancy issues or toxicities, oral cholestyramine 8 g three times daily can be administered for 11 days to adsorb and cause fecal excretion of the drug. Serum drug levels can be assessed through the manufacturer or in commercial laboratories; for certainty, two specimens obtained two weeks apart are recommended.

Monitoring

In addition to CBC and serum chemistries with emphasis on liver function and enzymes, hepatitis serologies should be obtained before the start of leflunomide therapy. Serial laboratory evaluations should be performed at least every 6 weeks or more frequently if there is evidence of hematological or liver abnormalities or when leflunomide is used concomitantly with methotrexate.

Azathioprine

Clinical Uses

Azathioprine is a versatile medication, used in a variety of autoimmune and inflammatory diseases diseases, including RA, SLE, myositis, inflammatory bowel diseases, spondyloarthropathies, uveitis, and systemic vasculitides. Other uses include immunosuppression for organ transplantation and the treatment of some malignancies. In the inflammatory disorders, azathioprine is commonly used in moderately severe but non-life-threatening situations, for maintenance therapy after disease control has been achieved with more potent medications, or when more toxic agents such as cyclophosphamide are not desired. In practice, azathioprine has generally occupied a position as a second-line agent.

Mechanism of Action

Azathioprine is a purine analogue that is converted to 6-mercaptopurine (6-MP), which in turn inhibits the de novo synthesis of purine nucleotides. Inhibition of purine synthesis is thought to decrease T and B cell proliferation and function and therefore affects both cellular and humoral immunity. Leukopenia is not necessary for immunosuppression, which is related to decreased circulating lymphocytes, decreased lymphocyte proliferation, inhibition of antibody formation, monocyte production, suppression of natural killer cell activity, and inhibition of cellular and humoral immunity.

Dosing and Administration

The usual maintenance dosage range of azathioprine is 2-3 mg/kg daily administered orally in two divided doses. Therapy is often initiated at lower dosages and then escalated over several weeks to maintenance dosages. Dose reduction is required with hepatic or renal insufficiency.

There are two important drug interactions with azathioprine. One is with allopurinol, which inhibits xanthine oxidase from metabolizing 6-MP. The dosage of azathioprine should be reduced by at least 75% when given concomitantly with allopurinol; this situation is common in the setting of organ transplantation. Similarly, sulfasalazine inhibits thiopurine methyltransferase, another enzyme involved in inactivating 6-MP. The concomitant use of azathioprine and sulfasalazine is associated with a significantly increased risk of leukopenia. Although no formal recommendations for dose reductions have been established, it is generally advisable to monitor the CBC closely when using this combination of medications.

Safety Issues and Adverse Effects

Nausea is common upon initiation of therapy but can be avoided with gradual dose escalation. Marrow suppression and immunosuppression are important potential adverse effects. Elevations in hepatic enzymes can occur but resolve with dose reduction and are rarely clinically relevant.

In patients with organ transplants, azathioprine has been associated with lymphoid and hematological malignancies, but oncogenicity has not been considered to be increased in the setting of the rheumatological diseases.

Studies of renal allograft recipients who have received azathioprine during pregnancy have not demonstrated an increase in birth defects (10), and azathioprine has been considered to be safe during pregnancy by many clinicians even though the medication is designated a class D drug.

As with any medication, however, the decision regarding whether it should be used during pregnancy should be made after weighing all of the potential risks and benefits.

Monitoring

Rapid falls in leukocyte counts and platelet counts can be seen, and CBC should be followed weekly for several weeks at the outset of azathioprine therapy or with dose escalations, then monthly after a maintenance dosage has been established.

Mycophenolate Mofetil

Clinical Uses

Mycophenolate mofetil is a recent addition to the rheumatological formulary but has had extensive use in organ transplantation medicine (11). Clinical settings in which mycophenolate mofetil has found use are similar to those for azathioprine. In particular, recent increased attention has been given to its use in the treatment of lupus nephritis. Small studies in the treatment of psoriasis, autoimmune hemolytic anemia, and vasculitis have also been published.

Mechanism of Action

Mycophenolate mofetil is hydrolyzed to mycophenolic acid, which is a reversible inhibitor of inosine monophosphate dehydrogenase, a critical enzyme in de novo purine synthesis. Mycophenolate mofetil is a potent inhibitor of T and B cell proliferation and functions.

Dosing and Administration

Mycophenolate mofetil is administered orally. Initial dosing is 250-500 mg twice daily, which can be escalated as clinically indicated to up to 1000 mg twice daily. Most of the medication and its metabolites are excreted renally, and so dose adjustment is required in the setting of renal insufficiency.

Safety Issues and Adverse Effects

Gastrointestinal intolerances, including mucosal ulcerations, nausea, vomiting, and diarrhea, are the most common adverse effects. Marrow suppression can be profound, and leukopenia and immunosuppression are important complications. Infections, especially those by opportunistic organisms, require early detection and treatment. Although not seen so far in the treatment of rheumatological disorders, there may be an increased incidence of lymphoproliferative and non-melanomatous cutaneous malignancies.

Monitoring

CBC should be followed weekly for several weeks at the outset of mycophenolate mofetil therapy and with dose escalations. Thereafter, monthly CBC should be obtained to monitor for myelosuppression.

Cyclophosphamide

Clinical Uses

Cyclophosphamide is the most potent immunosuppressive agent in common use in rheumatology (12). It is generally reserved for the most severe complications of rheumatic diseases such as glomerulonephritis, severe thrombocytopenia, or central nervous system involvement in SLE; systemic vasculitides (e.g., Wegener's granulomatosis, Churg-Strauss syndrome) and vasculitic complications of other primary illnesses such as SLE or RA; or interstitial lung disease in inflammatory myositis or diffuse scleroderma. Use in RA in the absence of vasculitis has largely been supplanted by less toxic medications with equal or better efficacy.

Mechanism of Action

Cyclophosphamide is metabolized into its active metabolite phosphoramide mustard, which alkylates and crosslinks DNA, resulting in breaks of DNA, decreased DNA synthesis, and cell death. Cyclophosphamide broadly affects immune cells throughout their cell cycle. T and B lymphocyte activation and proliferation are suppressed, resulting in both decreased cell-mediated immunity and antibody production.

Dosing and Administration

Cyclophosphamide is available as an oral preparation or as an intravenous infusion. Intravenous cyclophosphamide is a standard intervention for diffuse proliferative lupus nephritis. A typical regimen is monthly intravenous cyclophosphamide 0.5-1.0 g/m^2 for 6 to 12 months, followed by dosing every 3 months until remission is achieved and maintained for at least 1 year. The dosage should be adjusted to achieve a leukocyte count of 2500-$3000/mm^3$ measured 10 to 14 days after infusions; the absolute neutrophil count should be kept above $1500/mm^3$. Patients should be hydrated with 1-2 L of intravenous fluid before cyclophosphamide infusions to achieve a urine specific gravity of less than 1.020 and should receive additional intravenous hydration afterwards. Mercaptoethane sulfonate (mesna) can be given before intravenous cyclophosphamide to prevent bladder toxicity.

Intravenous cyclophosphamide is generally well-tolerated and associated with lower risks for adverse effects such as leukopenia and bladder toxicities than oral cyclophosphamide. Unfortunately, however, systemic vasculitides often do not respond as well to intravenous cyclophosphamide as to oral regimens. Oral cyclophosphamide is dosed at 2 mg/kg/d, again aiming for a leukocyte count between 2500-3000/mm^3. Patients receiving oral cyclophosphamide should be encouraged to maintain ample fluid intake to ensure adequate urine output and clearance of the drug.

Although the half-life of cyclophosphamide is increased in patients with hepatic insufficiency, its clinical toxicity is not increased, and no dose adjustment for liver disease is needed. Cyclophosphamide and its metabolites are cleared through renal excretion, but only mild dose adjustments are needed for renal dysfunction (25% dose reduction for creatinine clearance 25-50 cc/min and 50% reduction for creatinine clearance <25 cc/min). Cyclophosphamide is removed by hemodialysis, and, accordingly, doses should be given post-dialysis in patients with end-stage renal disease.

Safety Issues and Adverse Effects

Adverse effects range from mild to severe and potentially life threatening. Anorexia, nausea, weight loss, alopecia, and fatigue are commonly reported. Metabolic effects include hyponatremia, which can occasionally be severe. Marrow suppression and immunosuppression can be profound, especially during the early phases of therapy when concomitant high-dose corticosteroid therapy is usually employed. Opportunistic infections such as *Pneumocystis carinii* pneumonia and herpes zoster are notably common. Prophylactic antibiotics against *Pneumocystis* have been advocated by many clinicians, and patients with recurrent herpes zoster may require chronic antiviral therapy (13).

There are important fertility and pregnancy issues associated with the use of cyclophosphamide. Amenorrhea, ovarian failure, and azoospermia are genuine complications of therapy, and cryopreservation of sperm, unfertilized ova, ova fertilized in vitro, or ovarian tissue before treatment is appropriate in many patients (14,15). Patients receiving cyclophosphamide should be counseled to practice effective contraception. Twenty-five percent of a maternal dose crosses the placenta, and congenital abnormalities can occur, especially with exposure in the first trimester. Fortunately, studies have noted that patients who have undergone cancer treatment with cyclophosphamide in childhood have had no increase in genetic abnormalities in their offspring.

Exposure of the bladder to acrolein, a metabolite of cyclophosphamide, is responsible for the hemorrhagic cystitis and bladder cancer associated with cyclophosphamide use (16). These complications are more common with oral administration. In addition, cigarette smoking may act synergistically to increase the risk of bladder cancer. Cyclophosphamide is also associated with an increased risk for myelodysplastic syndrome, leukemia, and lymphoma (16).

Monitoring

CBC should be monitored every 2 to 3 weeks initially when starting oral cyclophosphamide and then monthly after a stable dose has been established. Urinalyses should also be obtained frequently to ensure early detection of microscopic hematuria.

With intravenous therapy, CBC, serum electrolytes, and urinalysis with specific gravity should be evaluated immediately before infusions and again 10 to 14 days afterwards to assess the leukocyte count nadir and renal function in order to adjust dosing if necessary.

Sulfasalazine

Clinical Uses

Sulfasalazine is used as monotherapy in mild-to-moderate RA or as part of a combination regimen in moderate-to-severe disease and has been shown to retard the progression of erosions. It is less widely prescribed in the United States than in Europe. Many clinicians also favor its use in the treatment of the seronegative spondyloarthropathies and in cases of inflammatory arthritis where differentiation between RA and spondyloarthropathy is unclear.

Mechanism of Action

Sulfasalazine is thought to be a weak inhibitor of folate metabolism, but unlike methotrexate, folinic acid does not reverse anti-proliferative effects, and therefore sulfasalazine probably acts by a separate mechanism. It suppresses inflammatory cell functions like superoxide generation and chemotaxis by neutrophils as well as granulocyte protease activity. It has also been demonstrated to be a potent scavenger of reactive oxygen radicals. In addition, sulfasalazine has immunomodulatory effects on T cells (reduced IL-2 and interferon-γ production), B cells (decreased immunoglobulin and rheumatoid factor synthesis), and monocytes (inhibition of IL-1 and TNF-α expression).

Dosing and Administration

Oral sulfasalazine therapy is started at 500 mg twice daily and then escalated over several weeks to 2-3 g/d in divided doses as dictated by clinical response and tolerability. Sulfasalazine is available as enteric-coated tablets to reduce gastrointestinal intolerance.

Safety Issues and Adverse Effects

Discontinuation rates of over 20% for sulfasalazine are largely due to significant upper gastrointestinal intolerance (e.g., anorexia, nausea, dyspepsia). Skin rashes occur in up to 5% of patients and are usually pruritic and maculopapular but occasionally urticarial. Although fetal abnormalities and prenatal morbidity or mortality have not been reported in the offspring of men and women taking sulfasalazine at the time of conception or during pregnancy, discontinuation of the drug is still preferable if possible. In men, sulfasalazine can cause reversible oligospermia. Sulfasalazine is a FDA category B drug during pregnancy but has been associated with hyperbilirubinemia in the neonate when administered in the third trimester.

Leukopenia is an important but uncommon (<3%) reversible adverse effect usually occurring within the first few months of therapy. Hemolytic anemia has been reported in patients taking higher doses of sulfasalazine for the treatment of inflammatory bowel diseases and in individuals with glucose-6-phosphate dehydrogenase (G6PD) deficiency. Sulfasalazine is contraindicated in patients with porphyria.

Monitoring

Some clinicians advocate assessing for G6PD deficiency before the start of sulfasalazine therapy. CBC and liver function and enzymes should be monitored weekly for one month and every four to six weeks thereafter, more frequently during dose escalations.

Antimalarial Agents: Hydroxychloroquine, Chloroquine, and Quinicrine

Clinical Uses

Antimalarial drugs are used for mild RA, non-visceral involvement in SLE (e.g., constitutional symptoms, skin disease, arthritis, serositis), and other mild manifestations of inflammatory diseases such as skin involvement in sarcoidosis. They are the least potent of the DMARDs and have not yet been demonstrated to limit the development of joint erosions in RA.

Due to its good tolerability and overall safety profile, hydroxychloroquine is the most commonly prescribed agent in this class of medications for the treatment of rheumatic diseases and is frequently used in combination with other DMARDs. Chloroquine and quinicrine are other options but are much less commonly used and are primarily prescribed for the treatment of mild SLE.

Mechanism of Action

The exact mechanism of action of antimalarial drugs is not known. They are known to affect lysosomal pH, protease activity, and membrane functions and may prevent antigen-presenting cells from processing pathogenic antigens.

Dosing and Administration

Hydroxychloroquine therapy is generally initiated at 400 mg daily, either as a single dose or as 200 mg twice daily. With disease control, the dose can be lowered to 200 mg daily. The usual daily dose of chloroquine is 150 mg, and the usual daily dose of quinicrine is 100 mg. These drugs should not be given in the setting of significant ophthalmological, hepatic, or renal disease.

Safety Issues and Adverse Effects

Discontinuation rates due to toxicities for antimalarial agents are generally less than 10% in clinical trials. The most frequently reported adverse effects are non-specific gastrointestinal complaints such as dyspepsia, nausea, and abdominal cramps. These often can be minimized by starting therapy at lower dosages or by giving the medication with meals or at bedtime. Rash is the most common adverse event resulting in discontinuation of the medication. Hemolytic anemia may rarely occur, particularly in patients with G6PD deficiency.

Ocular toxicity is the most clinically important adverse effect associated with antimalarial agents and is due to drug deposition on the retina. When detected early, the retinopathy is reversible with cessation of therapy, and so regular ophthalmological slit-lamp examinations are mandatory. Hydroxychloroquine is less apt to cause ophthalmological problems than the other agents. Overall, the incidence of retinal toxicity is extremely low and most commonly occurs in the setting of renal or hepatic insufficiency, when given in higher than recommended dosing, and in the elderly (17). Less frequent complications include ototoxicity, peripheral neuropathy, and myopathy, but these are more common with prolonged use. Chronic quinacrine therapy is notable for a reversible yellow skin discoloration.

Neither female nor male fertility appears to be affected by antimalarial agents. Although hydroxychloroquine is classified as a category C drug, several recent studies have not shown any adverse effects on fetal development and pregnancy (18). In fact, some clinicians believe that control of the underlying disease (notably SLE) with antimalarial agents may improve obstetrical outcomes for both mother and infant.

Monitoring

A baseline ophthalmological examination and serial examinations every 6 to 12 months is mandatory. CBC should be obtained every 4 to 6 months.

Cyclosporine

Clinical Uses

Approved indications for the use of cyclosporine include RA, organ transplantation, and psoriasis, but off-label use for a variety of autoimmune and systemic inflammatory diseases such as psoriatic arthritis, vasculitis, Behçet's disease, and membranous nephropathy is common. In the treatment of RA, cyclosporine has been shown to retard the evolution of erosions and can be used alone or in conjunction with other DMARDs, particularly methotrexate. However, despite proven effectiveness, significant side effects have limited its usefulness in the rheumatic diseases.

Mechanism of Action

Cyclosporine exerts its therapeutic effects largely by inhibiting early steps in T cell activation and proliferation. Binding of cyclosporine to intracellular proteins known as immunophilins results in the failure to transcribe early genes involved in T cell activation including many that encode pro-inflammatory cytokines and lymphokines such as tumor necrosis factor-α and interleukin-2. Because the site of action of cyclosporine occurs just distal to cell membrane receptor/ligand interaction, a broad range of downstream effects are affected, resulting in profound immunosuppression.

Dosing and Administration

For the treatment of rheumatoid arthritis, cyclosporine is administered orally and should be started at 2.5 mg/kg/d and may be increased slowly by 0.5 mg/kg/d at 4 to 8 weekly intervals to the maximum dose of 5.0 mg/kg/d. Although monitoring blood levels of cyclosporine is available, such monitoring has generally not been helpful in the management of rheumatic diseases.

Cyclosporine is poorly absorbed from the gut with a bioavailability of about 30%. Metabolism and elimination is controlled by two mechanisms that account for significant drug interactions: the drug efflux transporter P-glycoprotein (P-gp) clears cyclosporine through the gastrointestinal tract, the liver, and the kidneys, while the CYP3A cytochrome enzyme system metabolizes the drug. Inhibitors of P-gp such as diltiazem and verapamil and inhibitors of the CYP3A system such as grapefruit juice, macrolide antibiotics (erythromycin and clarithromycin), and azole antifungal drugs (fluconazole, itraconazole, and ketoconazole) increase serum cyclosporine concentrations. Conversely, inducers of P-gp such as rifampin and activators of the CYP3A system such as phenytoin, carbamazepine, and phenobarbital can lower levels of cyclosporine.

Safety Issues and Adverse Effects

Treatment with cyclosporine is associated with a significant risk of hypertension and renal dysfunction (19). Increase in blood pressure is the most common adverse effect of cyclosporine therapy, occurring in as many as one-third of patients. Approximately 20% of patients demonstrate a rise in serum creatinine, and of these only 50% will revert to their baseline levels when the dosage of cyclosporine is reduced. In one 12-month study, a 30% or greater rise in serum creatinine occurred in more than 50% of patients.

The immunosuppressive effects of cyclosporine are significant, and constant vigilance for infectious complications is required. Other side effects include gastrointestinal intolerance, hirsuitism, headaches, paresthesias, gingival hyperplasia, liver enzyme elevations, hyperkalemia, hyperuricemia, hypercholesterolemia, and hypomagnesemia.

Cyclosporine is a category C medication. Its effects on male and female infertility are not known, and no consistent effects on pregnancy outcomes have been documented (10). Breastfeeding is contraindicated in women taking the drug.

Monitoring

Two separate baseline blood pressure readings and serum creatinine levels should be assessed before the start of therapy. Guidelines suggest careful biweekly monitoring of both blood pressure and serum creatinine during the initial 3 months of treatment and during dose escalations. Dose reductions of 25% to 50% should be made for persistent hypertension or a 30% rise in the serum creatinine.

Gold Salts

Clinical Uses

Gold salts are among some of the older DMARDs. They can be administered orally or intramuscularly for the treatment of RA, juvenile chronic arthritis, and psoriatic arthritis. They can delay the evolution of joint erosions, but with the advent of many newer and generally more effective DMARDs, the use of gold salts has waned. However, they remain an important therapeutic option for select patients unresponsive to or intolerant of other DMARDs.

Mechanism of Action

In the laboratory, gold salts can be shown to affect many arms of the immune and inflammatory systems, including inhibition of T and B lymphocyte activation, monocyte and macrophage functions, neutrophil activities, cytokine production, angiogenesis, and the complement system. However, which of these properties are clinically relevant is not known.

Dosing and Administration

Only gold sodium thiomalate is currently available for intramuscular injections. Typically, a 10 mg test dose is given, and if tolerated, a 25 mg dose is administered a week later. Subsequently, a maintenance weekly 50 mg dose is administered until a therapeutic response is observed. This typically takes at least 2 months and as many as 6 months, at which time the medication should be discontinued if there is no effect, or the interval between injections increased to every 2 weeks if there is benefit. The interval can be adjusted according to the clinical response; doses every 4 to 6 weeks may be possible in the best scenarios.

Oral gold (auranofin) is initiated at 3 mg daily and increased to 9 mg daily as dictated by the clinical picture.

Safety Issues and Adverse Effects

Dermatitis and stomatitis are the most common side effects associated with intramuscular gold therapy; they resolve with discontinuation of the medication (20). Except in the very rare cases of exfoliative dermatitis, therapy at a reduced dose can be reinitiated. In up to 2% of patients, hematological abnormalities (thrombocytopenia, anemia, leukopenia, neutropenia, or rarely pancytopenia/aplastic anemia) can occur idiosyncratically (21), and gold should not be restarted in these cases. The other relatively common complication is proteinuria (22). Proteinuria of greater than 500 mg/d should prompt discontinuation of the drug, which can be reinstituted at a lower dose when the urinalysis normalizes. Rare nitritoid reactions due to the thiomalate component, including sweating, flushing, dizziness, nausea, and dyspnea, can be very uncomfortable and alarming to the patient and may be cause to consider alternative therapies.

The mucocutaneous, hematological, and renal toxicities are much less common with auranofin. However, oral gold has a higher incidence of gastrointestinal intolerances that include general abdominal discomfort and diarrhea.

Monitoring

Complete blood counts and urinalyses should be examined frequently, even as often as before every injection, with intramuscular gold therapy. Less frequent monitoring (every 4 to 6 weeks) is adequate with auranofin.

Tumor Necrosis Factor-α Antagonists: Etanercept, Infliximab, and Adalimumab

Clinical Uses

Etanercept, infliximab, and adalimumab are genetically engineered antagonists of tumor necrosis factor (TNF)-α and are commonly known as biological

DMARDs. The FDA has formally approved etanercept for the treatment of RA, psoriatic arthritis, and juvenile chronic arthritis, and infliximab has been approved for combination therapy with methotrexate in the treatment of RA and for the management of Crohn's disease. Adalimumab is the most recently approved DMARD for the treatment of RA.

In practice, these agents may be used as monotherapy or in combination with other DMARDs, and they do retard the progression of joint erosions in RA. Because of their overall effectiveness and safety, rheumatologists are increasingly using these agents successfully for the off-label treatment of a myriad of other inflammatory conditions, including myositis, seronegative spondyloathropathies, sarcoidosis, and uveitis (23).

Etanercept is a fusion protein created by the linkage of the ligand-binding region of the human p75 TNF-α receptor to the Fc portion of a human immunoglobulin G1 molecule. It has a longer biological half-life (72-96 hours) than the parental native p75 TNF-α receptor (half-life 7-8 hours), allowing for intermittent subcutaneous dosing. Infliximab is a chimeric monoclonal antibody composed of the Fc region of human IgG1κ coupled to the antigen-binding region of a high-affinity murine anti-human TNF-α antibody. Adalimumab (D2E7) is a fully humanized monoclonal antibody against human TNF-α.

Mechanism of Action

Although TNF-α was first described as a serum factor with the ability to cause necrosis of tumors, it has since been extensively characterized as a pleiotropic pro-inflammatory and immunomodulatory cytokine. Monocytes and macrophages are the major source of TNF-α. Acting synergistically with interleukin (IL)-1, TNF-α stimulates synovial fibroblasts in the rheumatoid joint to secrete matrix-degrading proteases, prostanoids, and other pro-inflammatory cytokines and induces increased expression of adhesion molecules on vascular endothelium. These events are responsible for the influx of neutrophils into the joint, the recruitment of lymphocytes into the subsynovial space, and the production of rheumatoid factor, all of which contribute to the chronic inflammatory response. Production of prostanoids and matrix metalloproteinases mediate destruction of cartilage as well as invasion of the rheumatoid pannus into subchondral bone resulting in irreversible damage to the joint. TNF-α and IL-1 also mediate many of the systemic constitutional symptoms of RA, like fatigue, anorexia, and weight loss.

The clinical benefits of etanercept, infliximab, and adalimumab are attributed to their ability to block the pro-inflammatory effects of TNF-α, resulting in not only retardation of local tissue destruction but also alleviation of systemic symptoms such as fatigue and cachexia.

Dosing and Administration

Etanercept 25 mg is administered subcutaneously twice weekly or 50 mg once weekly. For the treatment of RA, infliximab is initially administered intravenously over 2 hours at 3 mg/kg, with subsequent similar dosing 2 and 6 weeks later. Thereafter, maintenance infusions are given every 8 weeks. However, it has been the experience of many clinicians that the dosage may require increasing to as much as 10 mg/kg; alternatively, the maintenance interval may be decreased to as short as 4 weeks. The recommended dose of adalimumab is a 40 mg subcutaneous injection every 2 weeks. Some patients may experience further benefit with weekly injections.

Safety Issues and Adverse Effects

Injection site reactions, typically consisting of urticarial lesions, occur in up to 40% of patients treated with etanercept and usually occur early in the course of therapy. However, they are generally self-limited and resolve with repeated dosing. Injection site reactions also occur with adalimumab but less frequently than with etanercept. Infusion reactions occur in up to 20% of patients receiving infliximab and may include headache, nausea, back pain, palpitations, or low-grade fever. Slowing the rate of infusion and pretreatment with acetaminophen or antihistamines can prevent most of these reactions.

Infections are the most worrisome complication of anti-TNF-α therapies (24). TNF-α is an important factor in defense against, and containment of, infections. Of particular interest, TNF-α is essential in the formation of granulomas to wall off mycobacterial and fungal organisms. Although in clinical trials treatment with TNF-α blockers did not result in increased risks for serious infections when compared with placebo or methotrexate, postmarketing surveillance have revealed rare cases of severe fungal infections, *Pneumocystis carinii* pneumonia, listeriosis, and herpes zoster in the setting of anti-TNF-α therapies. In addition, more than 100 cases of tuberculosis in patients receiving infliximab and 17 cases in patients receiving etanercept have been reported. In those cases of tuberculosis associated with infliximab therapy, infections typically occurred within the first three infusions and were most likely to be reactivation of past infections. In clinical trials, adalimumab has also been associated with tuberculosis, frequently disseminated or extrapulmonary. The FDA has placed "Black Box" warnings for infliximab and adalimumab, requiring that all patients be prescreened with a tuberculin skin test, and the Centers for Disease Control has recommended treatment with isoniazid if the tuberculin test is positive (regardless of whether the patient has ever received bacillus Calmette-Guérin vaccination) before initiation of therapy. A chest X-ray is also recommended before treatment. It is probably prudent to follow these recommendations for all anti-TNF-α agents (25).

One intriguing, apparently paradoxical, consequence of anti-TNF-α therapy is the development of autoimmune phenomena. Patients receiving etanercept, infliximab, or adalimumab may develop anti-nuclear or anti-double stranded (ds) DNA antibodies. Although most of these patients are asymptomatic, a few develop a reversible mild SLE-like illness (26). These autoimmune effects may be related to the inhibition of immunoregulatory activities of TNF-α by these agents on lymphocytes, resulting in the loss of immune tolerance. A possibly related observation is the finding that the use of TNF-α antagonists in the treatment of multiple sclerosis (MS) has been associated with more frequent flares and general worsening of disease. Moreover, rare de novo cases of demyelinating disease (characterized by confusion, weakness, paresthesias, or optic neuritis) associated with MRI findings characteristic of MS and oligoclonal immunoglobulins on cerebrospinal fluid analysis have been reported in the context of anti-TNF-α therapy.

A conspicuous uncertainty that remains with the use of TNF-α antagonists is their effect on immune surveillance for malignancies. Although cases of lymphoma have been reported in the context of anti-TNF-α therapy, no definitively increased risk for the development of malignancies over that linked to RA itself has been observed. However, these potential risks are very legitimate concerns. At present, most clinicians will not recommend anti-TNF-α therapy in patients with concurrent or recently treated malignancies. Lastly, there are suggestive data that TNF inhibitors induce or exacerbate heart failure in some patients.

Monitoring

Prevention and early identification of infections are the most important aspects of long-term monitoring for complications in patients receiving anti-TNF-α therapies. As noted above, a tuberculin skin test and a chest X-ray should be done before the start of therapy to identify patients with past exposure to *Mycobacterium tuberculosis.* In clinical trials, several fatalities due to serious bacterial infections occurred after receiving TNF-α antagonists. Although the total number of deaths did not exceed that which would be expected in the study population, the deaths seemed to cluster in those patients with open draining wounds or other active infections. Therefore, vigilance for new or ongoing infections is essential, and discontinuation of therapy should be strongly considered when the patient is at increased risk for infection (e.g., perioperatively) or when severe infections are identified.

Cytopenias, including aplastic anemia, have been rarely reported in post-marketing surveillance, and complete blood counts are recommended at the outset of therapy and then every 2 to 3 months thereafter. Risks for the development of absolute neutropenia and severe infections are increased with concomitant anti-interleukin-1 therapy with anakinra.

Anakinra

Clinical Uses

Anakinra is a biological DMARD that specifically antagonizes interleukin (IL)-1. It can be given as a single agent for the treatment of RA but is commonly used in combination with methotrexate. Experience with anakinra in conditions other than RA is limited.

Mechanism of Action

IL-1β is produced by synovial fibroblasts and macrophages in the rheumatoid joint and can transform resting synovial cells to an activated phenotype. This results in the local increased production of metalloproteinases and other degradative enzymes and various pro-inflammatory chemokines. IL-1β is thought to be the most potent cytokine mediating cartilage and bone destruction in RA.

IL-1 receptor antagonist (IL-1Ra) is a structural homologue of IL-1β and is a naturally occurring competitive inhibitor of IL-1β binding to the IL-1 type 1 receptor. Anakinra is a recombinant form of IL-1Ra, which differs from the native protein by a single methionine residue at its amino terminus.

Dosing and Administration

The recommended dose for anakinra is 100 mg/d given by subcutaneous injection.

Safety Issues and Adverse Effects

Injection site reactions are the most common adverse effect associated with anakinra therapy, occurring in almost three-quarters of patients. Although most reactions are mild, they accounted for the majority of withdrawals from therapeutic trials. They may consist of erythema, ecchymosis, inflammation, or pain and typically last 1 to 2 weeks. Most injection site reactions occurred within the first month of therapy, and most patients who developed them did not continue to have them with subsequent continued treatment.

When compared with individuals receiving placebo in clinical trials, there was a 3-fold to 5-fold increase in serious bacterial infections in anakinra-treated groups (27,28). Asthma may be a co-morbid risk factor for serious infection; patients with asthma who received anakinra were five times more likely to develop a serious infection than anakinra-treated patients without asthma.

In clinical trials, up to 8% of patients receiving anakinra had significant reductions in the absolute neutrophil count (ANC) compared with 2% of patients receiving placebo, with 0.3% becoming absolutely neutropenic (ANC <1000/mm^3) in treatment groups. The clinical significance of mild neutropenia remains to be determined.

Concomitant use of anakinra and etanercept increases the risk of absolute neutropenia and also markedly increases the risk of serious infections. Such use should be considered only in exceptional circumstances and then extremely cautiously.

Thus far, the limited experience with anakinra has not demonstrated an increase in the frequency of mycobacterial, fungal, viral, or unusual opportunistic infections.

Monitoring

As with anti-TNF-α agents, anakinra therapy requires prevention of and vigilance for infectious complications. Because of the risk for neutropenia, current guidelines recommend monthly monitoring of the complete blood count for 3 months and then quarterly thereafter.

Intravenous Immunoglobulin

Clinical Uses

Intravenous immunoglobulin (IVIg) preparations are highly purified pooled polyvalent IgG from thousands of human volunteers that are increasingly being used for the treatment of a variety of autoimmune and inflammatory diseases (29). Conditions in which IVIg has been considered first-line or early adjunctive therapy include immune thrombocytopenia purpura (ITP), autoimmune hemolytic anemia, Kawasaki's disease, inflammatory myositis, myasthenia gravis, Guillain-Barré syndrome, inflammatory demyelinating polyneuropathy, and recurrent miscarriages in the anti-phospholipid syndrome (APS). IVIg is also occasionally used as a non-immunosuppressive approach to the treatment of systemic vasculitides.

Mechanism of Action

Many mechanisms of action have been proposed for the effectiveness of IVIg in the treatment of autoimmune and inflammatory diseases and likely vary from condition to condition. Blockade of immunoglobulin receptors by the Fc fragment of IVIg is probably responsible for its rapid clinical benefit in the treatment of ITP and Guillain-Barré syndrome. In other disorders in which the effects of IVIg occur over the long-term, immunoglobulins with specificity against pathogenic autoantibodies have been implicated in the down-regulation of autoreactive T and B cell activity.

Dosing and Administration

A variety of dosing schemes for IVIg have been employed for the treatment of autoimmune and inflammatory disorders. In general, dosages on the order of 2 g/kg in single or divided doses have been used. For example, a standard protocol for the treatment of ITP is 1 g/kg daily for 2 days, whereas Kawasaki's disease, myositis, Guillain-Barré syndrome, myasthenia gravis, and miscarriage prevention in APS are commonly treated with 0.4 mg/kg daily for 5 days. Courses of IVIg are typically repeated on a monthly basis as necessary.

Safety Issues and Adverse Effects

Minor early adverse effects, occurring within 1 hour of infusion, can include hypotension, flushing, headache, chest or back discomfort, fevers, chills, diaphoresis, or nausea. These reactions occur in as many as 15% of patients, are generally related to the rate of infusion, and respond to a decrease in flow rate. Premedication with acetaminophen and diphenhydramine may prevent some of these early effects. On rare occasions, anaphylaxis can occur in patients with complete IgA deficiency and circulating anti-IgA antibodies, which can react with IgA molecules found in the IVIg.

Delayed adverse effects that can occur after 24 hours post-infusion include serum sickness, aseptic meningitis, renal failure, hemolytic anemia, and hypercoagulability. Pulmonary edema may be an early or late complication and typically occurs in patients with pre-existing cardiomyopathy or cardiopulmonary disease.

Monitoring

Absolute deficiencies in IgA may predispose to anaphylaxis because of pre-existing anti-IgA antibodies and should be assessed before therapy. In patients with IgA deficiencies, immunoglobulin preparations that have depleted of IgA have been used safely (30). A thorough cardiopulmonary examination should be performed before infusions, and vital signs should be monitored every 30 minutes during treatment.

Fertility, Pregnancy, and Nursing Issues

Issues around family planning often arise in the context of DMARD use because many rheumatic illnesses, notably RA and SLE, commonly affect young women. Data regarding the effects of DMARDs on fertility and their safety during pregnancy and breastfeeding are variable and often incomplete (see Table 31-2) (31,32).

In general, it is fair to hold that, if possible, any medication should be discontinued before conception and avoided through pregnancy (particularly in the first trimester when the risk of teratogenicity is greatest) and during breastfeeding. For category X drugs such as methotrexate and leflunomide, it is absolutely necessary that patients be counseled to practice effective contraceptive techniques and to discuss with their physicians well in advance when they consider having children in order to make appropriate adjustments to their medical regimen. Notably, in the case of leflunomide, discontinuation of the medication for at least 4 months or elimination of the drug using cholestyramine is necessary before attempts at conception.

However, it is equally important to appreciate that maintaining disease control also contributes significantly to the outcome of pregnancy and in many cases outweighs potential obstetrical risks. For example, there are substantial data to suggest that, although hydroxychloroquine is classified as a category C drug, discontinuation of the drug in SLE during gestation can result in disease exacerbations, potentially affecting the pregnancy adversely (18). Similarly, many clinicians regard cyclosporine (category C) and azathioprine (category D) as reasonably acceptable agents to use during pregnancy in select patients who are at high risk for exacerbations and significant morbidities due to their systemic rheumatic diseases.

Cyclophosphamide (category D) is notable for its adverse effects on both female and male fertility, in addition to its potential abortifacient and teratogenic properties. One viable option for patients considering cyclophosphamide therapy is cryopreservation of sperm, unfertilized ova, ova fertilized in vitro, or ovarian tissue in order to leave open the possibility of future attempts at conception.

REFERENCES

1. **Case JP.** Old and new drugs used in rheumatoid arthritis: a historical perspective. Part 1: the older drugs. Am J Ther. 2001a;8:123-43.

2. **Case JP.** Old and new drugs used in rheumatoid arthritis: a historical perspective. Part 2: the newer drugs and drug strategies. Am J Ther. 2001b;8:163-79.

3. **van Everdingen AA, Jacobs JWG, Siewertsz van Reesema DR, Bijlsma JWJ.** Low-dose prednisone therapy for patients with early active rheumatoid arthritis: clinical efficacy, disease-modifying properties, and side effects: a randomized, double-blind, placebo-controlled clinical trial. Ann Intern Med. 2002;136:1-12.

4. **van Ede AE, Laan RF, Rood MJ, et al.** Effect of folic or folinic acid supplementation on the toxicity and efficacy of methotrexate in rheumatoid arthritis: a forty-eight week, multicenter, randomized, double-blind, placebo-controlled study. Arthritis Rheum. 2001;44:1515-24.

5. **West S.** Methotrexate hepatotoxicity. Rheum Dis Clinic North Am. 1997;23:883-915.

6. **Gutierrez-Urena S, Molina JF, Garcia CO, et al.** Pancytopenia secondary to methotrexate therapy in rheumatoid arthritis. Arthritis Rheum. 1996;39:272-6.

7. **Alarcon GS, Kremer JM, Macaluso M, et al.** Risk factors for methotrexate-induced lung injury in patients with rheumatoid arthritis: a multicenter, case-control study. Ann Intern Med. 1997;127:356-64.

8. **Kremer JM, Alarcon GS, Lightfoot RW Jr, et al.** Methotrexate for rheumatoid arthritis: suggested guidelines for monitoring liver toxicity. American College of Rheumatology. Arthritis Rheum. 1994;37:316-28.

9. **Cohen S, Cannon GW, Schiff M, et al.** Two-year, blinded, randomized, controlled trial of treatment of active rheumatoid arthritis with leflunomide compared with methotrexate. Arthritis Rheum. 2001;44:1984-92.

10. **Armenti VT, Radomski JS, Moritz MJ, et al.** Report from the National Transplantation Pregnancy Registry (NTPR): outcomes of pregnancy after transplantation. Clin Transpl. 2002;121-30.

11. **Furst DE.** Leflunomide, mycophenolic acid and matrix metalloproteinase inhibitors. Rheumatology. 1999;38(Suppl):14-8.

12. **Singer NG, McCune WJ.** Update on immunosuppressive therapy. Curr Opin Rheumatol. 1998;10:169-73.

13. **Singer NG, McCune WJ.** Prevention of infectious complications in rheumatic disease patients: immunization, *Pneumocystis carinii* prophylaxis, and screening for latent infections. Curr Opin Rheumatol. 1999; 11:173-8.

14. **Boumpas DT, Austin HA 3rd, Vaughan EM, et al.** Risk for sustained amenorrhea in patients with systemic lupus erythematosus receiving intermittent pulse cyclophosphamide therapy. Ann Intern Med. 1993;119:366-9.

15. **Masala A, Faedda R, Alagna S, et al.** Use of testosterone to prevent cyclophosphamide-induced azoospermia. Ann Intern Med. 1997;126:292-5.

16. **Radis CD, Kahl LE, Baker GL, et al.** Effects of cyclophosphamide on the development of malignancy and on long-term survival of patients with rheumatoid arthritis: a 20-year followup study. Arthritis Rheum. 1995;38:1120-7.

17. **Levy GD, Munz SJ, Paschal J, et al.** Incidence of hydroxychloroquine retinopathy in 1207 patients in a large multicenter outpatient practice. Arthritis Rheum. 1997;40: 1482-6.

18. **Costedoat-Chalumeau N, Amoura Z, Duhaut P, et al.** Safety of hydroxychloroquine in pregnant patients with connective tissue diseases: a study of 133 cases compared with a control group. Arthritis Rheum. 2003;48:3207-11.

19. **Kvein TK, Zeidler HK, Hannonen P, et al.** Long term efficacy and safety of cyclosporin versus parenteral gold in early rheumatoid arthritis: a three year study of radiographic progression, renal function, and arterial hypertension. Ann Rheum Dis. 2002; 61:511-6.

20. **van Gestel A, Koopman R, Wijnands M, et al.** Mucocutaneous reactions to gold: a prospective study of 74 patients with rheumatoid arthritis. J Rheumatol. 1994; 21:1814-9.

21. **Yan A, Davis P.** Gold induced marrow suppression: a review of 10 cases. J Rheumatol. 1990;17:47-51. Ann Rheum Dis. 2002;61(Suppl 2):70-3.

22. **Hall CL, Fothergill NJ, Blackwell MM, et al.** The natural course of gold nephropathy: long term study of 21 patients. Br Med J. 1987;295:745-8.

23. **Criscione LG, St Clair EW.** Tumor necrosis factor-alpha antagonists for the treatment of rheumatic diseases. Curr Opin Rheumatol. 2002;14:204-11.

24. **Kroesen S, Widmer AF, Tyndall A, Hasler P.** Serious bacterial infections in patients with rheumatoid arthritis under anti-TNF-alpha therapy. Rheumatology. 2003;42:617-21.

25. **Gardam MA, Keystone EC, Menzies R, et al.** Anti-tumour necrosis factor agents and tuberculosis risk: mechanisms of action and clinical management. Lancet Infect Dis. 2003;3:148-55.

26. **Rau R.** Adalimumab (a fully human anti-tumour necrosis factor alpha monoclonal antibody) in the treatment of active rheumatoid arthritis: the initial results of five trials. Ann Rheum Dis. 2002;61(Suppl 2):70-3.

27. **Nuki G, Bresnihan B, Bear MB, McCabe D.** Long-term safety and maintenance of clinical improvement following treatment with anakinra (recombinant human

interleukin-1 receptor antagonist) in patients with rheumatoid arthritis: extension phase of a randomized, double-blind, placebo-controlled trial. Arthritis Rheum. 2002;46:2838-46.

28. **Fleishmann RM.** Safety of anakinra, a recombinant interleukin-1 receptor antagonist (r-metHuIL-1ra), in patients with rheumatoid arthritis and comparison to anti-TNF-alpha agents. Clin Exp Rheumatol. 2002;20(5 Suppl 27):S35-41.

29. **Mandell BF.** Intravenous gamma-globulin therapy. J Clin Rheumatol.1996;2:317-24.

30. **Cunningham-Rundles C, Zhou Z, Mankarious S, Courter S.** Long-term use of IgA-depleted intravenous immunoglobulin in immunodeficient subjects with anti-IgA antibodies. J Clin Immunol. 1993;13:272-8.

31. **Janssen NM, Genta MS.** The effects of immunosuppressive and anti-inflammatory medications on fertility, pregnancy, and lactation. Arch Intern Med. 2000;160:610-9.

32. **Ramsey-Goldman R, Schilling E.** Immunosuppressive drug use in pregnancy. Rheum Dis Clin North Am. 1997;23:149-67.

APPENDICES

Appendix A

Generic and Trade Names of Disease-Modifying Anti-Rheumatic Drugs

Generic Name	Trade Name	Trade Name	Generic Name
Adalimumab	Humira	Aralen	Chloroquine
Anakinra	Kineret	Arava	Leflunomide
Auranofin	Ridaura	Atabrine	Quinacrine
Azathioprine	Imuran	Aurolate	Gold sodium thiomalate
Chlorambucil	Leukeran	Azulfidine	Sulfasalazine
Chloroquine	Aralen	CellCept	Mycophenolate mofetil
Cyclophosphamide	Cytoxan	Cuprimine	Penicillamine
Cyclosporine	Sandimmune, Neoral	Cytoxan	Cyclophosphamide
		Depen	Penicillamine
Etanercept	Enbrel	Dynacin	Minocycline
Gold sodium thiomalate	Myochrysine, Aurolate	Enbrel	Etanercept
		Humira	Adalimumab
Hydroxychloroquine	Plaquenil	Imuran	Azathioprine
Infliximab	Remicade	Kineret	Anakinra
Leflunomide	Arava	Leukeran	Chlorambucil
Mercaptopurine	Purinethol	Minocin	Minocycline
Methotrexate	Rheumatrex, Trexall	Myochrysine	Gold sodium thiomalate
Minocycline	Dynacin, Minocin	Neoral	Cyclosporine
		Plaquenil	Hydroxychloroquine
Mycophenolate mofetil	CellCept	Prosorba	Protein A immuno-adsorption column
Penicillamine	Cuprimine, Depen		
		Purinethol	Mercaptopurine
Protein A immuno-adsorption column	Prosorba	Remicade	Infliximab
		Rheumatrex	Methotrexate
Quinacrine	Atabrine	Ridaura	Auranofin
Sulfasalazine	Azulfidine	Sandimmune	Cyclosporine
Thalidomide	Thalomid	Thalomid	Thalidomide
		Trexall	Methotrexate

Appendix B

Generic and Trade Names of Drugs Used for Treatment of Metabolic Bone Disorders

Generic Name	Trade Name	Trade Name	Generic Name
Alendronate	Fosamax	Actonel	Risedronate
Calcitonin	Calcimar, Miacalcin	Aredia	Pamidronate
		Calcimar	Calcitonin
Etidronate	Didronel	Didronel	Etidronate
Pamidronate	Aredia	Evista	Raloxifene
Raloxifene	Evista	Forteo	Teriparatide
Risedronate	Actonel	Fosamax	Alendronate
Teriparatide	Forteo	Miacalcin	Calcitonin
Tiludronate	Skelid	Skelid	Tiludronate
Zoledronic acid	Zometa	Zometa	Zoledronic acid

Appendix C

Generic and Trade Names of Miscellaneous Drugs

Generic Name	Trade Name	Trade Name	Generic Name
Bosentan	Tracleer	Evoxac	Cevimeline
Cevimeline	Evoxac	Neurontin	Gabapentin
Cyclosporine (eyedrops)	Restasis	Restasis	Cyclosporine (eyedrops)
Gabapentin	Neurontin	Salagen	Pilocarpine
Pilocarpine	Salagen	Tracleer	Bosentan
Tramadol	Ultram	Ultram	Tramadol

Index